PSYCHOSOCIAL RESILIENCE AND RISK IN THE PERINATAL PERIOD

Bringing together experts in the field, this important book considers the underlying risk factors that create situations of psychosocial vulnerability and marginalisation for mothers, from their baby's conception up to a year after birth. Adopting a strengths-based approach, the book looks not only at the incidence and impact of disadvantageous circumstances on women but also explores protective factors at an individual, family, community and service level. It identifies promising evidence-based interventions and sources of resilience.

With a distinctive focus on social and cultural diversity, *Psychosocial Resilience and Risk in the Perinatal Period* considers a wide range of personal circumstances and social groups, including women's experiences of traumatic birth, domestic and family violence, drug and alcohol use and mothering by indigenous, same-sex and disabled women. Throughout, case studies and service user experiences are used to illuminate the issues and illustrate exemplary care practice.

International in scope, this book is particularly strong on the implications for care practices and health service delivery within Western models of maternity care. Its applied focus and evidence base makes it eminently suitable for study purposes and professional reference. Of relevance to midwives, health visitors and other health and social care practitioners, *Psychosocial Resilience and Risk in the Perinatal Period*'s final chapters focus on developing resilience amongst professionals and multiprofessional and interagency working.

Gill Thomson is Senior Research Fellow at the Maternal and Infant Nutrition and Nurture Unit, University of Central Lancashire, UK.

Virginia Schmied is Professor of Midwifery in the School of Nursing and Midwifery at the Western Sydney University, Australia, and co-leads the Mother Infant and Family Health (MIFam) Research Network.

PSYCHOSOCIAL RESILIENCE AND RISK IN THE PERINATAL PERIOD

Implications and Guidance for Professionals

Edited by Gill Thomson and Virginia Schmied

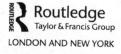

Routledge
Taylor & Francis Group

LONDON AND NEW YORK

First published 2017
by Routledge
2 Park Square, Milton Park, Abingdon, Oxon OX14 4RN

and by Routledge
711 Third Avenue, New York, NY 10017

Routledge is an imprint of the Taylor & Francis Group, an informa business

British Library Cataloguing-in-Publication Data
A catalogue record for this book is available from the British Library

Library of Congress Cataloging-in-Publication Data
Names: Thomson, Gill, editor. | Schmied, Virginia, editor.
Title: Psychosocial resilience and risk in the perinatal period : implications and guidance for professionals / edited by Gill Thomson and Virginia Schmied.
Description: Abingdon, Oxon ; New York, NY : Routledge, 2017. | Includes bibliographical references and index.
Identifiers: LCCN 2016057479| ISBN 9781138101579 (hardback) | ISBN 9781138101586 (pbk.) | ISBN 9781315656854 (ebook)
Subjects: | MESH: Pregnant Women--psychology | Mothers--psychology | Vulnerable Populations--psychology | Risk Factors | Resilience, Psychological | Psychosocial Support Systems
Classification: LCC RG560 | NLM WQ 200.1 | DDC 618.2/0651--dc23
LC record available at https://lccn.loc.gov/2016057479

ISBN: 978-1-138-10157-9 (hbk)
ISBN: 978-1-138-10158-6 (pbk)
ISBN: 978-1-315-65685-4 (ebk)

Typeset in Bembo
by Saxon Graphics Ltd, Derby

CONTENTS

FOREWORD
From Other to Us

Soo Downe

The design and delivery of health care has increasingly taken account of those who are marginalised in society. Programmes for refugees, for those experiencing domestic and family violence, and for those who have had mental health problems, are now part of mainstream maternity care provision in a number of countries. However, a fundamental issue remains to be addressed: what is called by sociologists 'Othering'.

> Otherness is a fundamental category of human thought. Thus it is that no group ever sets itself up as the One without at once setting up the Other over against itself.
>
> (Simone de Beauvoir, *The Second Sex*, 1949, p. 44)

Othering is a process whereby anyone that does not fit into particular social norms of what is, or what should be (practically, morally, clinically, socially, and in any other way) tends to be disregarded. At a deep social level, those who are stigmatised as Other are not accorded the same rights and provisions as those who are regarded as Us. Once someone is Othered, on the basis of their gender, race, sexual orientation, or their extreme experiences of grief, pain, and/or trauma, they are no longer seen clearly, and their legitimacy is diminished, in terms of what society believes it owes them.

With a wonderful mix of knowledge and wisdom, evidence and personal accounts, and hints and tips to enable deeper understanding and action, this book brings women who have been Othered in a range of ways back into sharp focus. It both addresses specific issues for the wide range of women who are included, and it offers insights into the experience of intersectional marginalisation, as many of the women have experiences that cover a range of domains of experience, and of discrimination. As well as providing a rich source of knowledge and evidence, the book offers insights into the visceral and lived experience of those on the other side of Othering, through the use of their quotes and stories.

The authors also resist the framing of women who are marginalised as victims. They offer examples of resilience, and of a positive, salutogenic orientation to addressing the issues identified. They raise the fundamental and urgent need for reform in the dominant global maternity care system in particular (and the health care system in general), making a strong case for maternity services to accommodate Maslow's 'powerful need to belong', as cited in Chapter 6 of the book. This goes beyond the need for the occasional specialist clinic. The text makes an argument for health care to shift from a neo-liberal consumerist model into one in which time, human rights, and positive collaborative relationships, are the bedrock: for equity as a way of addressing inequality; and for meaningfulness, manageability and comprehensibility to be built into maternity care for all of those using it. Ultimately, as the final chapter clearly illustrates, this has to be fractal. It has to happen at the macro (systems) level, the meso (service design) level, and at the micro (interpersonal) level. If you are interested in learning from the best, and in making change at any or all of these levels, this is the book for you.

CONTRIBUTORS

Susan Ayers is a Professor of Maternal and Child Health and leads the Centre for Maternal and Child Health Research at City University, London, UK. She specialises in women's mental health during pregnancy and after birth, with a particular focus on birth and post-traumatic stress disorder. She publishes and comments regularly on women's perinatal mental health issues and advises government. Susan is author of *Psychology for Medicine* (2011) and *The Cambridge Handbook of Psychology, Health and Medicine* (2007). She has given numerous invited lectures and workshops and was awarded the Annual Lecturer Prize by the Society of Reproductive and Infant Psychology in 2012.

Marie-Clare Balaam currently works as a Senior Research Assistant in the Research in Childbirth and Health Unit at the University of Central Lancashire, Preston, UK. Marie-Clare's background is in History and Women's Studies. She has worked as a lecturer and an academic and community-based researcher. Her research interests are migrant women's experiences of maternity care and childbirth in the UK and Europe; social support; and historical and socio-cultural perspectives on women's health particularly menopause. Her current research focuses on the experiences of asylum-seeking and refugee women and social support for marginalised women.

Cheryl Beck is a Distinguished Professor at the University of Connecticut, School of Nursing, Storrs, Connecticut, USA. She received her certificate in nurse-midwifery and master's degree in maternal-newborn nursing from Yale University. Her Doctor of Nursing Science degree is from Boston University. She is a fellow in the American Academy of Nursing. Cheryl has focused her research efforts on developing a research programme on postpartum mood and anxiety disorders. Cheryl developed the Postpartum Depression Screening Scale (PDSS) which is published by Western Psychological Services. She has published over 150 journal articles and seven books, three of which were named the *American Journal of Nursing* Book of the Year Awards.

Courtney Breen is a Research Fellow at National Drug and Alcohol Research Centre (NDARC) at the University of New South Wales in Sydney, Australia. She is interested in examining effective treatments for vulnerable populations including women with substance use disorders. Recent work has focused on examining treatment and support for women who are pregnant and use substances.

Lucinda Burns is Associate Professor at the National Drug and Alcohol Research Centre (NDARC) at the University of New South Wales in Sydney, Australia. She is manager of the Drug Trends Program that examines patterns of illicit drug use in Australia. Her other interests are in examining effective treatments for vulnerable populations including women with substance use disorders and people who are homeless.

Victoria Coleman-Cowger is a Clinical Psychologist and Principal Research Scientist with Battelle Public Health Center for Tobacco Research in Baltimore, Maryland, USA. Her research interests are in the areas of women's health, substance use, mental health, and health disparities. She has acted as Principal Investigator on grants from the National Institutes of Health focused on substance use among pregnant and postpartum women, holds a faculty appointment at the University of Maryland, Baltimore, has served on several expert panels related to perinatal substance use and has published widely on these topics

Melanie Haith-Cooper is a Senior Lecturer in Midwifery and Reproductive Health at the University of Bradford, Bradford, UK. She is a registered nurse and midwife with research interests predominantly around vulnerable migrants and health services. This has mainly focused on the health and well-being of pregnant asylum-seeking and refugee women, working closely with the voluntary sector on various projects. She co-leads the Maternity Stream charity and also designed the inclusive maternity model 'the pregnant woman within the global context' which is now widely used in different educational contexts alongside an educational film.

Susan Crowther is Professor of Midwifery at Robert Gordon University, Aberdeen, UK. Susan has worked as a midwife in many regions globally including UK and New Zealand. She has practised as a group practice midwife and a self-employed independent caseload midwife both in the UK and New Zealand. Susan was the first consultant midwife at Addenbrookes Hospital in Cambridge UK where she set up the midwifery-led unit before emigrating to New Zealand. Her research interests include relational models of care, sustainability and resilience in the midwifery workforce, rural and remote maternity care provision and spirituality in and around childbirth. Susan is editor on several peer-reviewed journals and publishes regularly.

Hannah Dahlen is the Professor of Midwifery in the School of Nursing and Midwifery at the Western Sydney University, Sydney, Australia. She has been a midwife for 26 years and still practises. Hannah has strong national and international research partnerships and has received 20 grants since 2000. She has over 120 publications and spoken at over 100 national/international conferences. She is also the National Media Spokesperson for Australian College of Midwives. Hannah is a past President of the Australian College of Midwives and received Life Membership in 2008 for her outstanding contributions. In November 2012 she was named in the *Sydney Morning Herald*'s list of 100 'people who change our city for the better'.

Soo Downe spent 15 years working as a midwife. In 2001 she joined University of Central Lancashire, Preston, UK where she is now the Professor of Midwifery Studies. Her main research focus is the nature of, and cultures around, normal birth. She is the editor of *Normal Birth, Evidence and Debate*, and, with Sheena Byrom, co-editor of the *Roar Behind the Silence* and the founder and Chair of the International Normal Birth Research Conference Series, now in its eleventh year. She is currently the Chair of EU COST Action (IS1405) including 31 countries and over 120 scientists from a wide range of disciplines. She is a member of the Board of Directors of the International MotherBaby Childbirth Organisation, and the Global Respectful Maternity Care Council of the White Ribbon Alliance, a member of the Steering Group for the Lancet Midwifery Series (2014), and of the Advisory Group for the Lancet Stillbirth Series (2016). She is also a member of the Technical Working Group of the current World Health Organisation antenatal guidelines development project and is a contributor to the new WHO Intrapartum and Reducing Caesarean Section guidelines.

Nancy Feeley is Associate Professor at Ingram School of Nursing, McGill University, Montreal, Québec, Canada, and has an appointment as a Senior Researcher at the Centre for Nursing Research and Lady Davis Research Institute of the Jewish General Hospital in Montréal. She holds a Senior Research Scholar Salary Award from the Fonds de la recherche du Québec – Santé. She is also Co-Director of the Québec Network on Nursing Intervention Research. Her programme of research focuses on the psychological adjustment and parenting of parents of children born preterm. She has expertise in approaches to intervention development and evaluation, including randomized controlled trials.

Susan E. Fleming earned her diploma of nursing at Los Angeles County School of Nursing, Los Angeles, California, USA, and her BSN from Washington State University Intercollegiate College of Nursing. In 2005, she received her MN from University of Washington, Seattle. She is a graduate of the PhD programme at Washington State University College of Nursing. She currently teaches Obstetrics for undergraduate nursing students at Seattle University, USA. Her research interest lies in studying technology and the American birth experience. Her goal is to improve nursing practice and health outcomes of mothers and their off springs for generations to come.

Cathrine Fowler is the Professor for the Tresillian Chair in Child and Family Health and is a member of the Centre for Midwifery, Child and Family Health at the University of Technology, Sydney, Australia. Cathrine is a child and family health nurse with midwifery qualifications who has extensive experience in the provision of professional, parent and community education. In 2009 she was appointed the Child Advocate for the Corrective Services NSW Mothers and Children programme. Her research and clinical focus is on working with families with complex and multiple vulnerabilities and child and family health nursing professional issues. Her recent research includes the Breaking the Cycle for Incarcerated Parents study that investigated parent education and support needs among incarcerated mothers and fathers.

Donna Hartz is a Research Fellow at the Poche Centre for Indigenous Health, University of Sydney, based at the Midwifery and Women's Health Research Unit, Royal Hospital for Women, Randwick, Sydney, Australia. Her main research focus has been continuity of midwifery care. Her current research supported by the Poche Centre is the evaluation of an urban Aboriginal community caseload model of midwifery care at Malabar, Sydney, Australia. She is also a board member of the Rhodanthe Lipsett Indigenous Midwifery Trust, a NFPO that provides scholarships and small grants to help Aboriginal and Torres Strait Islander people access midwifery education, complete studies and ongoing professional development. Donna identifies as a descendant from her grandmother's people Kamillaroi.

Brenda Hayman is a registered nurse and for the past 25 years has worked in both clinical and education environments. Brenda currently works as a lecturer in the School of Nursing & Midwifery at the Western Sydney University, Australia. Brenda's areas of expertise are aged care, palliative care, women's health, infection control, nurse education and qualitative research. The focus of her current research is lesbian mothering, mothering, lesbian ageing and lesbian mental health, using qualitative methods.

Leesa Hooker is a Maternal and Child Health nurse, midwife and academic at the La Trobe Rural Health School in Bendigo, Victoria, Australia. She has been working in the area of women's and children's health for the past 20 years. Her research interests include intimate partner violence, rural women's health and improving health care service response to abused women and children.

Julie Jomeen is Professor of Midwifery and Dean, Faculty of Health and Social Care at the University of Hull, Hull, UK. She leads a Research Group for Maternal, Reproductive and Sexual Health within the Faculty. A key focus of her work is exploring issues of perinatal mental health and psychological health outcomes in childbearing women. A programme of research which has led to a collaborations and publications in relation to national and international research, service development work and practitioner training initiatives. Julie is Chair of the Society for Reproductive and Infant Psychology.

Dineke Korfker is a midwife and a cultural anthropologist. At the beginning of her career she worked as a private midwife in Amsterdam in a disadvantaged neighbourhood. Thereafter she worked in Mozambique and Egypt for the United Nations Population Fund as chief technical adviser in reproductive and sexual health programmes. In Egypt she worked on an IEC (information, education, communication) strategy to combat female genital mutilation. From 2001 to 2016 she worked as a researcher in reproductive health for the research institute TNO in the Netherlands. She has recently moved to Rwanda to be involved in reproductive health projects.

Denise Lawler is a nurse, midwife and midwifery educator and is Head of the Discipline of Midwifery and Director of Midwifery Progammes in the School of Nursing and Midwifery, Trinity College, Dublin, Republic of Ireland. Her research activities can be categorised as (i) optimising access to maternity services for service users and (ii) theory generation. She is a reviewer for a number of peer-reviewed journals including the *International Journal of Childbirth*; *BMC Pregnancy and Childbirth*; *Midwifery* and the *Journal of Advanced Nursing*.

Leona McGrath is a proud Aboriginal woman from Queensland, Australia, and a descendant of the Woopaburra and Ku Ku Yalanji peoples. Leona is a midwife, artist, mother to three beautiful children and one gorgeous grandson. She is the Senior Advisor for the New South Wales Aboriginal Nursing and Midwifery Strategy. Leona is the Chair of the Australian College of Midwives Aboriginal and Torres Strait Islander Advisory Committee and also the co-Chair of the Rhodanthe Lipsett Indigenous Charitable Midwifery Trust Fund. Leona is passionate about increasing the Aboriginal and Torres Strait Islander midwifery workforce which will contribute to better health outcomes for Aboriginal and Torres Strait Islander women, babies and community

Colin R. Martin is Professor of Mental Health at Buckinghamshire New University, Middlesex, UK. He has published or has in press well over 200 research papers and book chapters. His books include *The Handbook of Behavior, Food and Nutrition* (2011), *Perinatal Mental Health: A Clinical Guide* (2012), *Nanomedicine and the Nervous System* (2012), *Comprehensive Guide to Autism* (2014), *Diet and Nutrition in the Menstrual Cycle, Periconception and Fertility* (2014), *Diet and Nutrition in Dementia and Cognitive Decline* (2015) and *Mental Health and Wellbeing in the Learning and Teaching Environment* (2016).

Kim Psaila is a nursing academic at the Western Sydney University, Sydney, Australia. She is a nurse with qualifications in neonatal nursing, midwifery, infant mental health, education and holds NIDCAP certification. Kim has significant experience as a registered nurse, predominantly working in the areas of neonatal nursing and nurse education. Her research interests include the parent–infant relationship, implementation of individualised, developmentally supportive care in the NICU and special care unit (SCN), collaboration, continuity and transition of care (TOC), particularly in relation to supporting families through TOC. Her main methodological expertise lies in qualitative and mixed methods design, and systematic reviews.

Chris Rossiter is a researcher at the Centre for Midwifery, Child and Family Health at the University of Technology, Sydney, Australia. She has worked as a social scientist, research manager and social policy analyst, and conducted qualitative and quantitative studies principally in the areas of health, education and community services. Her research has particularly focused on child and family health, and studies of families with complex needs, mothers with substance dependence issues and incarcerated parents. She has also participated in research into perinatal outcomes of different birth settings, obesity and nutrition, and preschool literacy.

Charles Savona-Ventura studied and trained in Malta, Leuven (Belgium), Warsaw (Poland), and Northern Ireland (UK). He currently works as a Consultant Specialist in Obstetrics and Gynaecology in the Public Health Service and serves also as Professor and Head of Department in the speciality of the University of Malta. He has published widely on issues relating to social reproduction particularly in terms of risk groups and in diabetes in pregnancy.

Virginia Schmied is Professor of Midwifery in the School of Nursing and Midwifery at Western Sydney University, Sydney, Australia, and co-leads the Mother Infant and Family Health (MIFam) Research Network. She is a registered midwife and a registered nurse with experience that extends across clinical practice, education, research and consultancy. She holds a Visiting Professorship at the University of Central Lancashire, Preston, UK. Her programme of scholarship, teaching and research is grounded in social science theory and methods and focuses on transition to motherhood, perinatal mental health, infant feeding, postnatal care, effective models to support vulnerable families, family centred care in NICU, strengthening the universal health services for families and children and the role of the child and family health nurse. She has published over 170 refereed journal articles, book chapters and published reports and regularly presents at national and international conferences. Her research has been translated to policy and practice.

Angela Taft is a public health social scientist, Professor and former Director of the Judith Lumley Centre for mother, infant and family health research at La Trobe University, Melbourne, Australia. For the last 15 years she has led the centre's competitively funded programme of research on intimate partner/ gender-based violence and sexual and reproductive health in Australia and in Timor-Leste. Her research is focused on improving the health system's response to partner violence in culturally diverse communities, promoting planned parenthood and reproductive rights and recently preventing and reducing alcohol-related partner violence.

Gill Thomson is a Senior Research Fellow working in the Maternal and Infant Nutrition and Nurture Unit at the University of Central Lancashire, Preston, UK. Gill has a psychology academic background and has worked within the public, private and voluntary sector. Over the last 20 years she has been involved in a number of research/evaluation-based projects funded by various Primary Care Trusts, Department of Health and the National Institute of Health Research to explore psychosocial influences and experiences of maternity services, infant feeding issues and support services. Gill's research interests relate to peer support models of care and psychosocial influences and implications of perinatal care, with a particular focus on factors that impact upon maternal mental health. She also has a particular specialism in interpretive phenomenological-based research.

1

INTRODUCING THE CHAPTERS AND FOCUS

Virginia Schmied and Gill Thomson

Globally there is increasing concern about women's health in the perinatal period (from pregnancy through to 12 months after birth). This concern is well-illustrated by the recent (2016) Lancet series on maternal health. Eminent authors argue that the burden of poor maternal health — mortality and severe morbidity — is concentrated among vulnerable populations. Across the globe many women miss out on quality maternity care particularly women who are marginalised including migrant, refugee and internally displaced women, Indigenous women, women living in poverty and women living in fragile states (McDougall, Campbell & Graham, 2016, p. 5). Less is said however, in this landmark series about the psychosocial health and well-being of women, their infants and families.

Psychosocial risk and resilience in the perinatal period is the focus of this edited book. The impetus for this has come from an increasing concern for the social and emotional health of women, their children and families in the perinatal period and how health professionals and maternity and child health services best respond to these needs.

This book aims to:

1   Provide in-depth insights into the risk factors, psychosocial concerns and support for women and families who are marginalised and/or experiencing complex life situations and experiences across the perinatal period.
2   Highlight individual, family, community and service system resilience (or protective) factors that can help to mitigate against adverse outcomes (for service users, families as well as professionals).
3   Identify 'promising', evidence-based interventions to respond to diversity and to address psychosocial issues and complex needs.
4   Consider implications for care practices and health service delivery within Western models of maternity care.

In the following sections we discuss why maternal psychosocial health matters. We then provide definitions into the key concepts of this book – 'risk' and 'resilience' – which have been considered in different population groups in the proceeding chapters. Finally, an outline of what is addressed in each of the chapters is provided.

Why maternal psychosocial health matters

Reports of maternal deaths in the United Kingdom (UK) indicate that suicide is one of the leading causes of mortality in the year after birth (Knight, Tuffnell, Kenyon, Shakespeare, Gray & Kurinczuk, 2015). In the UK, one in eleven women who died during or up to six weeks after pregnancy, died from mental health-related causes. However, almost a quarter of all maternal deaths between six weeks and a year after birth are related to mental health problems, and one in seven of the women who died in this period died by suicide (Knight *et al.*, 2015). The higher prevalence of late maternal deaths (between 43 days and one year after birth) is supported by Australian research where suicide and accidental injury are the two leading causes of death for women within one year of birth (Thornton, Schmied, Dennis, Barnett & Dahlen, 2013), International data suggest that the prevalence of maternal mental health problems have at best remained static over the past 20 years (Schmied *et al.*, 2013; Ibanez, Blondel, Prunet, Kaminski & Saurel-Cubizolles, 2015) or are increasing, particularly women diagnosed with anxiety disorders (Fairbrother, Young, Janssen, Antony & Tucker, 2015).

Recognising and addressing woman's social and emotional needs in the perinatal period is critical. Treatments and service design and delivery have typically been informed by either a biomedical or psychological approach focused on the individual (Davydov, Stewart, Ritchie & Chaudieu, 2010). More recently, models such as Developmental Origins of Behaviour, Health and Disease (Marmot, 2010) and socio-ecological model of development (Bronfenbrenner, 1979) that emphasise the significant and long-term consequences of maternal (and increasingly paternal) psychosocial health for the developing child, are informing interventions and service delivery for women, families and communities.

The *Developmental Origins of Behaviour, Health, and Disease* concept describes pregnancy and the early postnatal period as periods of opportunity and risk (Marmot, 2010). This is a time of 'developmental plasticity' when a number of physical, social, environmental, behavioural and psychological factors may influence the biology of the developing child (Moore, McDonald & McHugh-Dillon, 2015; Van den Bergh, Mulder, Mennes & Glover, 2005), and as a consequence affect a child's competence across a range of areas, from health and social behaviour to employment and educational attainment (Coles, Cheyne & Daniel, 2015; Tickell, 2011). A child's neurological development across the early stages of their life provides the foundations for future cognitive capacities. For example, the biological effects of birth weight on brain development interact with other social determinants to influence a child's cognitive development (Marmot, 2010).

Evidence has demonstrated that insults during sensitive developmental periods, such as pregnancy or in the early childhood period (up to three years of age), may trigger the reprogramming of genetic tissue which in turn, not only predisposes the individual to behavioural problems, learning difficulties, delayed cognitive development in childhood, but may also lead to early cognitive decline, psychopathology, cancer, cardio-metabolic, neuroendocrine and other diseases in adult life (Murgatroyd & Spengler, 2011). Disease processes such as diabetes, heart disease and cancer, previously thought to develop due to adult lifestyle behaviours, have now been linked to prenatal and early childhood experiences (Fairbrother *et al.*, 2015; Power, Kuh & Morton, 2013). Most recently Dahlen and colleagues (2013) have put forward the Epigenetic Impact of Childbirth (EPIIC) hypothesis. They argue that evidence is emerging that certain intrapartum and early neonatal interventions – specifically the use of synthetic oxytocin, antibiotics and caesarean section – affect the epigenetic remodelling processes and subsequent health of the mother and offspring (Dahlen *et al.*, 2013).

The social ecological model: Bronfenbrenner (1979) proposed an ecological model to explain influences on child development at all levels (see Figure 1.1). He placed the child at the centre and argued that the child's development was influenced not only by the more proximal, and relatively stronger influences, of the parents and family, peers, school and neighbourhood, but also by distal factors of the broader social context such as the media, parents' work arrangements and governmental policies. The social ecological model helps to understand the multifaceted and interactive effects of personal, family and environmental factors that determine behaviours, and for identifying behavioural and organisational touchpoints and mediators for promoting health and well-being. For example, a child whose mother is experiencing depression and has casual, low-paid work, and a father who is unemployed, living in a disadvantaged community is more likely to experience poor developmental outcomes.

Research based on the social ecological model demonstrates the impact of the parent–infant relationship and parenting quality as one of, if not the most important, proximal factor influencing child development. The quality of early parent–infant interactions directly affects the way the brain develops. Parental sensitivity and the quality of interactions with infants in the first three years of life predict the social and cognitive competence of children extending into adulthood (Raby, Roisman, Fraley & Simpson, 2015). Exposure to harsh and inconsistent discipline and limited cognitive stimulation and or exposure to stressors such as parental mental illness, substance abuse or family violence, poverty, unsafe communities, all interact to determine developmental outcomes for children in the short and long term (Fox, Southwell, Stafford, Goodhue, Jackson & Smith, 2015). Importantly, the presence of risk factors alone does not determine whether or not a child develops his or her potential in life, however the presence of risk factors make it more difficult.

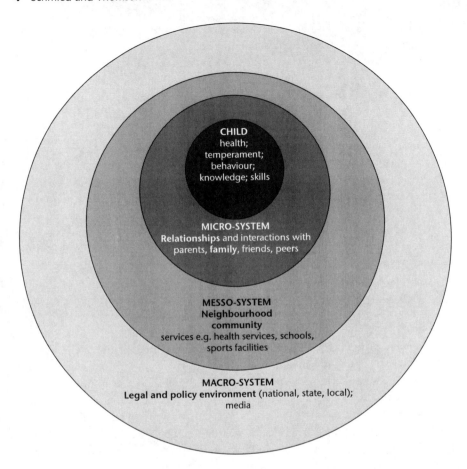

FIGURE 1.1 The social ecological model

Adapted from the Centers for Disease Control and Prevention (CDC), *The Social Ecological Model: A Framework for Prevention*, www.cdc.gov/violenceprevention/overview/social-ecologicalmodel.html

Risk and protective factors and the concept of resilience

A risk factor is defined as a 'measurable contributor to later negative developmental outcomes' (Loxley *et al.*, 2004, p. 72). Typically, this applies to risk factors known to impact on child development either in childhood or as an adult.

There are a number of known, identifiable risk factors for poor maternal (and infant) outcomes, including mental health problems (prior and current), domestic and family violence, drug and alcohol misuse, past history of abuse and situational factors such as quality of significant relationships (Schmied *et al.*, 2013), socio-economic circumstances, migrant or refugee status (O'Mahony, Donnelly, Raffin Bouchal & Este, 2013).

Children and adults alike are more vulnerable if exposed to more risk factors and less protective factors – when more protective factors are available this reduces exposure to, or the impact of risk factors.

Protective factors: Less is known about the protective factors for maternal mental health. Loxley *et al.* (2004, p. 73) conceptualises protective factors as 'characteristics that buffer, mediate or moderate the influence of risk factors, thereby reducing the likelihood that risk factors will lead to later problem outcomes'. Protective factors such as self-confidence, good social support, preparedness to utilise services may modify or mediate the relationship between risk factors and maternal and infant outcomes.

Resilience: At its most basic level resilience refers to 'positive adaptation, or the ability to maintain or regain mental health, despite experiencing adversity' (Herrman, Stewart, Diaz-Granados, Berger, Jackson & Yuen, 2011, p. 259). Resilience was first conceptualised as a personal trait, strengths or assets such as intellectual functioning that helped people survive adversity (Herrman *et al.*, 2011). Later, the concept expanded to include the contribution of systems (families, services, groups, and communities) in assisting people to cope with adversity. Broader definitions were introduced including 'the protective factors and processes or mechanisms that contribute to a good outcome, despite experiences with stressors shown to carry significant risk for developing psychopathology' (Herrman *et al.*, 2011, p. 260). The complexity of resilience and its value as a theory or concept in informing interventions is addressed in Chapter 2 in this book. Here Jomeen and colleagues argue as do others, that the theoretical evidence base for this term is limited and contentious.

Overview of the book

In this book we aim to provide insights into the risk factors, psychosocial concerns, resilience and strength based factors and support for women and families who are marginalised and/or experiencing complex life situations and experiences across the perinatal period. Maternal mental health and well-being is central to all chapters in this book and in Chapter 2, Julie Jomeen and colleagues, set the scene by examining the prevalence and risk factors for perinatal mental health problems and discussing the foundations of effective interventions for women.

As illustrated by the social ecological model (Figure 1.1), there are a number of situational factors that may impact on maternal well-being. Many women and families experience marginalisation and stigma, or as Soo Downe describes in the foreword to this book they are 'Othered', because of who they are, and isolated as a consequence. In Chapter 3, Marie-Claire Balaam and colleagues examine the experiences of refugee and asylum seeking women. For these women, pre-migration trauma and loss and separation from family contribute to the risk of developing mental health problems. Donna Hartz and Leona McGrath then examine in Chapter 4 the impact that colonisation has had on maternal and infant health amongst Indigenous communities in Australia, New Zealand and Canada.

Characteristics of positive policy and service responses and strategies aimed at promoting psychosocial resilience and optimising health outcomes for Indigenous childbearing women, their babies and families in these countries are explored.

In Chapter 5, Brenda Hayman talks about the challenges experienced by lesbian women when seeking maternity care and the limited understanding that maternity care professionals have of their specific needs. Denise Lawler in Chapter 6 offers an important theoretical lens on how mothers with a disability develop their sense of maternal identity and negotiate the stigma and discrimination they experience.

Some women experience significant complexities in their lives and these difficulties can impact on their capacity to parent effectively. Women who experience domestic and family violence (DFV) for example, are also likely to experience antenatal and postnatal anxiety, depression, and post-traumatic stress disorder (PTSD) and some will struggle to parent effectively (Howard, Oram, Galley, Trevillion & Feder, 2013). In Chapter 7, Angela Taft and Lessa Hooker review the prevalence and health impact of DFV in the perinatal period and describe women's experience and stages of women's pathways to safety. This chapter offers important information on how health professionals can respond effectively.

Drug and alcohol use in pregnancy are markers of complex pregnancies and women in this situation often experience multiple comorbidities with adverse fetal and infant outcomes. In Chapter 8, Lucy Burns and colleagues examine the nature, patterns, outcomes and treatments for the most commonly used substances in pregnancy in Australia and the United States. In Chapter 9, Cathrine Fowler and Chris Rossiter focus on the impact of incarceration on mothers and their children – yet this difficult and chaotic situation can be a catalyst for change for women. The authors describe the benefits of delivering relational parenting programmes based on attachment theory in prison with the aim to enhance the mother's knowledge of child development.

Maternal social and emotional health is also associated with a mother's physical health, with her birth experience, if she has breastfeeding difficulties, or her infant has a difficult infant temperament or is unwell. Having a premature baby for example is very stressful for parents and in Chapter 10, Canadian researcher Nancy Feeley, describes the numerous stressors experienced by mothers of preterm infants. This chapter highlights the higher risk for these mothers of developing depression and PTSD and the potential for parenting programs to support the development of the mother-infant relationship. In Chapter 11, eminent researchers – Gill Thomson, Cheryl Beck and Susan Ayers – examine the prevalence and associated risk factors for childbirth-related PTSD. While mental health problems and previous trauma are risk factors for birth related PTSD, disturbingly, birth trauma is often related to how a woman was treated by health professionals. Importantly, these authors demonstrate that health professionals who are attuned to women's needs can foster resilience in women with a subsequent birth. In Chapter 12 Hannah Dahlen generously shares her personal experience of grief and loss, having given birth to two babies who died soon after birth. This experience is offered as a way to assist health professionals to walk beside women and families, to guide them and protect them to ensure they have a safe and respectful care while they create precious memories of their baby.

Service delivery and support for professionals

Given the impact of maternal social and emotional health on outcomes for children, early identification of risk and early intervention is now a priority across services. Best practice for identifying risk and protective factors is addressed by the chapter authors discussed above. Implementing evidence-based treatments or programmes of support is essential to ameliorate the symptoms of poor mental health and in each chapter the authors discuss current evidence-based psychosocial interventions to support mothers and infants.

Finally, attention must be given to the needs of health and social care professionals who work closely with women, children and families with complex psychosocial needs. In Chapter 13, Susan Crowther discusses the emotional work of maternity care provision and highlights the complexity of contemporary maternity environments and the increasing stress experienced by perinatal health providers when supporting women. This chapter argues for more transdisciplinary long-term strategies to support maternity care professionals and explores the notions of resilience and sustainability.

In Chapter 14, Kim Psaila and Virginia Schmied emphasise the need for service integration and collaboration. They explore the characteristics of collaborative practice as a way to address the challenges women and families face when trying to access appropriate services within, what is currently in most countries, a fragmented system of health and social care.

Concluding remarks

In selecting the topics for this edited volume we do not intend to 'Other' individuals or to problematise women and families as 'vulnerable'; rather to introduce readers to the debates around psychosocial risk together with the challenges in understanding and identifying resilience amongst diverse groups of women and their families. We acknowledge that this book is not comprehensive in its coverage of topics. For example, we have not focused on fathers, and this is a limitation. Fathers, similar to mothers' experiences are diverse and complex. In some cases, we know little about fathers for example, the experiences of fathers of preterm infants. Many chapters, however, emphasise the need for health professionals to ensure fathers are included in services and recognise that fathers have particular needs.

Economic analyses have demonstrated that investment in the early years of a child's life is far more cost effective than instituting interventions at later periods (Heckman & Raut, 2016). The critical pre-birth and early childhood period therefore provides an opportunity to mitigate risk factors and improve the long-term health and well-being not only of individuals but also communities.

This book is designed to support and inform multi-disciplinary professionals, academics and researchers about the issues that a diverse group of women and families may face and to ensure that their needs are recognised, identified and appropriately supported.

References

Bronfenbrenner, U. (1979). *The ecology of human development: Experiments by nature and design*. Cambridge, MA: Harvard University Press.

Centers for Disease Control and Prevention (CDC). (2015) *The social ecological model: A framework for prevention*. Available from: www.cdc.gov/violenceprevention/overview/social-ecologicalmodel.html [Accessed 22 October, 2016].

Coles, E., Cheyne, H. & Daniel, B. (2015). Early years interventions to improve child health and wellbeing: What works, for whom and in what circumstances? Protocol for a realist review. *Systematic Reviews*, 4(79). doi: 10.1186/s13643-015-0068-5.

Dahlen, H.G., Kennedy, H.P., Anderson, C.M., Bell, A.F., Clark, A., Foureur, M., Ohm, J.E., Shearman, A.M., Taylor, J.Y., Wright, M.L. & Downe, S. (2013). The EPIIC hypothesis: Intrapartum effects on the neonatal epigenome and consequent health outcomes. *Medical Hypotheses*, 80(5), 656–662.

Davydov, D.M., Stewart, R., Ritchie, K. & Chaudieu, I. (2010). Resilience and mental health. *Clinical Psychology Review*, 30, 479–495.

Fairbrother, N., Young, A.H., Janssen, P., Antony, M.M. & Tucker, E. (2015). Depression and anxiety during the perinatal period. *BMC Psychiatry*, 15(2006). doi:10.1186/s12888-015-0526-6.

Fox, S., Southwell, A., Stafford, N., Goodhue, R., Jackson, D. & Smith, C. (2015). *Better systems, better chances: A review of research and practice for prevention and early intervention*. Canberra: Australian Research Alliance for Children and Youth (ARACY). Available from: www.community.nsw.gov.au/__data/assets/pdf_file/0008/335168/better_systems_better_chances_review.pdf [Accessed 28 September, 2016].

Heckman, J.J. & Raut, L.K. (2016). Intergenerational long-term effects of preschool-structural estimates from a discrete dynamic programming model. *Journal of Econometrics*, 191, 164–175.

Herrman, H., Stewart, D.E., Diaz-Granados, N., Berger, E., Jackson, B. & Yuen, T. (2011) What is resilience? *Canadian Journal of Psychiatry*, 56(5), 258–265.

Howard, L.M., Oram, S., Galley, H., Trevillion, K. & Feder, G. (2013). Domestic violence and perinatal mental disorders: A systematic review and meta-analysis. *PLOS Medicine*. Available from http://dx.doi.org/10.1371/journal.pmed.1001452 [Accessed 9 February 2017].

Ibanez, G., Blondel, B., Prunet, C., Kaminski, M. & Saurel-Cubizolles, M.J. (2015). Prevalence and characteristics of women reporting poor mental health during pregnancy: Findings from the 2010 French National Perinatal Survey. *Revue d'Epidémiologie et de Santé Publique*, 63(2), 85–95.

Knight, M., Tuffnell, D., Kenyon, S., Shakespeare, J., Gray, R. & Kurinczuk, J.J. (Eds.) (2014). *Saving lives, improving mothers' care – Surveillance of maternal deaths in the UK 2011–13 and lessons learned to inform maternity care from the UK and Ireland Confidential Enquiries into maternal deaths and morbidity 2009–13*. Oxford: National Perinatal Epidemiology Unit. Available from: www.npeu.ox.ac.uk/downloads/files/mbrrace-uk/reports/MBRRACE-UK%20Maternal%20Report%202015.pdf [Accessed 18 October, 2016].

Loxley, W., Toumbourou, J.W., Stockwell, T., Haines, B., Scott, K., Godfrey, C. & Williams, J. (2004). *The prevention of substance use, risk and harm in Australia: A review of the evidence.* Canberra Department of Health and Ageing, Australian Government. Available from www.health.gov.au/internet/main/publishing.nsf/Content/health-pubhlth-publicat-document-mono_prevention-cnt.htm [Accessed 16 September, 2016].

McDougall, L., Campbell, O.M.R. & Graham, W. (2016). *Maternal health: An executive summary for The Lancet's Series.* Available from: www.thelancet.com/pb/assets/raw/Lancet/stories/series/maternal-health-2016/mathealth2016-exec-summ.pdf [Accessed 19 October, 2016].

Marmot, M. (2010). *Fair Society, Healthy Lives: A strategic review of health inequalities in England.* Available from: www.instituteofhealthequity.org/projects/fair-society-healthy-lives-the-marmot-review [Accessed 18 October, 2016].

Moore, T., McDonald, M. & McHugh-Dillon, H. (2015). *Early childhood development and the social determinants of health inequities: A review of the evidence.* Parkville, Victoria: Centre for Community Child Health at the Murdoch Childrens Research Institute and the Royal Children's Hospital. Available from www.rch.org.au/uploadedFiles/Main/Content/ccch/151014_Evidence-review-early-childhood-development-and-the-social-determinants-of-health-inequities_Sept2015.pdf [Accessed 5 October, 2016].

Murgatroyd, C. & Spengler, D. (2011). Epigenetics of early child development. *Frontiers in Psychiatry* 2(16). doi:10.3389/fpsyt.2011.00016.

O'Mahony, J.M., Donnelly, T.T., Raffin Bouchal, S. & Este, D. (2013). Cultural background and socioeconomic influence of immigrant and refugee women coping with postpartum depression. *Journal of Immigrant and Minority Health*, 15(2), 300–314.

Power, C., Kuh, D. & Morton, S. (2013). From Developmental Origins of adult disease to Life Course Research on adult disease and aging: Insights from birth cohort studies. *Annual Review of Public Health*, *34*, 7–29.

Raby, K.L., Roisman, G.I., Fraley, R.C. & Simpson, J.A. (2015). The enduring predictive signify years. *Child Development*, 86(3), 659–708.

Schmied, V., Johnson, M., Naidoo, N., Austin, M-P., Matthey, S., Kemp, L., Mills, A., Meade, T. & Yeo, T. (2013). Maternal mental health in Australia and New Zealand: A review of longitudinal studies. *Women and Birth*, 26(3), 167–178.

Thornton, C., Schmied, V., Dennis, C.L., Barnett, B. & Dahlen, H.G. (2013). Maternal deaths in NSW (2000–2006) from nonmedical causes (suicide and trauma) in the first year following birth. *BioMed Research International*, 1–6. Available from http://dx.doi.org/10.1155/2013/623743 [Accessed 9 February 2017].

Tickell, C. (2011). *The early years: Foundations for life, health and learning: An independent report on the early years foundation stage to Her Majesty's Government.* Available from: www.educationengland.org.uk/documents/pdfs/2011-tickell-report-eyfs.pdf [Accessed 28 September, 2016].

Van den Bergh, B.R.H., Mulder, E.J.H., Mennes, M. & Glover, V. (2005). Antenatal maternal anxiety and stress and the neurobehavioural development of the fetus and child: Links and possible mechanisms. A review. *Neuroscience Biobehaviour Review*, *29*, 237–258.

2

WOMEN WITH A DIAGNOSED MENTAL HEALTH PROBLEM

Julie Jomeen, Susan E. Fleming and Colin R. Martin

Introduction

Globally many women will experience mental health problems. Though this is also true of men, there are significant differences in the way in which mental health problems both occur and impact on men and women's lives. Women are more likely to suffer health inequalities such as poverty or lone parenting; the low value often placed on women's work can have a negative impact on self-esteem and compound risk for mental illness. Certain groups such as black and ethnic minority, lesbian and bisexual women as well as women offenders are also more vulnerable to mental health problems (Price, 2007). Women's mental health, therefore, must be defined within the context of women's lives. A key defining context for women's mental health is the experience of pregnancy and childbirth. Approximately 80 per cent of women in high-income countries conceive and experience pregnancy and pregnancy occurs in a period (25–44 years) where mental health disorders in women have been identified as more prevalent (American College of Nurse Midwives [ACNM], 2013). Pregnancy and early motherhood is a psychological and social experience in a woman's life, which cannot be separated from her past and present experiences (Darvill, Skirton & Farrand, 2010). Hence, mental health disruption can occur in the perinatal period as the continuation, exacerbation or relapse of existing mental illness, or as a first episode in response to the stressors that the journey from conception to motherhood places on some women. Mental illness is not a personal failure of individual women, rather it is a failure of systems and care provision to effectively assess, identify and respond with adequate care provision, or offer and connect women with appropriate support. This chapter aims to identify the prevalence of perinatal mental health problems (PMHP) and the potential consequences associated with a failure to effectively identify and support those women at risk. Issues surrounding assessment and identification of PMHP will be explored and the utility of measures briefly deliberated. Risk factors will be examined and resilience will be discussed and critiqued in this context, raising thought provoking questions for practitioners and service providers about the foundations of effective interventions for women with PMHP.

Prevalence of PMHP

PMHP is best described as spectrum of disorders (depression, anxiety, obsessive-compulsive disorders, post-traumatic stress disorder [PTSD], postpartum psychosis) that can appear anytime throughout the pregnancy and/or the 12 months following the birth of a baby. In line with general population data, anxiety and depression occur more frequently than other PMHP (Brucker & King, 2015). Globally, rates for PMHP vary between 10 and 41 per cent. The variation in these figures being dependent on both definition used and the mental health condition or symptomology measured, as well as the assessment used to determine categorisation; figures for clinically significant non–psychotic PMHP, predominantly depression and anxiety, in high-income countries are cited as 10 per cent of pregnant women and 13 per cent of postnatal mothers and higher in middle- to low-income countries, with rates of 15.6 per cent and 19.8 per cent respectively (Fisher *et al.*, 2010). Evidence demonstrates that rates of anxiety are higher than those of depression with rates of around 21 per cent quoted across the antenatal and postnatal periods (Heron, O'Conner, Evans, Golding & Glover, 2004). It is noteworthy that differences often exist in prevalence between self-report assessment and diagnostic assessment (Fisher *et al.*, 2010) and definition may be a key issue to keep in mind when considering prevalence rates. A recent study of Dutch pregnant women using a composite construct of maternal distress – described as a spectrum consisting of a variety of psychological constructs excluding psychiatric pathology – cited rates of maternal distress as 22 per cent (Fontein-Kuipers, Ausems, Dude, van Limbeek, de Vries & Nieuwenhuijze, 2015a). It can be useful to work this out percentage wise in terms of national or local birth population to get a sense of the scale of the issue. Taking England as an example, if 700,000 women give birth each year, using the more conservative estimates of 10 and 13 per cent respectively at least 70,000 women will be affected, by depression and anxiety, antepartum and 91,000 postpartum. However, using a maternal distress construct, potentially 154,000 women may be at risk.

PMHP are, however, a spectrum of conditions, varying in severity. The figures above refer to the largest group of women who will be affected by distress and often mild to moderate depressive illness and anxiety states. The spectrum also includes (rates per 1000 maternities indicated here in brackets): severe depressive illness (30); PTSD (30), chronic serious mental illness (2) and postpartum psychosis (2) (Royal College of Psychiatrists, 2012), which affect smaller groups of women but can have more severe impact and consequences.

Impact and consequences of perinatal mental health problems

There is significant and continually accruing evidence of PMHP as predictors of negative birth outcomes, poorer maternal outcomes, implications for partners and societal impact. Evidence has demonstrated that the fetal environment can be compromised by a mother's mental health status, resulting in outcomes such as low birth weight and prematurity (Dunkel Schetter & Tanner, 2012). First trimester implications include low birth weight (Paarlberg Vingerhoets, Passchier, Dekker, & Van Geijn, 1995) as well as neurodevelopmental consequences that can lead to adverse cognitive and behavioural development of the child (Mennes, Stiers, Lagae & Van den Bergh, 2006). Third trimester PMHP have been associated with preterm uterine activity; second and third trimester risks include elevated incidence of affective disorders in children (Monk, Spicer & Champagne, 2012). Adverse short and long-term deleterious mental health outcomes have been identified for mothers (Heron *et al.*, 2004), their partners (Leigh & Milgrom, 2008) and their children through infancy to adulthood (Schuurmans & Kurrasch, 2013). Postpartum risks include the compromised mother–infant relationship as well as the quality of the family relationship more broadly (Leigh & Milgrom, 2008).

Suicide has been identified in the last decade as an alarming sequelae of severe PMHP. In the UK the 2004 UK Confidential Enquiries in Maternal and Child Health (CEMACH) report identified deaths from PMHP as the overall leading cause of maternal mortality (CEMACH, 2004). Subsequent reports (Centre for Maternal and Child Enquiries (CMACE, 2011; CEMACH, 2007) have continued to evidence PMHP as a significant cause of death and highlight no decrease in suicide rates in perinatal women. Of significance is that as a major cause of maternal mortality, it exceeds those more commonly acknowledged conditions such as haemorrhage and hypertensive disorders (American College of Obstetricians and Gynecologists [ACOG], 2015; ACNM, 2013). An Australian study demonstrated that deaths from non-medical causes peaked at around 9–12 months postpartum, with a comment that often services are focused on short-term rather than long-term support (Thornton, Schmied, Dennis, Barnett & Dahlen, 2013).

One important consideration is that women with existing depression who stop their antidepressant medication during pregnancy are at risk of a fivefold increase for a depression relapse compared with women who continue their medication (ACOG, 2009). Depression without medications has its own risks, which can result in poor engagement with prenatal care and the use of alcohol, nicotine and drugs as self-selected coping mechanisms.

The US provides one example of where substance use disorders experienced during the perinatal period are mounting and are a major and debilitating health, social and financial concern (Centers for Disease Control and Prevention, 2015). Anxiety as the most prevalent mental health disorder in the US, is often underreported and self-managed with alcohol, non-medical use of prescription drugs, or illicit drug use. Every year the US government investigates national trends occurring in those who are 12 years old or older and reports that in 2014 there was a decrease in non-medical pain relief use with a corresponding rise in marijuana use and an increase in illicit drug use such as heroin (Substance Abuse and Mental Health Services Administration, 2014). Similar to the rise of opiate use within the US general population, there has been a dramatic increase in pregnant women using opiates and the associated effects resulting from the use/abuse of alcohol and drugs, which include fetal alcohol spectrum, intrauterine growth restriction, placenta abruption and Neonatal Intensive Care Unit (NICU) admission for neonatal withdrawal (ACOG, 2009; Chaudron, 2013) (also refer to Chapter 8). NICU admissions from 2004 to 2013 have increased from 7 cases per 1,000 to 27 cases per 1,000 (also refer to Chapter 10). Likewise, the length of stay has increased from 13 to 19 days (Tolia *et al.*, 2015).

Recent UK evidence has also highlighted the burden in economic terms of a failure to identify and manage women with PMHP, citing a cost to UK society of about £8.1 billion for each one-year cohort of births (Bauer, Parsonage, Knapp, Iemmi & Adelaja, 2014); the majority of these costs relating to long-term child outcomes. Hence, the effective assessment of PMH is of growing concern to policy makers and practitioners globally. Clinical guidelines in the USA, Canada, Scotland and Australia (Darwin, McGowan & Edozien, 2015) recommend assessment of women at risk of PMHP.

Identifying, assessing and managing perinatal mental health problems

Whilst the range and type of PMHP might vary, they can present across the perinatal period. Practitioners will see women with existing mental health disorders who become pregnant, as well as women who develop PMHP when they have previously been well. The existing evidence base makes a distinction between those two groups of women and the associated differing approach to assessment; that is 'prediction' of the risk of a mental health disorder and attempts to 'detect' onset of a 'distress'/depression episode in previously well women.

A number of countries have developed approaches to assessing psychological health, and the literature shows a wide variability of screening tools (Paschetta *et al.*, 2014). In the UK the National Institute of Health and Clinical Excellence (NICE) guidelines for antenatal and postpartum mental health give all healthcare professionals working with pregnant and postpartum women a clearly defined remit for prediction and detection of PMHP (NICE, 2014) (refer to Box 2.1). The original guidance issued in 2007 focused on the detection of depression using the Whooley questions (NICE, 2007). The 2014 guidelines have responded to the increasing evidence base around perinatal anxiety and additionally sought to address assessment of the range and prevalence of anxiety disorders, using the Generalised Anxiety Disorder Scale-2 as part of routine assessment.

Australia has introduced psychosocial assessment and depression screening (using the Edinburgh Postnatal Depression Scale (EPDS)) alongside routine physical care in a maternity context, in recognition of the impact of psychosocial

BOX 2.1 NICE DETECTION AND PREDICTION QUESTIONS (ADAPTED FROM NICE, 2014)

Prediction questions

At the woman's first contact with services during pregnancy and the postpartum period, healthcare professionals (including midwives, obstetricians, health visitors and GPs) should ask about:

1   Past or present severe mental illness, including schizophrenia, bipolar disorder, psychosis in the postpartum period and severe depression.
2   Previous treatment by a psychiatrist/specialist mental health team, including inpatient care.
3   Family history of perinatal mental illness.

Detection questions (Whooley questions: PHQ-2)

At the woman's first contact with primary care, booking visit and postpartum (usually at four to six weeks and three to four months), healthcare professionals (including midwives, obstetricians, health visitors and GPs) should ask two questions to identify possible depression:

1   During the past month, have you often been bothered by feeling down, depressed or hopeless?
2   During the past month, have you often been bothered by having little interest or pleasure in doing things?

Also consider using the 2-item Generalized Anxiety Disorder scale (GAD-2):

1   Over the last two weeks, how often have you been bothered by feeling nervous, anxious or on edge?
2   Over the last two weeks, how often have you been bothered by not being able to stop or control worrying?

If a woman responds positively to either of the depression questions, is at risk of developing a mental health problem, or there is clinical concern, consider using the EPDS or the Patient Health Questionnaire (PHQ-9) as part of a full assessment or referring the woman to her GP or to a mental health professional.

If a woman scores three or more on the GAD-2, consider using the GAD-7 for further assessment or referring the woman to her GP or to a mental health professional.

If a woman scores less than three on the GAD-2 scale, but you are still concerned she may have an anxiety disorder, ask the following question:

1   Do you find yourself avoiding places or activities and does this cause you problems?

If she responds positively, consider using the GAD-7 scale for further assessment or referring the woman to her GP or to a mental health professional.

problems on maternal and child outcomes (Rollans, Schmied, Kemp & Meade, 2013). The American Congress of Obstetricians and Gynecologists (ACOG, 2015) and the ACNM (2013) recommend that universal mental health screening should commence during the perinatal period, using a standardised and validated tool, such as EPDS; Post-Partum Depression Scale (PPDS); Beck Depression Inventory (BDI) I or II, to screen for depression at least once during the perinatal period.

Whilst short self-report measures are undoubtedly attractive for use in clinical practice due to their ease of use and potential cut-off scores, which may help facilitate practitioner judgements (Alderdice et al., 2013), measures are not a panacea response. Numerous issues have been highlighted with PMHP assessment measures, false-positive rates (King, Pestell, Farrar, North & Brunt, 2012), threshold scores (Jomeen & Martin, 2005) and scoring methods (Spiteri, Jomeen & Martin, 2013) and a failure to be validated in perinatal populations (Jomeen, 2012).

It must be remembered that assessment tools are not diagnostic in nature and a score on a screening tool only serves to highlight possible or probable PMHP. While tools might be useful in underpinning mood assessment, they should not be considered a replacement for clinical skills and expertise (King et al., 2012). A recent review by Johnson and colleagues sought to critically evaluate measures assessing PMHP risk but concluded that none of the instruments met all of the requirements of psychometric properties defined within the review (Johnson et al., 2012).

It is also important to reflect that potential 'cases' can be missed due to under-disclosure (Darwin et al., 2015) linked to the social stigma that still surrounds mental illness, particularly in the childbearing context. Assessment can also be compounded by the overlap of the physical symptoms of pregnancy and those of PMHP, aspects such as changes in sleep architecture, appetite, energy levels and libido coalesce and hence can lead to misdiagnosis. However, they can have significant utility when used sensitively and considerately as part of a broader assessment and decision-making (Jomeen, 2012).

Improved identification of PMHP offers an opportunity for earlier intervention to address the illness and reduce the risk of longer-term problems for the mother, her baby and family. Interventions must be underpinned by both clear referral pathways and evidence-based care provision. Effective service provision for PMHP, requires joint working between mental health services, midwifery and

The PMHS is delivered through a hub and spoke model. As NICE (2014) guidance recommends the centre is part of a clinical care network:

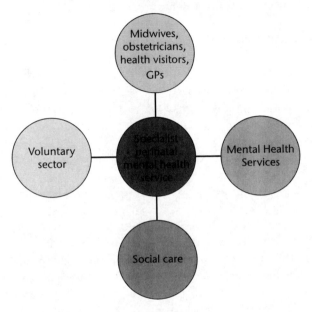

The hub is staffed by a psychiatrist, mental health nurses and a psychological therapist and provides/supports:

- early identification of mental health issues using NICE recommendations;
- early referrals to mental health services when required;
- specialist assessments;
- early interventions using the biopsychosocial approach;
- individualised care plans for management of PMHP;
- ensuring child protection and welfare of the family;
- woman and family-centred care;
- improved public health by endeavouring to reduce mental health morbidity in mothers;
- raised awareness and competence by delivering education and training events targeted at key professional groups;
- improved interagency working and communication;
- collaborative working.

The spokes are linked together and supported by:

- clear pathways of care;
- multiagency care planning with user involvement;
- training;
- directories of available services from the community and voluntary sectors;
- a maternal mental health advisory group to promote effective communication across services.

FIGURE 2.1 Hull and East Yorkshire Specialist Perinatal Mental Health Service (PMHS) – A UK practice example

Adapted from Jomeen & Martin, 2014.

obstetrics, acute care, primary care, children's services, paediatrics and the voluntary sector (NSPCC, 2013). Joint working within or across organisations must be facilitated by effective communication and provide a seamless perspective to care (also refer to Chapter 14 for insights into collaborative multi-agency practices). It is noteworthy that despite clear recommendations and guidelines for practice, support for women with PMHP often remains spasmodic and lacking. In the UK, for example, service mapping lucidly demonstrates that it remains a lottery whether women get access to services and the right help (Jomeen and Martin, 2014). Whilst some areas have specialist services, mental health specialist midwives and voluntary sector services (refer to Figure 2.1 for case example), other areas have little or no specialist service provision, which runs the risk of the service users 'dropping out' through gaps in the system, as demonstrated in the quote below:

> Then of course there was the CPN [community psychiatric nurse] but there was always a gap between GP [family doctor], health visitor and then CPN, that was certainly my experience … [refers to a previous experience] … they did one assessment and felt that it wasn't severe enough to warrant their input, but for me it was a bit more than I could help with, and there was nowhere to go really.
>
> (Jones, Jomeen, Glover, Garg & Marshall, 2015, p. 387)

Local strategies need to prioritise the development of pathways of care for women with PMHP at all levels, which are critical to optimise care for women and their families, but are also essential to support practitioners to confidently and proactively identify and assess women's PMHP (Jones et al., 2015). Such pathways of course need to lead to the provision of evidence-based interventions. Recent work has sought to try and identify and develop effective interventions to improve outcomes for women with PMHP – refer to Figure 2.1 for a case example.

Risk factors and resilience

Risk factors have been identified as predictors of PMHP but also potentially modifiable factors to mitigate against poorer emotional outcomes. Risk factors are best described as vulnerability, adverse factors or characteristics that are present in a woman's life and hence put them at greater risk of developing PMHP (Raynor & England, 2010). Using an example such as postnatal depression, it is readily accepted and evidence-based to state that there are significant, assessable and measureable antenatal risk factors and indeed, predictors, of postnatal depression (Martin, 2012). Of note is the recognition that risk factors, as independent causal variables, are not necessarily recommended to predict PMHP (NICE, 2014) because there is no inevitable cause and effect relationship. The presence of risk factors, however, may be utilised to determine an individual's vulnerability, particularly if the individual is subject to 'a cluster of these adverse factors' (Raynor & England 2010, p. 55). That the risk factors suggested have been found to be fairly globally consistent (see Box

---

BOX 2.2 POTENTIAL RISK FACTORS FOR PMHP

- Previous psychiatric disorder
- Family history of serious mental ill-health
- Social disadvantage and isolation
- Poverty
- Minority ethnic group
- Asylum seekers and refugees
- Late bookers and non-attenders
- Domestic violence
- Substance misuse
- Known to child protection services
- Employment status
- Physical ill health
- Life events
- Lack of support

Additional risk factors listed by NICE [2014]

- The woman's attitude towards the pregnancy, including denial of pregnancy
- The woman's experience of pregnancy/problems experienced by her, the fetus or the baby
- The mother–baby relationship
- Social networks/quality of interpersonal relationships
- Domestic violence and abuse, sexual abuse, trauma or childhood maltreatment
- Responsibilities as a carer for other children and young people or other adults

---

2.2), should support practitioner confidence in the consideration of these as part of the assessment of women's perinatal mental health status.

Resilience is an area gathering some focus in the perinatal literature, described as a process that allows people to adapt well in the face of adversity, trauma, tragedy, threats or significant sources of stress. Hence providing people with the psychological strength to cope with stress and calamity (also refer to Chapter 13 for further insights into resilience from a provider perspective). Increasingly research has focused on the impact of protective resilience factors to influence individual adaptation to life stressors and there is emergent, albeit relatively small body of literature in relation to psychological health in the perinatal period.

It is critical to be clear, however, that risk factors are not 'resilience' factors. The differentiating consideration being the predictive utility of risk factors and their integration within a vulnerability profiling framework, thus contributing to targeted care provision. This should then facilitate management of a woman's condition, which may include, where possible, avoidance of environmental risk factors and triggers and underpin informed choices about treatment options. Practitioners, therefore must be able to differentiate the subtle though important differences between risk factors, predictors and resilience in relation to PMHP and well-being.

It is suggested that low resilience can cause childbirth to be an especially stressful event (Takegata, Haruna, Matsuzaki, Sharaishi, Okano & Severinsson, 2014), and a history of mental illness, anxiety sensitivity and neurotic characteristics have all been associated with low stress resiliency (Takegata *et al.*, 2014), which in turn has been linked to, for example, fear of childbirth (Handelzalts, Zacks & Levy, 2016). Such evidence would suggest an association between resilience and PMHP, which raises the question of whether resilience-based interventions can offer benefits for women with PMHP.

Differing models of early intervention and treatment and limitations of the current evidence base

Evidence-based interventions which are underpinned by a coherent model of resilience applied to PMHP are sparse in the literature. Interventions that are generally used in the context of diagnosed perinatal mental illness fall into two groups, (i) pharmacotherapy and (ii) psychological therapies. These may be used in combination, which highlights the role of (i) biological and (ii) psychological/psychosocial factors in the manifestation of PMHP. Consideration of both groups is very useful as it provides an axis to consider how useful and effective a resilience model of intervention could be.

Biological models and resilience

Evidence of biological substrates implicated in perinatal mental illness include, hypothalamic-pituitary-adrenal axis dysregulation, inflammatory responses and genetic pre-dispositional factors (Yim, Tanner Stapleton, Guardino, Hahn-Holbrook & Dunkel Schetter, 2015). There is little evidence to support the suggestion of a biological model of resilience applied to PMH and therefore a resilience-based model is essentially discordant to any prevailing model of either pharmacological intervention, or the understanding of PMHP in relation to biological substrates. Modifiable biological domains where intervention might be more generally efficacious again does not accord with a resilience model, for example PMH and nutritional status (Leung & Kaplan, 2009). With regard to pharmacological treatments, risk versus benefits needs to be examined. Noteworthy is that pharmacology is neither appropriate nor effective for women with mild to moderate PMHP, meaning alternative approaches are required.

Psychological approaches and resilience

A suggestion of a resilience model might be reconciled within the arena of psychological intervention and it is this approach that has currently attracted some attention in the field of PMHP. There is a danger of confusing an evidence-based approach to mental illness intervention such as CBT with a resilience-defined intervention. Resilience has been investigated as a personal protective resource, against PTSD in particular, and results demonstrate that women with high resilience show significantly less depression and better mental quality of life in the postpartum period compared to women with low resilience (Mautner *et al.*, 2013). The construct of resilience has also been used in recent work as a framework on which to base interventions for women with PTSD (Turkstra *et al.*, 2013), though with more efficacious effects demonstrated in women without existing mental illness (further insights into PTSD onset following childbirth are discussed in Chapter 11). The studies that utilise a resiliency based framework in a perinatal context predominantly focus on modifying internal assets – that is those things that reside within the individual – such as coping skills and self-efficacy (Reed, Fenwick, Huack, Gamble & Creedy, 2014). Other studies suggest that Antonovsky's sense of coherence theory (in that individuals with high levels of comprehensibility, meaningfulness and manageability are more able to face and resolve stressors and remain in positive health), works as a resiliency factor to help women cope with the stress of childbirth and may be modifiable to positively impact pregnancy related distress (Staneva, Morawska, Bogossian & Wittkowski, 2015), though this is yet to translate in to a testable intervention. Attempts to modify and improve the women's external resources, such as social support (Easterbrooks, Kotake, Raskin & Bumgarner, 2016), do seem to offer some promising findings in terms of limiting the enduring nature of depression but whether this is a resilience-based approach or an attempt to modify an identified risk factor, remains questionable.

This evidence base for resilience interventions in PMHP, at present remains somewhat tenuous. It seems to suggest that impacting resilience is more effective as a protective factor for women at risk, rather than a treatment approach for women with a diagnosed PMHP, who appear more disposed to have low resilience. This demands consideration of whether the most effective focus remains on early identification and treatment approach to address the PMHP, using evidence-based therapies, alongside models of care which address modifiable risk factors such as social support. This seems supported by Turkstra and colleagues (2013) findings; their intervention offered counselling to women with PTSD, based on cognitive-behavioural principles, with a focus on individual situational supports for the present and future. One additional challenge here is that whilst theoretically based interventions such as CBT, PSI (psychosocial intervention), IPT (interpersonal therapy) and mindfulness (MFN) may have demonstrated effectiveness in other defined clinical populations, their efficacy in relation to PMHP in the prenatal period remains unconfirmed (Wadephul, Jones & Jomeen, 2016) – though some evidence suggests that women with higher baseline symptoms/higher risk do seem more likely to benefit (Wadephul *et al.*, 2016). Despite a lack of quantitative evidence of efficacy of psychological approaches in reducing low level symptomology, women and their partners qualitatively report benefits, mainly in terms of peer support and shared experiences, as the quotes below demonstrate (Wadephul *et al.*, 2016, pp. 16–17):

> Being able to talk to someone and listen to advice.

> It was great being around women who were in a similar situation to me and I liked being able to talk about my own experience.

> I learned that this is a shared human experience, and I'm not the only one who suffers.

> I have learned how to better understand my thoughts and my body. How my thoughts can trigger feelings and how these thoughts are not always factual.

Theoretical issues and considerations

One of the issues in relation to resilience and PMH might be the conceptual clarity of the term. Though 'resilience' has become widely accepted as a domain of importance and relevance to mental health, some authors claim the theoretical evidence base for the term is both lacking and indeed contentious (Atkinson, Martin & Rankin, 2009). The studies cited above all focus on differing 'resilience' variables, making definition of the construct difficult but also comparisons across studies challenging.

A note of caution must then be offered about what this means for the woman with a PMHP. Are we engendering her with the responsibility for her PMHP because she is not resilient enough? Resilience should not be used to fill a void that should be met by evidenced-based clinical services. The use of the term as linked to behaviours, thoughts and actions, which if lacking, may result in mental distress, engenders the woman with PMHP with accountability for her mental distress, at a time when she may be at her most vulnerable. Reflecting on the notion of resilience and the confounding conceptual issues highlighted above, it is crucial that health professionals consider the limitations of the term resilience and moreover what may be more practically useful, aligned to practice and rooted in the evidence base. Reconciling these shortcomings in resilience the health professional is directed to consider, pragmatically, the utility of modifiable risk factors.

The way forward and implications for practice and research

The poor definition of the term resilience is a fundamental issue to be borne in mind in terms of service provision for women with PMHP. The integration of non-evidence-based interventions into specialist PMH services is not tenable (Jomeen & Martin, 2014). Effective clinical decision-making and clinical practice must be underpinned by an evidence-based framework with the linkage of theory to practice being assessable, measureable and auditable (Jefford, Jomeen & Martin, 2016).

Whilst targeted psychological approaches demonstrate limited efficacy, there are multiple known factors that are linked to the development of PMHP, which include past and present circumstances, the context of women's lives, obstetric factors, coping behaviours and social and professional support. Factors such as knowledge, skills, attitude and self-efficacy and an environment that facilitate coping behaviours can be critical (Fontein-Kuipers, van Limbeek, Ausems, de Vries & Nieuwenhuijze, 2015b), further research to consider how to support these for women is required. The difficulty with many interventions is that they seek to target PMHP from one theoretical perspective aligned to improvement of often uni-dimensional outcomes, albeit associated, such as depression or anxiety, when for many women their psychological status is in fact much more composite and multi-dimensional (Jomeen, 2005). A more valuable and essential first step for women may be the ability to recognise their own personal contributing factors to PMHP, in order to underpin the process of disclosure and help-seeking and/or self-management (Fontein-Kuipers *et al.*, 2015b). Whilst recognition is knowledge based, help-seeking may require behaviour change modification and needs to occur within a context of adequate and effective social and/or professional support. Resources and facilities are then necessary to enable childbearing women to cope in an effective way and will probably include available and supportive maternity, early years and psychological services, as well a peer support groups which enable women to address their own modifiable variables. Examples of good practice exist along the continuum of the perinatal period. Interventions in the prenatal period will inevitably differ in their focus to those in the postpartum, which may focus more on supporting the mother–infant relationship (refer to Box 2.3 for a case example).

BOX 2.3 MINDING THE BABY: A GOOD PRACTICE EXAMPLE (ADAPTED FROM NSPCC, 2013)

Programmes that have been shown to be successful in improving mothers' reflective functioning (parental reflective functioning refers to how they use an understanding of mental states – intentions, feelings, thoughts, desires, and beliefs – to make sense of and, even more importantly, to anticipate their child's actions), can be used alongside or as part of therapeutic services. One example of a programme that appears to be successful in this area is the *Minding the Baby* programme, developed by experts at Yale University, in which social workers and nurses work with new mothers to enhance attachment relationships by developing reflective functioning capacities and supporting positive parent behaviours.

Approaches which aim to optimise the context from which women can engage in effective behaviours to promote more positive mental health may not be at odds with the concept of resilience as currently posited. However, if the notion of resilience is to become a useful one in this context, then further definition of the concept is required in relation to PMHP. The task is entirely feasible within contemporary research paradigms; good examples of the measurement and quantification of abstract concepts such as quality of life are abundant in the literature and have been applied extensively to pregnancy and maternity care (e.g. Jomeen & Martin, 2005) where these concepts are seen as relevant and important to women and their perinatal care and well-being (Jomeen & Martin, 2012). Adopting such an approach to resilience would allow the concept to be understood contextually and also with transparency, thus tacit agreement on the term, its use and the development of coherent theoretical framework from which truly evidence-based interventions based on the concept could be developed, utilised and evaluated.

Conclusion

International literature and policy continues to focus on psychological morbidity. Pregnancy, birth and the postpartum period is inherently dynamic for women and will inevitably represent both a physical and psychological challenge (Jomeen & Martin, 2008). Supporting women to manage that challenge requires a multifaceted approach, which begins with effective assessment of a women's needs, in order to intervene appropriately and from an evidence-based perspective. The evidence base for resilience in terms of women with a diagnosed PMHP means that it, as yet, cannot offer a solution for treatment. However, supporting women with PMHP may lend itself to an approach which addresses risk factors by capturing and utilising the presence of women's positive capabilities and emotions to support women in achieving a sense of enhanced well-being.

References

Alderdice, F., Ayers, S., Darwin, Z., Greenwood, J., Jomeen, J., Kenyon, S., Martin, C.R., Morrell, C.J., Newham, J.J., Redshaw, M., Savage-McGlynn, E. & Walsh, J. (2013). Measuring psychological health in the perinatal period: Workshop consensus statement, 19 March 2013. *Journal of Reproductive and Infant Psychology, 31*(5), 431–438.

American College of Nurse Midwives. (2013). *ACNM position statement: Depression in women*. Washington, DC: American College of Nurse Midwives.

American Congress of Obstetricians and Gynecologists. (2009). *Depression during pregnancy treatment recommendations: A joint report from APA and ACOG*. Washington, DC: American Congress of Obstetricians and Gynecologists.

American Congress of Obstetricians and Gynecologists. (2015). *ACOG committee opinion number 630: Screening for perinatal depression*. Washington, DC: American Congress of Obstetricians and Gynecologists.

Atkinson, P.A., Martin, C.R. & Rankin, J. (2009). Resilience revisited. *Journal of Psychiatric and Mental Health Nursing 16*(2), 137–145.

Bauer, A., Parsonage, M., Knapp, M., Lemmi, V. & Adelaja, B. (2014). *Costs of perinatal mental problems*. London: London School of Economics and Political Science.

Brucker, M.C. & King, T.L. (2015). *Pharmacology for women's health*. 2nd edition. Burlington, MA: Jones and Bartlett Publishers.

Centers for Disease Control and Prevention. (2015). *Morbidity and mortality weekly report: Vital signs: Demographic and substance use trends among Heroin users – United States, 2002 –2013. 64*(26), 719–725.

Centre for Maternal and Child Enquiries. (2011). Saving mothers' lives: Reviewing maternal deaths 2006–2008. *British Journal of Obstetrics and Gynaecology, 118* (Suppl. 1), 1–203.

Chaudron, L.H. (2013). Complex challenges in treating depression during pregnancy. *American Journal of Psychiatry, 3*(170), 12–20.

Confidential Enquiry into Maternal and Child Health (CEMACH). (2004). *Why mothers die (2000–2002)*. London: Royal College of Obstetricians & Gynaecologists.

Confidential Enquiry into Maternal and Child Health (CEMACH). (2007). *Saving mothers' lives: Reviewing maternal deaths to make motherhood safer (2003–2005)*. London: Royal College of Obstetricians & Gynaecologists.

Darvill, T., Skirton, H. & Farrand, P. (2010). Psychological factors that impact on women's experiences of first-time motherhood: A qualitative study of the transition. *Midwifery, 26*, 357–366.

Darwin, Z., McGowan, L. & Edozien, L.C. (2015). Antenatal mental health referrals: Review of local clinical practice and pregnant women's experiences in England. *Midwifery, 31*(3), e17–e22.

Dunkel Schetter, C. & Tanner, L. (2012). Anxiety, depression and stress in pregnancy: Implications for mothers, children, research and practice. *Current Opinion Psychiatry, 25*, 141–148.

Easterbrooks, M.A., Kotake, C., Raskin, M. & Bumgarner, E. (2016). Patterns of depressions among adolescent mothers: Resilience related to father support and home visiting program. *American Journal of Orthopsychiatry 86*, 61–68.

Fisher, J., de Mello, M., Patel, V., Rahman, A., Tran, T., Holton, S. & Holmes, W. (2010). Prevalence and determinants of common perinatal mental disorders in women in low- and lower-middle-income countries: A systematic review. *Bulletin of the World Health Organisation, 90*, 139–149. Available from: www.who.int/bulletin/volumes/90/2/11-091850/en/ [Accessed 12 January 2016].

Fontein-Kuipers, Y., Ausems, M., Bude. L., van Limbeek, E., de Vries, R. & Nieuwenhuijze, M. (2015a). Factors influencing maternal distress among Dutch women with a healthy pregnancy. *Women and Birth, 28*, 36–43.

Fontein-Kuipers, Y., van Limbeek, E., Ausems, M., de Vries, R., & Nieuwenhuijze, M. (2015b). Using intervention mapping for systematic development of a midwife-delivered intervention for prevention and reduction of maternal distress during pregnancy. *International Journal of Women's Health and Wellness, 1*:008. Available from: http://clinmedjournals.org/articles/ijwhw/international-journal-of-womens-health-and-wellness-ijwhw-1-008.pdf [Accessed 4 January 2016].

Handelzalts, J.E., Zacks, A. & Levy, S. (2016). The association of birth model with resilience variables and birth experience: Home versus hospital birth. *Midwifery, 36*, 80–85.

Heron, J., O'Conner, T., Evan, J., Golding, J. & Glover, V. (2004). The course of anxiety and depression thourhg pregnancy and the postpartum in a community sample. *Journal of Affective Disorders, 80*, 65–73.

Jefford, E., Jomeen, J. & Martin, C.R. (2016). Determining the psychometric properties of the enhancing decision-making assessment in midwifery (EDAM) measure in a cross cultural context. *BMC Pregnancy and Childbirth*, 16, 95. doi:org/10.1186/s12884-016-0882-3.

Johnson, M., Schmied, V., Lupton, S.J., Austin, MP., Matthey S.M., Kemp L., Meade, T. & Yeo A.E. (2012). Measuring women's perinatal mental health risk. *Archives of Women's Mental Health*, 15, 375–386.

Jomeen, J. (2005). The importance of assessing psychological status during pregnancy, childbirth and the postnatal period as a multidimensional construct: a literature review. *Clinical Effectiveness in Nursing*, 8, 143–155.

Jomeen, J. (2012). Women's psychological status in pregnancy and childbirth – measuring or understanding? *Journal of Reproductive and Infant Psychology*, 30(4), 337–340.

Jomeen, J. & Martin, C.R. (2005). The factor structure of the SF-36 in early pregnancy. *Journal of Psychosomatic Research*, 59(3), 131–138.

Jomeen, J. & Martin, C.R. (2008). Reflections on the notion of post-natal depression following examination of the scoring pattern of women on the EPDS during pregnancy and in the post-natal period. *Journal of Psychiatric and Mental Health Nursing*, 15(8), 645–648.

Jomeen, J. & Martin, C.R. (2012). Perinatal quality of life: Is it important for childbearing women? *The Practising Midwife*, 15, 30–34.

Jomeen, J. & Martin, C.R. (2014). Developing a specialist perinatal mental health service: Overcoming challenges and promoting success. *The Practicing Midwife*, 17(3), 18–21.

Jones, C., Jomeen, J., Glover, L., Garg, D. & Marshall, C. (2015). Exploring changes in health visitors' knowledge, confidence and decision making for women with perinatal mental health difficulties following a brief training package. *European Journal for Person Centred Healthcare*, 3(3), 384–391.

King, L., Pestell, S., Farrar, S., North, N. & Brunt, C. (2012). Screening for antenatal psychological distress. *British Journal of Midwifery*, 20, 396–401.

Leigh, B. & Milgrom, J. (2008). Risk factors for antenatal depression, postnatal depression and parenting stress. *BMC Psychiatry*, 8, 24. doi:10.1186/1471-244X-8-24.

Leung, B.M. & Kaplan, B.J. (2009). Perinatal depression: Prevalence, risks, and the nutrition link–A review of the literature. *Journal of the America Diet Association*, 109(9), 1566–1575.

Martin, C.R. (2012). *Perinatal mental health: A clinical guide*. Keswick: M&K Update.

Mautner, E., Stern, C., Deutsch, M., Nagele, E., Greimel, E., Lang, U. & Cervar-Zivkovic, M. (2013). The impact of resilience on psychological outcomes in women after preeclampsia: An observational cohort study. *Health Quality of Life Outcomes*, 11:194. doi:10.1186/1477-7525-11-194.

Mennes, M., Stiers, P., Lagae, L. & Van den Bergh, B. (2006). Long-term cognitive sequealae of antenatal maternal anxiety: Involvement of the orbitofrontal cortex. *Neuroscience and Biobehavioural Reviews*, 30, 1076–1086.

Monk, C., Spicer, J. & Champagne, F. (2012). Linking prenatal maternal adversity to developmental outcomes in infants: The role of epigenetic pathways. *Developmental Psychology*, 24, 1361–1376.

National Institute for Clinical Excellence. (2007). *Antenatal and postnatal mental health: Clinical management and service guidance*. London: Department of Health.

National Institute for Clinical Excellence. (2014). *Antenatal and postnatal mental health: Clinical management and service guidance*. London: Department of Health.

NSPCC. (2013). *Prevention in Mind. All babies count: Spotlight on perinatal mental health.* Available from: www.nspcc.org.uk/Inform/resourcesforprofessionals/underones/spotlight-mental-health-landing_wda96578.html [Available from 9 March, 2016].

Paarlberg, K.M., Vingerhoets, A.J.J.M., Passchier, J., Dekker, G.A. & Van Geijn, H.P. (1995). Psychosocial factors and pregnancy outcome: A review with emphasis on methodological issues. *Journal of Psychosomatic Research, 39*(5), 563–595.

Paschetta, E., Berrisford, G., Coccia, F., Whitmore, J., Wood, A., Pretlove, S. & Khaled, I. (2014). Perinatal psychiatric disorders: An overview. *American Journal of Obstetrics and Gynaecology, 210*(6), 501–509.

Price, S. (2007). *Mental health in pregnancy and childbirth.* Philadelphia, PA: Churchill Livingstone; Elsevier.

Raynor, M. & England, C. (2010). *Psychology for midwives: Pregnancy, childbirth and puerperium.* Maidenhead: Open University Press.

Reed, M., Fenwick, J., Huack, Y., Gamble, J. & Creedy, D.K. (2014). Australian midwives' experiences of delivering a counselling intervention for women reporting a traumatic birth. *Midwifery, 30*, 200–275.

Rollans, M., Schmied, V., Kemp, L. & Meade, T. (2013). 'We just ask some questions …': The process of antenatal psychosocial assessment by midwives. *Midwifery, 29*, 935–942.

Royal College of Psychiatrists. (2012). *Guidance for commissioners of perinatal mental health services.* Available from: www.jcpmh.info/resource/guidance-perinatal-mental-health-services/ [Accessed 10 January 2016].

Schuurmans, C. & Kurrasch, D. (2013). Neurodevelopmental consequences of maternal distress: What do we really know? *Clinical Genetics, 83*, 110–117.

Spiteri, C.M., Jomeen, J. & Martin, C.R. (2013). Reimagining the general health questionnaire as a measure of emotional wellbeing: A study of postpartum women in Malta. *Women and Birth, 26*(4), e105–e111.

Staneva, A., Morawska, A., Bogossian, F. & Wittkowski, A. (2015). Pregnancy-specific distress: The role of maternal sense of coherence and antenatal mothering orientations. *Journal of Mental Health, 11*, 1–8. doi:10.3109/09638237.2015.1101425.

Substance Abuse and Mental Health Services Administration. (2014). *Results from the 2013 national survey on drug use and health: Summary of national findings.* Rockville, MD: US Department of Health and Human Services, Substance Abuse and Mental Health Services Administration. NSDUH Series H-48, HHS Publication No. (SMA) 14–4863.

Takegata, M., Haruna, M., Matsuzaki, M., Sharaishi, M., Okano, T. & Severinsson, E. (2014). Antenatal fear of childbirth and sense of coherence among healthy pregnant women in Japan: A cross-sectional study. *Archives of Women's Mental Health, 17*, 403–409.

Thornton, C., Schmied, V., Dennis, C.-L., Barnett, B. & Dahlen, H.G. (2013). Maternal deaths in NSW (2000–2006) from nonmedical causes (suicide and trauma) in the first year following birth. *Biomed Research International, 623743*, doi:org/10.1155/2013/623743.

Tolia, V., Patrick, S., Bennett, M., Murthy, K., Sousa, J., Smith, B., Clark, R. & Spitzer, A. (2015). Increasing incidence of the neonatal abstinence syndrome in U.S. neonatal ICUs. *New England Journal of Medicine, 372*, 2118–2126.

Turkstra, E., Gamble, J., Creedy, D.K., Fenwick, J., Barclay, L., Buist, A., Rydiing, E.L. & Scuffham, P.A. (2013). PRIME: Impact of previous mental health problems on health related quality of life in women with childbirth trauma. *Archives of Women's Mental Health, 16*, 561–564.

Wadephul, F., Jones, C. & Jomeen, J. (2016). The impact of antenatal psychological group interventions on psychological well-being: A systematic review of the qualitative and quantitative evidence. *Healthcare*, *4*(2), 32. doi:10.3390/healthcare4020032.

Yim, I.S., Tanner Stapleton, L.R., Guardino, C.M., Hahn-Holbrook, J. & Dunkel Schetter, C. (2015). Biological and psychosocial predictors of postpartum depression: Systematic review and call for integration. *Annual Reviews of Clinical Psychology*, *11*, 99–137.

3

ASYLUM SEEKERS AND REFUGEES

A cross-European perspective

Marie-Clare Balaam, Melanie Haith-Cooper, Dineke Korfker and Charles Savona-Ventura

Introduction

In this chapter we explore issues of psychosocial resilience and risk related to asylum seeking and refugee women during the perinatal period, drawing on experiences from three diverse European countries; the United Kingdom (UK), Malta and the Netherlands. First we define the terms asylum seekers and refugees to allow us to focus on the issues that pertain specifically to women experiencing this form of migration. We also note the prevalence of migration in contemporary society. We explore recent research on asylum seeking and refugee women in the perinatal period to identify; the barriers women face in accessing care in their reception countries and their experiences of perinatal care. The challenges faced by healthcare professionals to provide culturally appropriate and high quality care to these women who face a range of psychosocial challenges are also highlighted. We suggest possible ways to address some of these challenges including how health professionals can actively build on the resilience of asylum seeking and refugee women to improve their perinatal experiences. We conclude by focusing on the implications of these findings, drawing on examples of good practice from the UK, the Netherlands and Malta to provide recommendations for practice and service development.

Definitions and prevalence

Contemporary society is characterised by an increasingly mobile global population with over 232 million people living outside their country of origin in 2013 (United Nations Department of Economic and Social Affairs [UN-DESA], 2014). This migrant population is diverse and includes people deemed to be legal as well as those considered illegal or undocumented. It also includes people who migrate voluntarily, such as economic migrants and students as well as people forced to migrate including refugees, asylum seekers and trafficked individuals.

This chapter focuses on forced migration, in particular asylum seeking and refugee women using the terms as defined by the United Nations (UN). Refugees are individuals who are outside their country of nationality 'owing to a well-founded fear of being persecuted for reasons of race, religion, nationality, membership of a particular social group or political opinion ... and are seeking in accordance with international conventions refuge in another country' (United Nations High Commissioner for Refugees [UNHCR], 1952, p. 14). Asylum seekers are individuals whose claim for refugee status has not been definitively decided by the country they seek refuge in (UN, 2014). In 2014 it was estimated there were more than 15 million refugees across the world, four-fifths of which were resident in low income counties, most commonly countries adjacent to their home countries; with the remaining fifth seeking refuge in higher income countries (UN, 2014). There has been a sharp escalation in the number of refugees with almost 60 million people displaced at the end of 2014 (UNHCR, 2015) and it is expected this will significantly increase with the intensification of the current conflict in Syria. Around four million people (one-fifth of Syria's population) have fled the country since 2011. Of the three European countries this chapter focuses on, the Netherlands has received the largest numbers of asylum seekers to date with numbers almost doubling in 2014–2015, reaching 57,000 by the end of 2015. In the UK, there were 25,771 claims for asylum between June 2014–2015. Malta had the smallest number of asylum applicants with 1,692 in 2015 (Home Office, 2015; Statistics Netherlands Statline, 2016; UNHCR, 2016).

The impact of forced migration on pregnant women and infants

The UNHCR (2015) estimates that around half of the population of forced migrants are women and girls. Research indicates that asylum seeking and refugee women are particularly likely to experience high levels of socioeconomic and financial disadvantage and physical and mental ill health in the countries in which they seek to settle (Porter & Haslam, 2005; Yelland et al., 2015). Pregnancy and early motherhood commonly exacerbate these issues (Aspinall & Watters, 2010; Shortall et al., 2015; UNHCR, 2015) with women and infants at risk due to malnourishment, anaemia, communicable diseases and psychiatric disorders (Burnett & Fassil, 2004). Although there is a dearth of data specifically around asylum seeking and refugee women, migrant women in general are at a disproportionately higher risk of a poor pregnancy outcome including low birth weight, preterm birth, perinatal and maternal morbidity and mortality (Bollini, Pampallona, Wanner & Kupelnick, 2009; Centre for Maternal & Child Enquiries [CMACE], 2011; National Institute for Health & Clinical Excellence [NICE], 2010). This is thought to be partly due to stress associated with the migration process, leading to conditions such as diabetes, raised blood pressure and chronic anxiety and depression (Brunner & Marmot, 2006).

Barriers and challenges to perinatal care

Research around asylum seeking and refugee women in the perinatal period has predominantly taken a risk-focused approach. As discussed above, this work has focused on the prevalence of poor pregnancy outcomes (Bakken, Skjeldal & Stray-Pedersen, 2015; Bollini et al., 2009; Bradby, Humphris, Newall & Phillimore, 2015; Gibson-Helm et al., 2014; Gissler et al., 2009; Goosen, 2014). Other work has highlighted the challenges faced by maternity care providers in meeting the needs of asylum seeking and refugee women within existing restrictive legal and bureaucratic structures (Boerleider, Francke, Manniën, Wiegers & Devillé, 2013; Feldman, 2006; Suurmond, Rupp, Seeleman, Goosen & Stronks, 2013). Research has also identified the challenges women face in accessing optimal care that meets their specific needs (Da Lomba & Murray, 2014; Médecins du Monde, 2007; Platform for International Cooperation on Undocumented Migrants [PICUM], 2011; Shortall et al., 2015). These challenges are explored further below using reference to existing literature and the voices of asylum seeking and refugee women.

Cultural constructions of health, illness and care

Evidence suggests that asylum seeking and refugee women may lack an understanding of the health services available to them due to their cultural construction of health and illness (Chauvin, Simonnot, Douay & Vanbiervliet, 2014; Phillimore, 2016) or a lack of health literacy (Chauvin et al., 2014; Riggs, Yelland, Duell-Piening & Brown, 2016) (see Chapter 4 for discussion of similar issues in relation to Indigenous populations). For example, one woman explained how she was unfamiliar with the term 'midwife':

> And my experience when I got a midwife here is what is a midwife because back home in my country they say nurse.
>
> (Maternity Stream of Sanctuary, 2015)

The woman therefore may either not understand the role of a midwife or see midwifery based care as inferior to more familiar medicalised care (Bryant, 2011; Inspectie voor de Gezondheidszorg, 2014). She may not understand the concept of preventative health care and thus not see the importance of attending antenatal or screening appointments (Carolan & Cassar, 2010; Feldman, 2014). One Somali women explained:

> What would my friends in Somalia say if I went a long way to hospital for a check-up, knowing that everything was OK with the pregnancy?
>
> (Essen, Johnsdotter, Hovelius, Gundmundsson, Sjoberg & Friedman, 2000, p. 1509)

A lack of understanding of health care provision more generally may inhibit access to maternity care in a number of ways. For example, in the UK, asylum seeking and refugee women frequently experience difficulties registering with a family doctor (GP). For some this is due to a lack of knowledge that in the UK, GPs are the initial contact point for care. Other women may hold the perception that they have the wrong documents to register with a GP (Lephard & Haith-Cooper, 2016; Psarros, 2014; Shortall et al., 2015). In the UK the GP is the gateway to the National Health Service (NHS) and not registering limits women's ability to access maternity and other health care (Bryant, 2011).

Charging for services

Uncertainty around the financing of maternity services for asylum seeking and refugee women can have serious implications for women seeking health care. For example, the fear of being charged is reported to be a key barrier (Chauvin et al., 2014; Feldman, 2014; Psarros, 2014). In the UK, maternity care is deemed 'immediately necessary' care and must not be withheld based on the ability to pay. However, while maternity care is free to all women who are 'ordinarily resident' in the UK and some migrants, other women may be charged including refused asylum seekers and undocumented migrants. Recent changes to legislation to restrict entitlement to free NHS care have caused confusion amongst health professionals and women. One woman described how she:

> Met a lady there that was telling me that you have to register and ... before you register you have to pay for your treatment ... if I don't pay they are going to report me to the United Kingdom Border Agency (Home Office).
> (Maternity Stream of Sanctuary, 2015)

Currently in the UK, asylum seeking and refugee women who are supported by the Home Office, as well as trafficked women (brought into a country for the purposes of forced labour or sexual exploitation) are exempt from all healthcare charges. However, women who have exhausted the asylum process (this relates to women who have been refused asylum and are awaiting deportation) may be charged for some healthcare and while maternity care must not be withheld, these women can and have been charged (Shortall et al., 2015).

In the Netherlands, no women, regardless of immigration status should be charged for care (Goosen, Uitenbroek, Wijsen & Stronks, 2009). However many health professionals are not aware of the reimbursement procedures and subsequently request payment from women who have been refused asylum (de Jonge, et al., 2011).

By contrast there is little uncertainty around charging for care in Malta. Public health care is free at the point of contact for all residents including asylum seekers and refugees. Thus they have legal rights to access and receive state medical care and services as required. While there is no official legislation for undocumented migrants, the reality is that these individuals receive all their health care needs including access to free medications (Health Care for Undocumented Migrants and Asylum Seekers, 2009; Ministry for Justice and Home Affairs, 2005).

Dispersal in pregnancy

In the UK, the government has a policy of dispersal. This is the 'no choice' movement of asylum seekers to different accommodation usually in different towns and which can occur frequently and with little notice. Pregnant women are exempt from dispersal during their pregnancy. However, research has shown that women are frequently dispersed close to their due date and also on postnatal hospital discharge (Bryant, 2011; Feldman, 2014; Lephard & Haith-Cooper, 2016; Phillimore, 2014) as reflected in the following quote:

> I was put in the coach with a lot of people and my baby is just the youngest one there (2 weeks) ... I ended up in Leeds [a city in the UK] in the night ... I don't know anybody.
>
> (Maternity Stream of Sanctuary, 2015)

Dispersal can interrupt perinatal care, often for several weeks as women struggle to access care in their new location (Feldman, 2014). In the Netherlands dispersal during pregnancy is also problematic, with women potentially being moved to a different centre for asylum seekers and refugees every few weeks. In 2015 guidelines were revised to facilitate a smooth transfer between centres; however, a report of the Dutch Inspectorate found that not all centres acted according to the guidelines (Inspectie voor de Gezondheidszorg, 2014). As a result of this report, health care providers revised the guidelines to include a verbal handover to prevent loss of health information which had often occurred to the detriment of women's care (Royal Dutch Organisation of Midwives, 2015). Dispersal is not an issue for women in Malta who once settled in accommodation outside their initial arrival location will not be relocated in this way.

Destitution

In the UK, poverty and destitution faced by asylum seeking and refugee women can be a real barrier to accessing maternity services (Phillimore, 2016). Research has found that many women struggle to access the limited benefits they are entitled to. In addition, women who are refused asylum in the UK but receive Home Office support are given vouchers with no access to cash to spend on public transport and consequently can miss health appointments (Feldman, 2014; Lephard & Haith-Cooper, 2016; Phillimore, 2016; Waugh, 2010). This issue is reflected in this woman's quote:

After I had my baby it was difficult to go to my appointment for my baby's immunisation because it was difficult to walk and the voucher was difficult to exchange for cash.

(Maternity Stream of Sanctuary, 2015)

Asylum seeking and refugee women on low incomes can claim travel to appointments but this is only retrospective; many women and health professionals are also unaware of this policy (Phillimore, 2016). One study reported that midwives often give women their own money to help them attend appointments (Bryant, 2011).

Deportation

Some women may fear being deported as a result of accessing health services believing that health professionals are connected to immigration services and attending appointments may lead to them being traced, deported or having their babies removed (Bryant, 2011; Phillimore, 2016; Shortall *et al.*, 2015). This fear being explicitly recounted within women's narratives:

I was scared that if I registered with the doctor … they would find out and deport me. When I was 12 weeks pregnant I was told at that there was a doctor for the homeless and that if you went there they would not give your details to the Home Office.

(Maternity Action & Refugee Council, 2013, p. 43)

Language barriers

It is well documented that language barriers inhibit women's access to maternity services (Chauvin *et al.*, 2014; Cross-Sudworth, Williams & Gardoski, 2015; Tobin, Murphy-Lawless & Tetano Beck, 2014; Waugh, 2010). Language difficulties can affect women's abilities to understand services available to them, book appointments and negotiate public transport to attend appointments (Phillimore, 2016). The quality and availability of interpreting services is also a key issue. Lack of, poor quality or inappropriate interpretation services may mean that women do not attend subsequent appointments, lack confidence in those chosen to interpret for them, particularly if these are family members, or are not provided with interpreters for key events such as during labour (Feldman, 2014; Haith-Cooper, 2014). One woman described how:

I overheard that I was getting an epidural … I was asking my friend what is an epidural?

(Tobin, Murphy-Lawless & Beck, 2014, p. 836)

Appropriate and effective provision of interpreters has been problematic in the UK and the Netherlands with limited access to services due to budget cuts and changes to service organisation. For example, in the UK midwives have reported not being able to access interpreters, particularly in less common languages and for unplanned encounters (Haith-Cooper, 2014; Phillimore, 2016). While in the Netherlands changes in funding has led to some health professionals being unaware of the availability of services and therefore not using interpreters when caring for asylum seeking and refugee women (Inspectie voor de Gezondheidszorg, 2014).

Poor experiences of maternity care

There is an increasing body of evidence that some asylum seeking and refugee women experience poor care when accessing maternity services and that this and a lack of continuity of carer can be a barrier to attending for subsequent appointments (Lephard & Haith-Cooper, 2016; Phillimore, 2014). This poor care includes prejudicial or negative staff attitudes, a lack of understanding of and empathy for the life situations of asylum seeking and refugee women, poor communication and discrimination, as well as poor co-ordination of specialist services such as referrals to doulas and Female Genital Mutilation (FGM) clinics (Shortall et al., 2015). In a study by Robertson one woman described how:

> They should have asked in a friendly way if we needed help … it was a very unpleasant experience, I felt like an idiot, as totally incompetent.
>
> (Robertson, 2015, p. 63)

The way forward: implications and recommendations for practice

In the following section we discuss three key areas that can contribute to improving the quality of maternity care offered to asylum seeking and refugee women. We discuss the role of specialist services, the promotion of resilience among asylum seeking and refugee women and the need to support staff to allow them to provide optimal care.

Specialist perinatal services

In the UK, NICE highlight the need for appropriate and accessible antenatal care for vulnerable women including asylum seeking and refugee women. This includes improved service organisation, information provision and communication and training to ensure cultural competence amongst service providers (NICE, 2010). Despite this there are currently no specific pathways for maternity care for asylum seeking and refugee women within the NHS. Although some specialist services that provide innovative practice exist in the UK, the availability varies between areas (Cross-Sudworth et al., 2015) and they are often provided by non-statutory and voluntary agencies (Balaam, Kingdon, Thomson, Finlayson & Downe, 2016;

Da Lomba & Murray, 2014). In the UK, the Haamla service is an example of a specialist maternity service for vulnerable migrant women in Leeds in the North of England. Community-based midwives lead a team which provides continuity of care during the antenatal and postnatal period, specialist education and a doula service. They also provide an FGM clinic for pregnant women (The Leeds Teaching Hospitals NHS, 2015) (examples of collaborative multiagency practice are also discussed in Chapter 14).

In the Netherlands pregnant asylum seeking and refugee women attend a specialist health care centre. Their maternity care pathway is similar to that of other Dutch women in that they are referred to a contracted midwifery practice, only seeing a doctor if there are medical problems. However, they are not allowed to give birth at home due to poor housing conditions, even though this birth choice is still relatively common for native Dutch women.

Malta on the other hand has established an exemplary unified statutory provision of care. In 2008 the Migrant Health Unit (MHU) was established to help migrants, including asylum seeking and refugee women access health services. The unit provides interpreting services, translated educational material and also undertakes community based health education initiatives to familiarise migrants with various aspects of their health needs, including sexual health and contraception, FGM clinics and specialist antenatal education based in the state hospital. In addition, the MHU trains health professionals in culture and diversity issues (Department of Primary Health Malta, 2008). Women are further supported by a unified social service structure, covering their social needs in the community and within the health service. In a small island community, this allows for easier communication between various branches of the service. There is also good communication between state and voluntary non-governmental organisations. Thus, perinatal migrant women with specific social needs are regularly referred to the hospital social worker services who liaise with the outreach social worker programme to help improve the woman's social situation outside the hospital.

Promoting resilience in asylum seeking and refugee women

As demonstrated above, research on asylum seeking and refugee women has highlighted the challenges women face in accessing optimal perinatal care. While it is crucial that health professionals and researchers recognise the complex psychosocial, economic and cultural challenges and 'structural constraints' (Robertson, 2015) faced by asylum seeking and refugee women there needs to be a broader approach to understanding this topic. Recently there has been an increased interest in taking a salutogenic approach which, following the work of Antonovsky (1987), rejects the traditional risk-focused, bio-medical paradigm, considering instead how health and well-being can be promoted through addressing issues such as resilience, capability and facilitating maternal coping strategies to overcome challenges to well-being (Lindström & Eriksson, 2010; Viken, Balaam & Lyberg, 2016; Viken, Lyberg & Severinsson, 2015).

Health professionals need to acknowledge the existent knowledge and skills of asylum seeking and refugee women, including past experiences of pregnancy and birth and actively engage, support and develop women's capabilities and resilience in responding to the situations they face (Balaam et al., 2016; Ngum Chi Watts, Liamputtong & McMichael, 2015; Robertson, 2015). A more holistic approach considering asylum seeking and refugee women's position within their new societies has been proposed (Haith-Cooper & Bradshaw, 2013; Viken et al., 2015) in which the migratory and post migratory stressors experienced by women are acknowledged but attention is directed to the ways in which women react to these stressors by acknowledging the resilience, skills and capabilities they demonstrate.

Research has identified that early intervention may positively promote maternal well-being in perinatal asylum seeking and refugee women (Gagnon, Carnevale, Mehta, Rousseau & Stewart, 2013; Viken et al., 2015). Interventions need to be designed to 'seek to increase and nurture social support networks' and build on 'the evident resilience and resourcefulness of migrant and asylum seeking and refugee women' (Ngum Chi Watts et al., 2015, p. 10). Examples of such interventions can be seen at both local and national levels. In Malta, following public debate over the standards of health and living conditions of asylum seekers in detention centres (Médecins du Monde, 2007) the government now ensures that asylum and refugee women are offered alternative more suitable housing within the community during the perinatal period. Not only does this ensure better living conditions, it acts to promote a sense of community cohesion and social support among women who often assist each other during the perinatal period.

Other interventions that promote resilience amongst pregnant asylum seeking, refugee and other migrant women are provided by non-statutory organisations at a more local level. For example, the health befriending project and the Maternity Stream of the City of Sanctuary in the UK have provided asylum seeking and refugee women with opportunities to build upon their own resilience whilst also improving maternity care for others in a similar situation. These projects have provided opportunities for training and voluntary work enabling women to provide peer befriending support, contribute to service development and maternity education as users, as well as presenting and chairing at national and international conferences (Haith-Cooper & McCarthy, 2015; McCarthy & Haith-Cooper, 2014).

Preparing health professionals

It can be argued that health professionals' lack of knowledge of the life experiences and care needs of asylum seeking and refugee women contributes to many of the difficulties faced by these women in the perinatal period. In light of this it is vital that professionals are both trained on issues of culture and diversity as well enabled to develop an understanding of the complexities of the lives of asylum seeking and refugee women and how to meet their holistic needs (Goosen, van Oostrum & Essink-Bot, 2010; Haith-Cooper & Bradshaw, 2013; Suurmond et al., 2013). A tool that can be used in training is the evidence based model 'The pregnant woman within the global context'. This tool is designed to enable health professionals to consider the asylum seeker and refugee woman at the centre of her care and consider how challenges within her reception and her home country will impact on her health and social care needs (see Haith-Cooper & Bradshaw, 2013 for a more detailed explanation of this model). The model can be used in conjunction with a film which considers some of the issues in more depth, discussing the experiences of asylum seeking and refugee women living in England (Maternity Stream of Sanctuary, 2015).

There is also a need to provide resources for midwives so they can support asylum seeking and refugee women to overcome the language barriers they face thus increasing their health literacy and understanding of health services in the reception country (Bennett & Scammell, 2014; Haith-Cooper & Bradshaw, 2013; Lyberg, Viken, Haruna & Severinsson, 2012; Riggs, Yelland, Duell-Piening & Brown, 2016). Measures to help facilitate effective communication between health professionals and women include the provision of adequate interpreting services (Grech & Cheng, 2010), the development of picture-based resources for women who have limited literacy in their own language (Bryant, 2011) as well as the increased use, where appropriate, of mobile applications which may help address language barriers (Haith-Cooper, 2014).

Box 3.1 below provides some prompts for health professionals to consider in their interactions with asylum seeking and refugee women.

BOX 3.1 TIPS FOR HEALTH PROFESSIONALS IN THEIR EVERYDAY PRACTICE

- **Communication**: Feeling safe and trusting the caregiver is vital. Use professional interpreters. Speak slowly. Using 'safe' open questions such as: 'Tell me about yourself?' and 'How does this compare to back home?' Listen if she wants to talk; if she doesn't, reassure her that this is OK. Explain how confidentiality works within the maternity services.
- **History taking**: Consider the woman's social situation. Has she got the resources to access maternity care? Is she receiving the financial support she is entitled to?
- **Advocacy**: Support the woman in challenges she faces such as lobbying to avoid dispersal and to access appropriate housing.
- **Signposting**: To local refugee organisations, support groups, specialist services such as FGM support, peer/doula support schemes.
- **Cultural context**: Explain the organisation of healthcare services. Discuss woman's expectations of childbirth and how any cultural requests can be met.

Conclusion

Drawing on current evidence and examples from the UK, Malta and the Netherlands this chapter has examined aspects of the perinatal care of asylum seeking and refugee women. We have identified as key the need for a clearer understanding of the socio/cultural/economic and legislative factors which effect both the nature of the care that health professionals can currently provide asylum seeking and refugee women and the ability of women to access care within existing care settings.

There is a need for change in mainstream health services to ensure they meet asylum seeking and refugee women's needs. Health professionals need training to ensure they feel confident to provide care which meets the complex needs of asylum seeking and refugee women. Women need to be able to access care without the fear of being charged for services. The good practice of an integrated, rather than piecemeal approach to health and social care in Malta through the migrant health unit could be adopted elsewhere. In addition, the provision of specialist perinatal services would appear more effective than mainstream statutory services. A fast track system for women booking late for antenatal care would ensure they can access services (Phillimore, 2016). Alongside these services, peer support interventions including befriending are a relatively inexpensive but an effective means of building resilience in asylum seeking and refugee women.

There is a need for ongoing research in this area including the impact of the wider political/social/cultural and economic situation on perinatal asylum seeking and refugee women's health and well-being, including pregnancy outcomes. This research needs to include a variety of both quantitative and qualitative approaches, to be specifically focused on asylum seeking and refugee women, rather than subsumed within broader research on migrant women, and to adopt a salutogenic approach focusing on building resilience to address the complexity and heterogeneity of women's lives.

Acknowledgement

This chapter is based upon work from the COST Action IS1405 BIRTH: 'Building intrapartum research through health – An interdisciplinary whole system approach to understanding and contextualising physiological labour and birth' (www.cost. eu/COST_Actions/isch/IS1405), supported by COST (European Cooperation in Science and Technology).

References

Antonovsky, A. (1987). *Unraveling the mystery of health: How people manage stress and stay well.* London: Jossey-Bass.
Aspinall, P. & Watters, C. (2010). *Refugees and asylum seekers: A review from an equality and human rights perspective.* Available from: www.equalityhumanrights.com/en/

publication-download/research-report-52-refugees-and-asylum-seekers-review-equality-and-human-rights [Accessed 2 February 2016].

Bakken, K., Skjeldal, O. & Stray-Pedersen, B. (2015). Immigrants from conflict zone counties: An observational comparison study of obstetric outcomes in a low risk maternity ward in Norway. *BMC Pregnancy & Childbirth*, *15*, 163. doi:10.1186/s12884-015-0603-3.

Balaam, M., Kingdon, C., Thomson, G., Finlayson, K. & Downe, S. (2016). 'We make them feel special': The experiences of voluntary sector workers supporting asylum seeking and refugee women during pregnancy and early motherhood. *Midwifery*, *34*, 133–140.

Bennett, S. & Scammell, J. (2014). Midwives caring for asylum seeking women: Research findings. *Practising Midwife*, *17*, 9–12.

Boerleider, A., Francke, A., Manniën, J., Wiegers, T. & Devillé, W. (2013). A mixture of positive and negative feelings: A qualitative study of primary care midwives' experiences with non-western clients living in the Netherlands. *International Journal of Nursing Studies*, *50*(12), 1658–1666.

Bollini, P., Pampallona, S., Wanner, P. & Kupelnick, B. (2009). Pregnancy outcomes of migrant women and integration policy: A systematic review of the international literature. *Social Science & Medicine*, *68*(3), 452–461.

Bradby, H., Humphris, R., Newall, D. & Phillimore, J. (2015). *Public health aspects of migrant health: A review of the evidence on health status for refugees and asylum seekers in the European Region*. Available from: www.euro.who.int/__data/assets/pdf_file/0004/289246/WHO-HEN-Report-A5-2-Refugees_FINAL.pdf [Accessed 15 January 2016].

Brunner, E. & Marmot, M. (2006). Social organisation, stress and health. In M. Marmot & R. Wilkinson (Eds.), *Social determinants of health*. 2nd edition (pp. 6–30). Oxford: Oxford University Press.

Bryant, H.B. (2011). *Improving care for refugees and asylum seekers: The experiences of midwives*. Available from: www.maternityaction.org.uk/wpcontent/uploads/2014/03/TheExperiencesofMidwivesReport-2011.pdf [Accessed 7 March 2016].

Burnett, A. & Fassil, Y. (2004). *Meeting the health needs of refugees and asylum seekers in the UK: An information and resource pack for health workers*. London: National Health Service.

Carolan, M. & Cassar, L. (2010). Antenatal care perceptions of pregnant African women attending maternity services in Melbourne. *Midwifery*, *26*, 189–201.

Chauvin, P., Simonnot, N., Douay, C. & Vanbiervliet, F. (2014). *Access to healthcare for the most vulnerable in a Europe in social crisis 2014: Focus on women and children*. Available from: http://issuu.com/dotw/docs/mdm_2014_eu_report_access_to_care [Accessed 19 January 2016].

CMACE. (2011). *Saving mothers' lives: Reviewing maternal deaths to make motherhood safer: 2006–2008. The eighth report on confidential enquiries into maternal deaths in the United Kingdom*. Available from: www.centreformidwiferyeducation.ie/news/cmace-2011-saving-mothers-lives [Accessed 10 February 2016].

Cross-Sudworth, F., Williams, M. & Gardoski, J. (2015). Perinatal deaths of migrant mothers: Adverse outcomes from unrecognised risks and substandard care factors. *British Journal of Midwifery*, *23*(10), 734–739.

Da Lomba, S. & Murray, N. (2014). *Women and children first? Refused asylum seekers' access to and experiences of maternity care in Glasgow*. Available from: www.scottishrefugeecouncil.org.uk/assets/0000/7924/Women__Children_First_Final.pdf [Accessed 10 March 2016].

de Jonge, A., Rijnders, M., Agyemang, C., van der Stouwe, R., den Otter, J., Muijsenbergh, M.E. & Buitendijk, S. (2011). Limited midwifery care for undocumented women in the Netherlands. *Journal of Pyschosomatic Obstetrics & Gynecology, 32*(4), 182–188.

Department of Primary Health Malta. (2008). *Migrant health unit.* Available from: https://health.gov.mt/en/phc/mhlo/Pages/mhlo.aspx. [Accessed 19 February 2016].

Essen, B., Johnsdotter, S., Hovelius, B., Gundmundsson, S., Sjoberg, N-O. & Friedman, J. (2000). Qualitative study of pregnancy and childbirth experiences in Somalian women resident in Sweden. *British Journal of Obstetrics and Gynaecology, 107*, 1507–1512.

Feldman, R. (2006). Primary health care for refugees and asylum seekers: A review of the literature and a framework for services. *Public Health, 120*, 809–816.

Feldman, R. (2014). When maternity doesn't matter: Dispersing pregnant women seeking asylum. *British Journal of Midwifery, 22*(1), 22–28.

Gagnon, A., Carnevale, F., Mehta, P., Rousseau, H. & Stewart, D. (2013). Developing population interventions with migrant women for maternal–child health: A focused ethnography. *BMC Public Health, 13*(1). doi:10.1186/1471-2458-13-471.

Gibson-Helm, M., Teede, H., Block, A., Knight, M., East, C., Wallace, E., & Boyle, J. (2014). Maternal health and pregnancy outcomes among women of refugee background from African countries: A retrospective, observational study in Australia. *BMC Pregnancy and Childbirth, 14*(392). doi:10.1186/s12884-014-0392-0.

Gissler, M., Alexander, S., MacFarlane, A., Small, R., Stray-Pedersen, B., Zeitlin, J., Zimbeck, M. & Gagnon, A. (2009). Stillbirths and infant deaths among migrants in industrialized countries. *Acta Obstetricia et Gynecologica Scandinavica, 99*(2), 134–148.

Goosen, S. (2014). A safe and healthy future? Epidemiological studies on the health of asylum seekers and refugees in the Netherlands. PhD, University of Amsterdam, Netherlands. Available from: http://dare.uva.nl/record/1/417931 [Accessed 10 March 2016].

Goosen, S., Uitenbroek, D., Wijsen, C., & Stronks, K. (2009). Induced abortions and teenage births among asylum seekers in the Netherlands: Analysis of national surveillance data. *Journal of Epidemiology & Community Health, 63*, 528–533.

Goosen, S., van Oostrum, I. & Essink-Bot, M. (2010). Obstetric outcomes and expressed health needs of pregnant asylum seekers: A literature survey. *Ned. Tijdschr. Geneeskd, 154*(47), 2170–2176.

Grech, H. & Cheng, L. (2010). Communication in the migrant community in Malta. *Folia Phoniatrica et Logopaedica, 62*, 246–254.

Haith-Cooper, M. (2014). Mobile translators for non-English speaking women accessing maternity services. *British Journal of Midwifery, 22*(11), 795–803.

Haith-Cooper, M. & Bradshaw, G. (2013). Meeting the health and social care needs of pregnant asylum seekers; Midwifery students' perspectives: Part 3; 'The pregnant woman within the global context'; An inclusive model for midwifery education to address the needs of asylum seeking women in the UK. *Nurse Education Today, 33*(9), 1045–1050.

Haith-Cooper, M. & McCarthy, R. (2015). Striving for excellence in maternity care: The maternity stream of the city of sanctuary. *British Journal of Midwifery, 23*(9), 648–652.

Health for Undocumented Migrants and Asylum Seekers Network (HUMA). (2009). *Access to health care for undocumented migrants and asylum seekers – Law and Practice: Malta.* Available from: www.epim.info/wp-content/uploads/2011/02/Legislative-Rapport-HUMA-Network.pdf [Accessed 17 January 2016].

Home Office. (2015). *National statistics asylum.* Available from: www.gov.uk/government/publications/immigration-statistics-april-to-june-2015/asylum#key-facts [Accessed 10 March 2016].

Inspectie voor de Gezondheidszorg. (2014). *Inzet professionele tolken en overdracht bij overplaatsing moetenbetervoor verantwoorde geboortezorg aan asielzoekers*. Available from: www.igz.nl/Images/2014-02%20Geboortezorg%20aan%20asiekzoekers_tcm294-3515 17.pdf [Accessed 16 March 2016].

Lephard, E. & Haith-Cooper, M. (2016). Pregnant and seeking asylum: Exploring experiences 'from booking to baby'. *British Journal of Midwifery*, 24(2), 130–136.

Lindström, B. & Eriksson, M. (2010). *The hitchhiker's guide to salutogenesis: Salutogenic pathways to health promotion*. Helsinki: Folkhälsan Research Centre, Health Promotion Research.

Lyberg, A., Viken, B., Haruna, M. & Severinsson, E. (2012). Diversity and challenges in the management of maternity care for migrant women. *Journal of Nursing Management, 20*, 287–295.

McCarthy, R. & Haith-Cooper, M. (2014). Evaluating the impact of befriending for pregnant asylum seeking and refugee women. *British Journal of Midwifery, 21*(6), 406–409.

Maternity Action & Refugee Council. (2013) When maternity doesn't matter: Dispersing pregnant women seeking asylum. Available from: www.refugeecouncil.org.uk/ assets/0002/6402/When_Maternity_Doesn_t_Matter_-_Ref_Council__Maternity_Act ion_report_Feb2013.pdf [Accessed 16 March 2016].

Maternity Stream of Sanctuary. (2015). Childbirth in the UK: Stories from refugees. Available from: http://maternity.cityofsanctuary.org/films [Accessed 5 January 2016].

Médecins du Monde. (2007). *Access to health care and human rights of asylum seekers in Malta – Experiences, results and recommendations*. Available from: https://issuu.com/ medecinsdumonde/docs/access-to-health-care-and-human-rig [Accessed 11 December 2015].

Ministry for Justice and Home Affairs. (2005). Irregular migrants, refugees and integration – Policy document. Malta: Ministry of Justice and Home Affairs and Ministry for the Family and Social Security. Available from: www.refworld.org/pdfid/51b197484.pdf [Accessed 11 December 2015].

Ngum Chi Watts, M., Liamputtong, P. & McMichael, C. (2015). Early motherhood: A qualitative study exploring the experiences of African Australian teenage mothers in greater Melbourne, Australia. *BMC Public Health, 15*, 873. doi:10.1186/s12889-015–2215-2212.

NICE. (2010). *Pregnancy and complex social factors: A model for service provision for pregnant women with complex social factors*. Available from: www.nice.org.uk/guidance/cg110 [Accessed 18 December 2015].

Phillimore, J. (2014). Delivering maternity services in an era of superdiversity: The challenges of novelty and newness. *Ethnic and Racial Studies, 38*(4). doi:10.1080/014198 70.2015.980288.

Phillimore, J. (2016). Migrant maternity in an era of superdiversity: New migrants' access to, and experience of, antenatal care in the West Midlands, UK. *Social Science & Medicine, 148*, 152–159.

PICUM. (2011). *Preventing undocumented women and children from accessing healthcare: Fostering Health inequalities in Europe*. Available from: http://picum.org/en/publications/ conference-and-workshop-reports/25872/ [Accessed 16 March 2016].

Porter, M. & Haslam, N. (2005). Predisplacement and postdisplacement factors associated with mental health of refugees and internally displaced persons: A meta-analysis. *Journal of the American Medical Association, 294*(5), 602–612.

Psarros, A. (2014). *Women's voices on health: Addressing barriers to accessing primary care.* Available from: www.betterhealth.org.uk/sites/default/files/consultations/responses/Access-to-Primary-Care-report-FINAL(1).pdf [Accessed 10 February 2016].

Riggs, E., Yelland, J., Duell-Piening, P. & Brown, S. (2016). Improving health literacy in refugee populations. *Medical Journal of Australia, 204* (1), 9–10.

Robertson, E. (2015). 'To be taken seriously': Women's reflections on how migration and resettlement experiences influence their healthcare needs during childbearing in Sweden. *Sexual and reproductive Health, 6,* 59–65.

Royal Dutch Organisation of Midwives. (2015). *Geboortezorg Asielzoekster.* Available from: www.knov.nl/fms/file/knov.nl/knov_downloads/2327/file/Bijlage_5_Ketenrichtlijn_geboortezorg_definitieve_versie_augustus_2015.pdf?download_category=richtlijnen-prak tijkkaarten [Accessed 9 February 2017].

Shortall, C., McMorran, J., Taylor, K., Traianou, A., Gracia de Frutos, M., Jones, L. & Mur-will, P. (2015). *Experiences of pregnant migrant women receiving ante/peri and postnatal care in the UK: A doctors of the world report on the experiences of attendees at their London drop in clinic.* Available from: http://b.3cdn.net/droftheworld/c8499b817f90db5884_iym6bthx1.pdf. [Accessed 7 March 2016].

Statistics Netherlands Statline. (2016). Twice as many asylum seekers and following family members in 2015 as in 2014. Available from: www.cbs.nl/en-gb/news/2016/04/twice-as-many-asylum-seekers-and-following-family-members-in-2015-as-in-2014 [Accessed 19 February 2016].

Suurmond, J., Rupp, I., Seeleman, C., Goosen, S. & Stronks, K. (2013). The first contacts between healthcare providers and newly-arrived asylum seekers: A qualitative study about which issues need to be addressed. *Public Health, 127*(7), 668–673.

The Leeds Teaching Hospitals NHS. (2015). *HAAMLA Service.* Available from: www. leedsth.nhs.uk/a-z-of-services/leeds-perinatal-centre/what-we-do/haamla-service/ [Accessed 11 March 2016].

Tobin, C., Murphy-Lawless, J. & Tetano Beck, C. (2014). Childbirth in exile: Asylum seeking women's experience of childbirth in Ireland. *Midwifery 30,* 831–838.

UN-DESA. (2014). *Number of international migrants rises above 232 million.* Available from www.un.org/en/development/desa/news/population/number-of-international-migrants -rises.html. [Accessed 19 February 2016].

UNHCR. (1952). *Refugee convention.* Available from: www.unhcr.org/pages/49c3646c137. html [Accessed 6 March 2016].

UNHCR. (2015). Women, particular risks and challenges. Available from: www.unhcr. org/pages/49c3646c1d9.html [Accessed 6 March 2016].

UNHCR. (2016). *Malta asylum trends.* Available from: www.unhcr.org.mt/charts/ [Accessed 26 November 2015].

United Nations. (2014). *Refugees/forced displacement overview.* Available from: www.un.org/ en/globalissues/briefingpapers/refugees/overviewofforceddisplacement.html [Accessed 26 November 2016].

Viken, B., Balaam, M. & Lyberg, A. (2016). A salutogenic perspective on maternity care for migrant women. In S. Church, S. Downe, L. Frith, M. Balaam, M. Berg, V. Smith, C. Van der Walt & E. Van Teijlingen (Eds.), *New thinking on improving maternity care: International perspectives* (pp. 107–122). London: Pinter & Martin.

Viken, B., Lyberg, A. & Severinsson, E. (2015). Maternal health coping strategies of migrant women in Norway. *Journal of Nursing Research and Practice 2015*: 1–11. doi:10.1155/2015/878040.

Waugh, M. (2010). *The mothers in exile project: Women asylum seekers' and refugees' experiences of pregnancy and childbirth in Leeds*. Leeds: Women's Health Matters.

Yelland, J., Riggs, E., Szwarc, J., Casey, S., Dawson, W., Vanpraag, D., East, C., Wallace, E., Teale, G., Harrison, B., Petschel, P., Furler, J., Goldfeld, S., Mensah, F., Biro, M.A., Willey, S., Cheng, I.H., Small, R. & Brown, S. (2015). Bridging the gap: Using an interrupted time series design to evaluate systems reform addressing refugee maternal and child health inequalities. *Implementation Science*, *10*(62). doi:10.1186/s13012-015-0251-z.

4

WORKING WITH INDIGENOUS FAMILIES

Donna Hartz and Leona McGrath

Introduction

In Australia, Aotearoa New Zealand and Canada, the impact of colonisation has resulted in profound disparities in health and social well-being between the Indigenous and non-Indigenous populations (Jackson Pulver *et al.*, 2010). Colonisation decimated Indigenous communities who were dispossessed of their traditional lands and forced onto reserves or missions. There was widespread genocide, incarceration and the forced removal of children into institutional or non-Indigenous family care in Australia (Human Rights and Equal Opportunity Commission, 1997) and Canada (The Truth and Reconciliation Commission of Canada, 2015). This has resulted in persistent intergenerational grief and loss compounded by government policy and societal ignorance around the effects of colonisation in fragmenting traditional norms. Current inequities between Indigenous and non-Indigenous peoples are multifaceted and are reflected in lower education levels, higher unemployment, poor housing and poorer physical and mental health (Jackson Pulver *et al.*, 2010).

In this chapter we discuss the perinatal health of Indigenous women and babies with a focus on three countries: Australia, New Zealand and Canada. First we emphasise the impact of colonisation on the health of Indigenous populations and describe disparity in social and health outcomes for Indigenous peoples compared with non-Indigenous people including perinatal outcomes. We then discuss the key characteristics of positive policy and service responses and identify the strategies aimed at promoting psychosocial resilience and optimising health outcomes for Indigenous childbearing women, their babies and families in these countries.

Colonisation and the impact on health

In this section of the chapter we provide a brief overview of the colonisation processes and impact in Australia, New Zealand and Canada. It is important to stress that all Indigenous populations are diverse within countries, with different languages and cultures and large geographical dispersion (Jackson Pulver *et al.*, 2010) and consequently individual experiences differ.

Australia Aboriginal and Torres Strait Islander peoples

Australian Indigenous people include both mainland Aboriginal and Torres Strait Islanders. They comprise a diversity of Aboriginal nations, each with their own language and traditions. The Torres Strait Islanders are a distinct group of Indigenous people from the mainland Aboriginal clans located to the very north of eastern Australia between Australia and Papua New Guinea. Aboriginal Australians are the oldest continuous culture in the world with archaeological evidence suggesting between 60,000 to 120,000 years of tenure. Australia was colonised by the British in 1778 and became a penal colony. The health of Aboriginal Australians was reported to be good prior to colonisation but the arrival of the British introduced disease and the ensuing genocide rapidly reduced the population (Sherwood & Geia, 2014).

Indigenous Australians make up three per cent of the population. The majority of Indigenous Australians (79 per cent) live in urban and regional areas and 21 per cent live in remote and very remote areas where access to health and social services is limited. Prior to 2006, there was a 17-year difference in the life expectancy of Australian Indigenous and the non-Indigenous population (Australian Institute of Health and Welfare & Australian Bureau of Statistics, 2005). More recent reports demonstrate an improvement in life expectancy with the gap narrowing to ten years (Australian Institute of Health and Welfare, 2015a). However, this reported improvement is challenged by some, stating that the change is in the approach to measurement and not in real life expectancy (Holland, 2016).

The Māori people of New Zealand

The Māori people are the traditional owners of New Zealand. New Zealand became a British colony in 1840. The Declaration of Independence in 1835 and the Treaty of Waitangi in 1840 between the British Government and the Māori was intended to promote a mutually beneficial relationship, based on the three principles of partnership, participation and protection. However, at the same time, there was a significant loss of Māori traditional lands, fuelling a loss of economic independence and decision-making. Haywood (2012) proposes that a Eurocentric worldview persisted, underpinned by the economic, education and health systems designed primarily for non-Māori. Consequently, inequities in health, housing, incarceration, employment and life expectancy appeared. This disparity was formally recognised by the government in 1961. However, strategies to address this, such as the movement of the predominantly rural Māori population to urban areas to assist assimilation into western culture, further eroded Māori cultural ways. Social reforms introduced in 1988 based on the three principles of the Treaty of Waitangi, now underpin many social and health reforms in New Zealand – and unlike other Indigenous peoples discussed in this chapter, New Zealand is a truly bicultural nation (Haywood, 2012).

Māori people make up 14.9 per cent of the population with a life expectancy that is less than non-Māori people by 7.1 years, although the expectancy has been increasing since the late 1990s at the same rate as non-Māori people. The majority of Māori people reside in urban areas and also endure similar health and social disparities as Australian Aboriginals (discussed below). In 2012 it was reported that nearly 30 per cent of Maoris were subjected to racial discrimination (New Zealand Ministry of Health, 2015a).

Canadian Indigenous peoples

The original inhabitants of Canada, the Aboriginal people, are three culturally distinct groups. They include First Nation (either on reserve and off reserve status), Inuit, and Métis people. In 2011 there were 851,560 people identified as First Nations people (75 per cent registered Indians) with 630 distinct First Nation communities and approximately 60 different languages. There were also 59,445 people identifying as Inuit that predominantly live in the remote Artic regions and mostly speak one language (Inuktituk) and approximately 451,795 (a third) identified as Métis (Statistics Canada, 2013). Like Australia, a higher proportion of Canadian First Nation people live in remote areas, in particular the Inuit people, and hence access to service provision is compromised. Colonisation by the French and English occurred from the early 1600s and again this occupation did not benefit the traditional owners. Canadian disparities reflect an inferior health status and more challenging living conditions. Life expectation is less than non-Indigenous Canadians, with Inuit people having 10 to 15 years, and Métis and First Nations 3 to 5 years less (National Collaborating Centre for Aboriginal Health, 2012; Statistics Canada, 2013).

The social determinants of health

The Indigenous peoples of Australia, New Zealand and Canada and other countries such as the United States endure a high burden of non-communicable (diabetes, obesity, heart disease, kidney disease) and infectious diseases all associated with premature death (Australian Institute of Health and Welfare, 2014; New Zealand Ministry of Health, 2013; Statistics Canada, 2013). The social determinants of disease are well documented and explain the devastating impact of poverty, poor food security and nutrition, poor housing, low education, and unemployment on the health of Indigenous peoples in these three countries. These circumstances are often intergenerational. The Aboriginal and Torres Strait Islander people, the Māori and Aboriginal Canadian people all demonstrate higher rates of smoking, binge drinking and alcohol dependence and drug misuse and incarceration (Australian Institute of Health and Welfare, 2015a; National Collaborating Centre for Aboriginal Health, 2012; New Zealand Ministry of Health, 2015a). These communities report earlier onset and higher levels and severity of mental health problems as well as domestic violence and suicide (Department of Health and Ageing, 2013; National Collaborating Centre for Aboriginal Health, 2012; New Zealand Ministry of Health, 2015a). Consequently, Indigenous peoples have a high level of need for appropriate health and social support services (Jackson Pulver *et al.*, 2010).

The perinatal health of Indigenous mothers and babies

In Australia, Canada and New Zealand, Indigenous mothers compared with non-Indigenous mothers are younger, have a higher birth rate, and are more likely to live in remote areas and/or areas of social deprivation. They are more likely to smoke and have comorbidities such as obesity, diabetes and hypertension and as a consequence have higher mortality rates (Australian Institute of Health and Welfare, 2015b; New Zealand Ministry of Health, 2015b; Smylie, 2014). Correspondingly, Indigenous babies also have higher morbidity rates than non-Indigenous babies, including low birth weight, prematurity and admission to special care nurseries at birth (further insights into mothers who have a premature baby are discussed in Chapter 10). Perinatal mortality rates are also higher, with higher rates of stillbirth and Sudden Infant Death Syndrome (SIDS) (Smylie, Crengle, Freemantle & Taualii, 2010).

Factors such as lower education, young motherhood, poverty, poor access to health services, and single parenthood often without the support of the extended community predispose Indigenous women to greater levels of common mental health disorders such as depression, anxiety, alcohol and drug problems (Smylie, 2014). The prevalence of perinatal mental health problems in Australian Indigenous women is unknown (Prandl, Rooney, & Bishop, 2012). In the general perinatal population, 10 to 16 per cent of women will experience depression and/or anxiety in pregnancy and approximately 14 to 16 per cent develop postnatal depression and or anxiety (beyondblue, 2011) (also refer to Chapter 2). One service evaluation in the state of New South Wales in Australia, indicated that approximately 40 per cent of Aboriginal women accessing the service had a history of mental health problems (Homer, Foureur, Allende, Pekin, Caplice & Catling-Paull, 2012). In the Christchurch area of New Zealand, it was reported that one in three young mothers (16–24 years) had experienced at least one mental health issue (New Zealand Ministry of Health, 2012) and Canadian Aboriginal women are twice as likely to be depressed than non-Aboriginal women (Daoud, Smylie, Urquia, Allan, & O'Campo, 2013). Indigenous mothers also have higher reported rates of domestic and family violence (Smylie, 2014) (also refer to Chapter 7).

Poor perinatal health is exacerbated by the lack of appropriate services to meet the women's expressed or cultural needs (Dietsch, Shackleton, Davies, McLeod & Alston, 2010) or the racist attitudes of care providers (Josif, Barclay, Kruske & Kildea, 2013). In both Australia and Canada, western biomedicine has replaced traditional birthing ways and many Aboriginal women living in rural and remote communities are required to leave their families and communities to give birth in hospitals that may be hundreds or thousands of miles from home (Perinatal Mental Health Consortium, 2008). This means access to culturally safe maternity care is very limited (Smylie, 2014).

In addition, due to the historical intergenerational removal of children from parents and communities (Silburn *et al.*, 2006) together with the increased incidence of mental health problems and drug and alcohol use, there are heightened fears of removal of babies into state custody. This is well-founded with data indicating that in Australia in 2014–2015, Indigenous children were ten times more likely to be in and out of home care (e.g. looked-after status) than non-Indigenous children (Australian Institute of Health and Welfare, 2016). Similarly, in Canada there are high levels of out of home care with half the children cared for in foster care being Aboriginal – four per cent of Aboriginal children live in foster care which is 13 times more than non-Aboriginal children (Statistics Canada, 2013).

Barriers to accessing antenatal care

There are many structural and personal life circumstances that impact on Indigenous women's ability or likelihood to attend antenatal care. A number of these barriers are summarised in Box 4.1.

Health literacy is also an important concept influencing health service use. Health literacy has been defined as 'the degree to which individuals can obtain, process, and understand the basic health information and services they need to make appropriate health decisions' (Australian Human Rights Commission, 2011, p. 123). It is more than being able to read information leaflets and successfully make appointments. Low levels of health literacy impede an individual's ability to engage with health care (Nielsen-Bohlman, Panzer & Kindig, 2011).

Resilience and Indigenous perinatal health

There are protective factors that can impact positively on the psychological emotional and social well-being of Indigenous communities. These include connectedness with family, community, traditional land, culture, spirituality and ancestry that include living on or near traditional lands. These important characteristics of well-being are related to self-determination and community governance and the passing on of cultural ways (beyondblue Support Service, 2016). The 'wordle' displayed in Figure 4.1 below was developed from a focus group discussion conducted by the authors with Australian Aboriginal elders, midwives, nurses, students and community members. It demonstrates the qualities of Australian Aboriginal and Torres Strait Islander communities that build resilience.

BOX 4.1 BARRIERS TO ACCESSING ANTENATAL CARE

Structural and personal barriers to antenatal care include:

- Poverty – affects ability to pay for health services, transportation, childcare, medicines, adequate housing.
- Remoteness – local services not available, lack of transportation, lack of childcare, lack of privacy in small community.
- Low education – influences ability to understand the importance of antenatal care or how to navigate funding or service provision.
- Lack of social support, strained/absent relationship with partner or family leading to social isolation and difficulty in attending appointments.
- Substance abuse, mental health issues and domestic violence may all pose more urgent priorities for women, preventing them from attending care.
- Mistrust of health professionals especially where there is previous removal of children due to welfare issues or a reputation for lack of racial/cultural understanding or presence of discrimination.
- Lack of language or culturally specific services or staff.
- Unwanted pregnancy that may be shameful in the community or from unwanted sexual encounter.
- Concurrent health issues/morbidities e.g. anaemia, heart disease, kidney disease, poor nutrition.

(Best Start Resource Centre, n.d.)

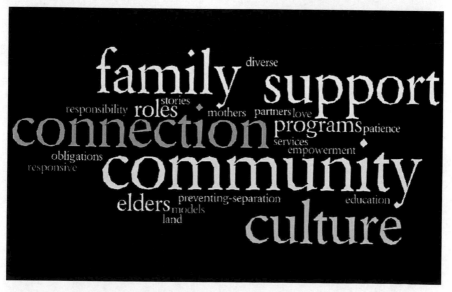

FIGURE 4.1 Factors that build resilience in Indigenous women. (Hartz & McGrath 2015)

Strengthening perinatal health services for Indigenous women

Access to culturally appropriate antenatal care, birthing services and maternal and child health services can reduce the risk of poor health outcomes for Indigenous mothers and their babies, children and families. Support needs to come from all levels including government policy, systems to identify women with additional needs and referral to appropriate services, availability of appropriate models of care, improving health literacy and health professionals with appropriate training in cultural safety and competency. A number of these issues are discussed in more depth below.

Government policy and resource allocation

Australia and New Zealand provide government funded universal health care to all citizens irrespective of ethnicity as well as funding for specific initiatives for maternal infant health in Aboriginal communities (New Zealand Ministry of Health, 2016; The Department of Health, 2016). Policy has played an important role in instilling principles such as equity, responsiveness and public participation in the development of Indigenous health initiatives and there has been a shift from centralised governmental control to community participation and ownership of health provision. However, despite focused policy and funding, significant gaps still exist in the provision of health services to Indigenous people in these three countries (Jackson Pulver *et al.*, 2010).

In Canada health policy and funding for service provision to the Indigenous population has been described as a 'patchwork' because funding arises from various sources including federal government and own-source revenue from Indigenous groups. Service provision and funding may vary from one province to the next and may be dependent on the Indigenous person status e.g. First Nation people may have 'status' as an Indian or live 'on-reserve' that dictates whether they are eligible for funding. The level of primary care on reserves is less than that provided to Canadians through the provincial/territorial health care systems (National Collaborating Centre for Aboriginal Health, 2011). Thus while Indigenous women are likely to be aware of the benefits of antenatal care some may not be eligible for care under existing health service provision arrangements in their region (Best Start Resource Centre, n.d.).

Identifying social and emotional problems in the perinatal period

Universal psychosocial assessment and depression screening is a recommendation for all pregnant women in Australia (Australian Health Ministers' Advisory Council, 2012) and New Zealand (New Zealand Guidelines Group, 2008). Considering the complex issues that many Indigenous women face, screening and assessment and early engagement in services is imperative to ensure timely and appropriate referral and collaboration with supporting services such as social work, mental health and drug and alcohol services if indicated.

The Edinburgh Postnatal Depression Scale (EPDS) is one of the most commonly recommended and utilised screening tools for depression in pregnancy (also refer to Chapter 2). However, its validity and reliability in Indigenous populations is unknown (2011). In Australia, a language-specific EPDS was developed and compared with the standard EPDS and this revised tool was found to be more suitable for some women. The language-specific EPDS did not appear to alter the overall EPDS score or change the response to the suicidal ideation question. The authors also concluded that the presence of Indigenous health workers during screening for psychosocial issues in pregnancy can enhance the women's understanding of screening tools, questions and to also provide information and access to support services (Campbell, Hayes & Buckby, 2008; Hayes, Beia, Buckby, Egan & McCulley, 2005).

Improving health literacy

As noted above low health literacy can be a significant barrier to service utilisation (also discussed in Chapter 3). Solutions to improve health literacy must come from three perspectives that complement each other, the individual woman, the health care practitioner and the health organisation: to improve the perinatal health literacy of Indigenous women, health professionals and health organisations. Nielsen-Bohlman et al. (2011) suggest the following:

- Support individuals to find information and services.
- Provide useful health promotion and healthcare.
- Understand what people are asking for particularly when there is a language or cultural barrier.
- Confirm with the community which information and services work best for different situations and people (p. ES-1).

A further important and effective strategy to improve health literacy is utilising trained Indigenous health workers to support the learning needs of their community (Nielsen-Bohlman et al., 2011).

Cultural safety and competency in health services

Undertaking cultural awareness and safety training for all health professionals is essential to improve outcomes for Indigenous women. When services are culturally safe Indigenous people are more likely to utilise them (Berkman et al., 2011). The term cultural safety is drawn from the work of Māori nurses and has been described by Williams (1999, p. 213) as:

> An environment that is spiritually, socially and emotionally safe, as well as physically safe for people; where there is no assault, challenge or denial of

their identity, of who they are and what they need. It is about shared respect, shared meaning, shared knowledge and experience of learning together.

A culturally safe environment promotes resilience amongst Indigenous peoples by promoting the feeling of safety in their identity, culture and community. A culturally competent workforce is essential in cultural safety. Cultural competency 'is the set of behaviours, attitudes, and policies that come together to enable a system, agency, or professionals to work effectively in cross-cultural situations' (Bainbridge, McCalman, Clifford & Tsey, 2015, p. 2). See Box 4.2 for an overview of characteristics of a culturally competent maternity service.

With these characteristics in mind you may now like to consider your workplace and answer the following practice questions:

Culturally safe care:

How do you and how does your service know that the care provided is culturally safe? Who determines what cultural safety is in your service?

BOX 4.2 KEY CHARACTERISTICS OF CULTURALLY COMPETENT MATERNITY CARE

- Physical environment is culturally appropriate and acceptable.
- Specific Indigenous maternal health programmes and initiatives.
- Indigenous workforce inclusion and development.
- Continuity of care and carer.
- Collaborating with Indigenous organisations and other agencies promoting integrated care and health networks.
- Effective and privileged communication, information-sharing and transfer of care between health services.
- Staff attitudes are respectful and cross-culturally aware and sensitive.
- Cultural education and competency programmes.
- Supportive relationships with Indigenous individuals, co-workers and partnership with the community.
- Informed choice and right of refusal.
- Tools to measure cultural competence.
- Culture specific guidelines.
- Culturally appropriate and effective health promotion and behaviour change activities.
- Engaging with the Indigenous community consumers and inclusion in clinical governance processes.

(Adapted from Kruske, 2011, p. 8)

Cultural awareness and safety training:

What do you know about your local Indigenous history and health?

What training courses are there to support you in the care of the local Indigenous peoples' health?

In organisations providing bi or multilingual culturally appropriate information, both signage or written/graphic material can support an individual to physically navigate the environment and understand their service options, and to create the feeling that they belong. It is important that local Indigenous communities are involved in the development of appropriate signage and service information. Consider the following practice question.

Signage and written material in your service:

Have the local Indigenous community been consulted on the cultural appropriateness and readability of these?

Do they make their experience at the service easier and more comfortable?

Building capacity in the health workforce

Indigenous communities are underrepresented within the health workforce (Australian Institute of Health and Welfare, 2013; New Zealand Council of Midwives, 2014; Van Wagner, Osepchook, Harney, Crosbie & Tulugak, 2012). Indigenous healthcare workers of all categories and all roles have long been recognised as integral to the success of health care initiatives and the healing of communities. Indigenous health care workers have the social, environmental and ethnic qualities of their culture and an understanding of verbal and non-verbal language, health beliefs and barriers to accessing care (Giblin, 1989). West, Usher and Foster (2010, p. 121) propose that:

Indigenous nurses bring a set of unique skills, knowledge and understanding to health service delivery and propose that their contribution has the potential to enhance future outcomes for Indigenous people by improving access to health services, ensure services are culturally appropriate and respectful, and assist non-Indigenous nurses to deliver culturally appropriate care.

Complementary to this is that through capacity building initiatives of the individual, the community further benefit through addressing social determinants of health including increased education levels, employment levels and subsequently housing and health standards (Jackson Pulver *et al.*, 2010).

Practice examples: initiatives to improve perinatal health for Indigenous women

In this final section we describe two innovative services for Indigenous women, one in Canada and one in Australia. A summary of strategies to help reverse the inequalities amongst Indigenous populations is then offered.

Inuit Indigenous birth on traditional lands: the Inuulitsivik midwifery service and midwifery education programme

The Inuulitsivik Birth Centres midwifery service and midwifery education programme is an exemplar of traditional community development that promotes improved health standards and the recognition of the importance of traditional lands to First Nation people in the perinatal period. During the late 1970s health policy introduced the evacuation of all childbearing women at 36–37 weeks gestation or earlier from the northern areas of Canada to regional hospitals to give birth. Women who were in good health were housed in hostels and could spend weeks or months away from home (Epoo, Stonier, Van Wagner & Harney, 2012). This practice continued for many years. In Puvirnituq (1986) and then Inukjuat (1998) and Salluit (2004), community-controlled services were implemented by the Nunavimmiut Inuits which enabled the return of childbirth services to the Nunavik region's Hudson Bay coastal communities, in the remote Inuit region of Northern Quebec, Canada. The key features of this service are detailed in Box 4.3.

BOX 4.3 THE INUULITSIVIK MIDWIFERY SERVICE

Key features of the Inuulitsivik midwifery service:
- Inuit leadership.
- Community involvement.
- Midwifery-led care.
- Broad scope of practice.
- Local education of midwives ensuring that care is provided within culture and language, and is sustainable.
- Using local students.
- Seeing local birth as an improved health outcome in and of itself.
- Integrating Indigenous and non-Indigenous approaches to birth.
- Local culture of normal birth supported by midwifery with use of technology.
- Collaboration with 'southern' (non-Inuit) midwives, midwifery organisations and the health care team, i.e. local and tertiary physicians and local nurses.
- Risk assessment in a cultural and social context.

(Kildea & Van Wagner, 2013, p.9)

Inuit midwifery and knowledge, and birthing within the community is reported to have provided a platform for cultural regeneration, greater family cohesion and the intergenerational exchange of traditional knowledge, all of which had been damaged post Western colonisation (Olson & Couchie, 2013). These culturally safe and culturally competent services have been evaluated as safe for all women, irrespective of their risk status (Van Wagner et al., 2012), and to have immeasurable community benefits:

> The establishment of the birth centres has been fundamental for community healing, and marks a turning point for many families who suffered from family violence in Nunavik. Male elders told the men that if they witnessed their partner giving birth, they would see that she has been through enough and respect and care for her.
>
> (JAG Films, 2002; Van Wagner, Epoo,
Nastapoka & Harney, 2007, p. 370)

Integrated Indigenous continuity of care in an urban context

The Malabar Community Midwifery Link Service in Sydney Australia provides continuity of care for Indigenous childbearing women. Midwives, an Aboriginal health education officer, a child and family health nurse, a social worker and an Aboriginal administrative assistant work in partnership with each other and the local community to provide an individualised, accessible and culturally appropriate service. An obstetrician, a paediatrician as well as specialised allied health professions also provide dedicated services. The service fosters community participation with a focus on Aboriginal and Torres Strait Islander families. The Aboriginal health workers who already have an identity in their community are pivotal to the process of engagement with the service at a community level (Homer et al., 2012). In a service evaluation, Homer et al. (2012) reported that women found this service provided ease of access, continuity of care and caregiver and trust and trusting relationships. Women and their babies have access to and are often referred to the local La Perouse community centre where ongoing care is provided including paediatric, family and child health nurses, drug and alcohol services. A case study of a woman who accessed the service is reported below.

Case study

Jasmine is a 16-year-old Aboriginal pregnant woman who has been raised by her grandmother (Nana) in South Eastern Sydney. Jasmine finds out from her friends and Aunties in the community that there is a local maternity service available for Aboriginal and Torres Strait Islander women. Jasmine books in with care with The Malabar Community Midwifery Link Service. At her first visit she meets with a midwife and an Aboriginal health education officer who co-ordinate her care needs. During the course of her pregnancy she meets the social worker who ensures she has financial support, a female doctor who monitors her health due to her age and a psychiatrist who she is able to discuss issues of previous childhood neglect with. She finds the local community clinic convenient and private. She is also able to meet other young mums and takes part in culturally based art group where she paints her story in traditional art on a plaster cast of her pregnant belly. When she is in labour her Nana and Aunties come with her to the local hospital and stay with her throughout the birth. A midwife she knows provides care during the birth of her baby girl and then visits her post birth in hospital and then at home. She plans to attend the mothers' group at the clinic after she gives birth where a child and family health nurse is available to provide ongoing support her and her baby girl. She knows that here she can also receive information about baby care, practical advice and assistance with breastfeeding, nutrition and parenting, monitoring of the baby's developmental milestones, immunisation status and infections, and health checks before starting school. She is excited that since the birth of her baby she has been able to attend the mother's exercise group with her new friends.

In summary, strategies to reverse the inequities experienced by Indigenous peoples have emerged and at the core of these is a worldview that positions the Indigenous communities as integral, legitimate, authoritative and valued (Thorpe, Arabena, Sullivan, Silburn & Rowley, 2016). Lifelong physical, mental, emotional and spiritual well-being begins before birth and therefore fostering psychosocial resilience during the perinatal period is imperative to improving the health of mothers, babies, families and the community (Marriot & Ferguson-Hill, 2014). From the insights highlighted in this chapter and work by Herceg (2005), a number of strategies to enhance psychosocial resilience amongst Indigenous women in the perinatal period have been identified:

- Offering culturally specific services.
- Incorporating psychosocial screening in pregnancy. Language or culture specific tools may be valuable. Indigenous health professionals can provide an added layer of cultural safety and support to interpret language differences.
- Developing, promoting and advocating community based and/or community-controlled services within the local area.
- Providing integrated continuity of care and a broad spectrum of services.
- Providing efficient appropriate communication with the women and between services, especially outreach services.
- Integration with other support services (e.g. Indigenous liaison, drug and alcohol, social work).
- Offering outreach cultural specific activities to promote community connection and health promotion.
- Providing or offering home visiting (as feasible).
- Providing a welcoming and safe service environment.
- Providing flexibility in service delivery and appointment times.
- A focus on communication, relationship building and development of trust.
- Demonstrating respect for Indigenous people and their culture.

- Demonstrating respect for family involvement in health issues and child care.
- An appropriately trained workforce.
- Valuing Aboriginal and Torres Strait Islander staff and female staff.
- Providing or subsidising transportation modes.
- Providing childcare or playgroups.
- If evacuated from her community for birth provide facilitate familial support for her in the referral centre and support for her partner and children in her local community when she is gone.

Conclusion

The threads of Indigenous traditional ways of being have been broken in British colonised communities, leading to unacceptable disparities in social determinants and health status. Australia, Aotearoa New Zealand and Canada all currently have Indigenous specific programmes/services, government policies and funding models that have attempted to address inequities. However, gaps in the health and perinatal outcomes of Indigenous communities remain. Promoting resilience in childbearing women and her family is an important foundation to improve individual and community health. Integral to this is the embracing of Indigenous peoples' worldview in the development, ownership and implementation of health promotion strategies. These include the enhancement of strategies to improve health literacy and cultural safety and capacity building of the Indigenous health workforce. Strategies such as Indigenous specific maternity and primary health care services, birth service provision in traditional communities and overarching health frameworks based on traditional knowledge and community law have started to reverse the inequities. Individual health professionals have a key role in providing culturally safe care and ensuring that they are culturally competent based on the expressed and traditional/cultural need of their Indigenous community/ies.

Acknowledgement

The authors of this chapter wish to acknowledge the extensive inquiry that has been undertaken by, with and on behalf of Indigenous peoples across the globe including those presented in this chapter. The authors do not speak on their behalf except where indicated but make reference to published works examining the impact of the social determinants of health on Indigenous populations and childbearing women and families in particular.

References

Australian Health Ministers' Advisory Council. (2012). *Clinical practice guidelines: Antenatal care – Module 1*. Available from: www.health.gov.au/antenatal [Accessed 5 January 2016].

Australian Human Rights Commission. (2011). *Social justice report 2011: Aboriginal and Torres Strait Islander Social Justice Commissioner*. Available from: www.humanrights.gov.au/sites/

default/files/content/social_justice/sj_report/sjreport11/pdf/sjr2011.pdf [Accessed 5 January 2016].

Australian Institute of Health and Welfare. (2013). *Nursing and midwifery workforce 2012.* Available from: www.aihw.gov.au/WorkArea/DownloadAsset.aspx?id=60129545314 [Accessed 5 January 2016].

Australian Institute of Health and Welfare. (2014). *Mortality and life expectancy of Indigenous Australians: 2008 to 2012.* Available from: www.aihw.gov.au/publication-detail/ ?id=60129548470 [Accessed 5 January 2016].

Australian Institute of Health and Welfare. (2015a). *The health and welfare of Australia's Aboriginal and Torres Strait Islander peoples 2015. Cat. no. AIHW 147.* Canberra: AIHW.

Australian Institute of Health and Welfare. (2015b). *Australia's mothers and babies 2013—in brief. Perinatal statistics series no. 31. Cat no. PER 72.* Available from: www.aihw.gov.au/ WorkArea/DownloadAsset.aspx?id=60129554140 [Accessed 10 January 2016].

Australian Institute of Health and Welfare. (2016). *Child protection Australia 2013–2014.* Available from: www.aihw.gov.au/publication-detail/?id=60129550762&tab=2 [Accessed 10 January 2016].

Australian Institute of Health and Welfare & Australian Bureau of Statistics. (2005). *The health and welfare of Australia's Aboriginal and Torres Strait Islander peoples 2005.* Available from: www.aihw.gov.au/WorkArea/DownloadAsset.aspx?id=6442458575 [accessed 9 February 2017].

Bainbridge, R., McCalman, J., Clifford, A. & Tsey, K. (2015). *Issue Paper no.13. Cultural competency in the delivery of health services for Indigenous people.* Available from: www.aihw. gov.au/uploadedFiles/ClosingTheGap/Content/Our_publications/2015/ctgc-ip13.pdf [Accessed 5 January 2016].

Berkman, N.D., Sheridan, S.L., Donahue, K.E., Halpern, D.J., Viera, A., Crotty, K., Holland, A., Brasure, M., Lohr, K.N., Harden, E., Tant, E., Wallace, I. & Viswanathan, M. (2011). Health literacy interventions and outcomes: an updated systematic review. *Evidice Report/Technology Assessment, 199,* 1–941.

Best Start Resource Centre. (n.d.). *Reducing the impact: Working with pregnant women who live in difficult life situations.* Available from: www.beststart.org/resources/anti_poverty/pdf/ REDUCE.pdf [Accessed 1 August 2016].

beyondblue (2011). *Guidelines expert advisory committee. Clinical practice guidelines for depression and related disorders – anxiety, bipolar disorder and puerperal psychosis – in the perinatal period. A guideline for primary care health professionals.* Available from: http://cope.org.au/ wp-content/uploads/2013/12/Perinatal-Mental-Health-Clinical-Practice-Guidelines.pdf [Accessed 1 August 2016].

beyondblue Support Service. (2016). *Aboriginal and Torres Strait Islander: Protective and risk factors.* Available from: www.beyondblue.org.au/who-does-it-affect/aboriginal-and-torres-strait-islander-people/risk-factors [Accessed 1 August 2016].

Campbell, A., Hayes, B. & Buckby, B. (2008). Aboriginal and Torres Strait Islander women's experience when interacting with the Edinburgh postnatal depression scale: A brief note. *Australian Journal of Rural Health, 16*(3), 124–131.

Daoud, N., Smylie, J., Urquia, M., Allan, B. & O'Campo, P. (2013). The contribution of socio-economic position to the excesses of violence and intimate partner violence among aboriginal versus non-Aboriginal women in Canada. *Canadian Journal of Public Health, 104*(4), e278–283.

Department of Health and Ageing. (2013). *National Aboriginal and Torres Strait Islander suicide prevention strategy.* Available from: www.health.gov.au/internet/main/publishing.nsf/

Content/305B8A5E056763D6CA257BF0001A8DD3/$File/IndigenousStrategy.pdf [Accessed 10 January 2016].

Dietsch, E., Shackleton, P., Davies, C., McLeod, M. & Alston, M. (2010). 'You can drop dead': Midwives bullying women. *Women and Birth, 23*(2), 53–59.

Epoo, B., Stonier, J., Van Wagner, V. & Harney, E. (2012). Learning midwifery in Nunavik: Community-based education for Inuit midwives. *Pimatisiwin: A Journal of Aboriginal and Indigenous Community Health, 10*(3), 283–300.

Giblin, P.T. (1989). Effective utilisation and evaluation of indigenous health care workers. *Public Health Reports, 104*(4), 361–368.

Hartz, D.L., & McGrath, L. (2015). Factors that build resilience in Indigenous women. Congress of Aboriginal and Torres Strait Islander Nurses and Midwives. Available from: http://catsinam.org.au/static/uploads/files/catsinam-pd-conference-2015-draft-program-190815-wfslfcpgqxiu.pdf [Accessed 24 February, 2017]

Hayes, B., Beia, L., Buckby, B., Egan, M. & McCulley, J. (2005). *Queensland intervention initiative: Indigenous women's project: Report of process and preliminary results.* In *The beyondblue national postnatal depression program prevention and early intervention 2001–2005 final report. Volume II: State-based antenatal intervention initiativ.* Available from: www.beyondblue. org.au/docs/default-source/8.-perinatal-documents/bw0076-report-beyondblue-national-research-program-vol2.pdf?sfvrsn=2 [Accessed 1 August 2016].

Haywood, J. (2012). *Biculturalism – From bicultural to monocultural, and back. Te Ara – the encyclopedia of New Zealand.* Available from: www.teara.govt.nz/en/biculturalism [Accessed 9 February 2017].

Herceg A. (2005). *Improving health in Aboriginal and Torres Strait Islander mothers, babies and young children: A literature review.* Available from: www.health.gov.au/internet/main/publishing.nsf/Content/A5665A1E705D14BACA257. [Accessed 15 August 2016].

Holland C. (2016). *Close the gap: Progress and priorites report.* Available from: www.humanrights.gov.au/our-work/aboriginal-and-torres-strait-islander-social-justice/publications/close-gap-progress [Accessed 10 July 2016].

Homer, C.S., Foureur, M.J., Allende, T., Pekin, F., Caplice, S. & Catling-Paull, C. (2012). 'It's more than just having a baby': Women's experiences of a maternity service for Australian Aboriginal and Torres Strait Islander families. *Midwifery, 28*(4), E449–455.

Human Rights and Equal Opportunity Commission. (1997). *Bringing them home: Report of the national inquiry into the separation of Aboriginal and Torres Strait Islander children from their Families.* Available from: www.humanrights.gov.au/sites/default/files/content/pdf/social_justice/bringing_them_home_report.pdf [Accessed 1 August 2016].

Jackson Pulver, L., Haswell, M.R., Ring, I., Waldon, J., Clark, W., Whetung, V., Kinnon, D., Graham, C., Chino, M., LaValley, J. & Sadana, R. (2010). *Indigenous Health – Australia, Canada, Aotearoa New Zealand and the United States – Laying claim to a future that embraces health for us all. World Health Report. Background Paper, 33.* Available from: www.who.int/healthsystems/topics/financing/healthreport/IHNo33.pdf. [Accessed 12 May 2016].

JAG Films (Producer). (2002). Birth rites. [Videorecording]: Australia. As cited in Van Wagner, V., Epoo, B., Nastapoka, J. & Harney, E. (2007). Reclaiming birth, health, and community: Midwifery in the Inuit villages of Nunavik, Canada. *Journal of Midwifery & Women's Health, 52*(4), 384–391, p. 390.

Josif, C.M., Barclay, L., Kruske, S. & Kildea, S. (2013). 'No more strangers': Investigating the experiences of women, midwives and others during the establishment of a new model of maternity care for remote dwelling aboriginal women in northern Australia. *Midwifery, 30*(3), 317–323.

Kildea, S., & Van Wagner, V. (2013). 'Birthing on Country' maternity service delivery models: an Evidence Check rapid review brokered by the Sax Institute (www.saxinstitute.org.au) on behalf of the Maternity Services Inter-Jurisdictional Committee for the Australian Health Ministers' Advisory Council.

Kruske, S. (2011). *Characteristics of culturally competent maternity care for Aboriginal and Torres Strait Islander women. Maternity Services Inter-jurisdictional Committee for the Australian Health Ministers Advisory Council.* Available from: www.health.gov.au/internet/main/publishing.nsf/Content/77F5B09BC281577ACA257D2A001EE8CD/$File/cultur.pdf [Accessed 9 February 2017].

Marriot, R. & Ferguson-Hill, S. (2014). Perinatal and Infant Mental Health and Wellbeing. In P. Dudgeon, H. Milroy & R. Walker, R. (eds.), *Working together: Aboriginal and Torres Strait Islander mental health and wellbeing principles and practice.* 2nd Edition. Available from: http://aboriginal.telethonkids.org.au/media/746839/Working-Together-Aboriginal-and-Wellbeing-2014.pdf. [Accessed 10 August 2016].

National Collaborating Centre for Aboriginal Health. (2011). *Looking for Aboriginal health in legislation and policies, 1970–2008: A policy sythesis project.* Available from: www.nccah-ccnsa.ca/Publications/Lists/Publications/Attachments/28/Looking%20for%20Aborig inal%20Health%20in%20Legislation%20and%20Policies%20(English%20-%20Web).pdf [Accessed 9 February 2017].

National Collaborating Centre for Aboriginal Health. (2012). *The state of knowledge of Aboriginal health: A review of Aboriginal public health in Canada.* Available from: www.nccah-ccnsa.ca/Publications/Lists/Publications/Attachments/52/SOK_report_EN_web.pdf [Accessed 9 February 2017].

New Zealand Council of Midwives. (2014). *2014 Midwifery workforce survey.* Available from: www.midwiferycouncil.health.nz/sites/default/files/site-downloads/WorkforceSurvey 2014.pdf [Accessed 10 June 2016].

New Zealand Guidelines Group. (2008). *Identification of common mental disorders and management of depression in primary care: An evidence-based best practice guideline.* Available from: www.health.govt.nz/system/files/documents/publications/depression_guideline. pdf [Accessed 1 May 2016].

New Zealand Ministry of Health. (2012). *Healthy beginnings: Developing perinatal and infant mental health services in New Zealand.* Available from: www.health.govt.nz/publication/healthy-beginnings-developing-perinatal-and-infant-mental-health-services-new-zealand [Accessed 1 May 2016].

New Zealand Ministry of Health. (2013). *The health of Māori adults And Children.* Available from: www.health.govt.nz/system/files/documents/publications/health-māori-adults-children-summary.pdf [Accessed 1 February 2016].

New Zealand Ministry of Health. (2015a). *Tatau Kahukura Māori Health Chart Book 2015.* 3rd edition. Available from: www.health.govt.nz/system/files/documents/publications/tatau-kahukura-maori-health-chart-book-3rd-edition-oct15.pdf [Accessed 10 May 2016].

New Zealand Ministry of Health. (2015b). *Report on Maternity 2014.* Available from www.health.govt.nz/publication/report-maternity-2014. [Accessed 1 February 2016].

New Zealand Ministry of Health. (2016). *Guide to eligibility for publicly funded health services.* Available from: www.health.govt.nz/new-zealand-health-system/eligibility-publicly-funded-health-services/guide-eligibility-publicly-funded-health-services?mega=NZ healthsystem&title=Guide to eligibility. [Accessed 8 July 2016].

Nielsen-Bohlman, L., Panzer, A.M. & Kindig, D.A. (Eds.). (2011). *Health literacy: A prescription to end confusion.* Available from: www.nap.edu/catalog/10883/health-literacy-a-prescription-to-end-confusion [Accessed 9 February 2017].

Olson, R. & Couchie, C. (2013). Returning birth: The politics of midwifery implementation on First Nations reserves in Canada. *Midwifery*, *29*(8), 981–987.

Perinatal Mental Health Consortium. (2008). *Perinatal mental health national action plan 2008– 2010 full report*. Available from: www.beyondblue.org.au/docs/default-source/8.-perinatal-documents/bw0125-report-beyondblues-perinatal-mental-health-(nap)-full-report.pdf?sfvrsn=2. [Accessed 16 May 2016].

Prandl, K.J., Rooney, R. & Bishop, B.J. (2012). Mental health of Australian Aboriginal women during pregnancy: Identifying the gaps. *Archives of Women's Mental Health*, *15*(3), 149–154.

Sherwood, J. & Geia, L. (2014). Historical and current perspectives on the health of Aboriginal and Torres Strait Islander people. In O. Best & B. Fredericks (Eds.), *Yatdjuligin: Aboriginal and Torres Strait Islander nursing and midwifery care*, (pp, 7–30). Melbourne: Cambridge University Press.

Silburn, S.R., Zubrick, S.R., Lawrence, D.M., Mitrou, F.G., De Maio, J.A., Blair, E., Cox, A., Dalby, R.B., Griffin, G.P. & Hayward, C. (2006). The intergenerational effects of forced separation on the social and emotional wellbeing of Aboriginal children and young people. Available from: https://aifs.gov.au/sites/default/files/ss(2).pdf [Accessed 1 June 2016].

Smylie, J. (2014). *Strong women, strong nations: Aboriginal maternal health in British Columbia*. Available from: www.nccah-ccnsa.ca/Publications/Lists/Publications/Attachments/129/2014_07_09_FS_2421_MaternalHealth_EN_Web.pdf [Accessed 1 June 2016].

Smylie, J., Crengle, S., Freemantle, J. & Taualii, M. (2010). Indigenous birth outcomes in Australia, Canada, New Zealand and the United States – An overview. *The Open Women's Health Journal*, *4*, 7–17. doi:10.2174/1874291201004010007.

Statistics Canada. (2013). *Aboriginal peoples in Canada: First Nations People, Métis and Inuit, national household survey, 2011*. Available from: www12.statcan.gc.ca/nhs-enm/2011/as-sa/99-011-x/99-011-x2011001-eng.pdf.

The Department of Health. (2016). *Indigenous health*. Available from: www.health.gov.au/Indigenous. [Accessed 1 May 2016].

The Truth and Reconciliation Commission of Canada. (2015). *Honouring the truth, reconciling for the future: Summary of the final report of the Truth and Reconciliation Commission of Canada*. Available from: http://nctr.ca/assets/reports/Final%20Reports/Executive_Summary_English_Web.pdf. [Accessed 1 May 2016].

Thorpe, A., Arabena, K., Sullivan, P., Silburn, K. & Rowley K. (2016). *Engaging First Peoples: A review of government engagement methods for developing health policy*. Available from: www.lowitja.org.au/sites/default/files/docs/Engaging-First-Peoples.pdf [Accessed 15 June 2016].

Van Wagner, V., Epoo, B., Nastapoka, J. & Harney E. (2007). Reclaiming birth, health, and community: Midwifery in the Inuit villages of Nunavik, Canada. *Journal of Midwifery & Women's Health*, *52*(4), 384–391.

Van Wagner, V., Osepchook, C., Harney, E., Crosbie, C. & Tulugak, M. (2012). Remote midwifery in Nunavik, Quebec, Canada: Outcomes of perinatal care for the Inuulitsivik health centre, 2000–2007. *Birth*, *39*(3), 230–237.

West, R., Usher, K. & Foster, K. (2010). Increased numbers of Australian Indigenous nurses would make a significant contribution to 'closing the gap' in Indigenous health: What is getting in the way? *Contemporary Nurse*, *36*(1–2), 121–130.

Williams, R. (1999). Cultural safety: What does it mean for our work practice? *Australian and New Zealand Journal of Public Health*, *23*(2), 213–214.

5

LESBIAN WOMEN BECOMING MOTHERS

Brenda Hayman

Introduction

This chapter discusses the experiences of partnered lesbian women who choose motherhood with particular emphasis on access to and experiences of perinatal services. It explores the process of making the decision to have a baby, the various methods of conceiving, pregnancy and birth, and the complexities of same-sex parenthood. Much of the information presented in this chapter is drawn from the findings of a qualitative, Australian study carried out by the author and colleagues (Hayman, Wilkes, Halcomb & Jackson, 2015) that aimed to examine the experiences of lesbian women who chose motherhood. A case study based on the women's stories is offered to highlight some of the challenges experienced by lesbian women when accessing maternity services. Some of the therapeutic strategies that health professionals can implement, such as reflecting on personal attitudes, raising awareness of heteronormative assumption in the clinical setting, reducing homophobia (overt and hidden) and the use of inclusive language, as approaches that can have a significant impact on the quality of perinatal care delivered to lesbian women are also presented.

Background

It is becoming increasingly acceptable for lesbian women to have children and become parents in Australia, and in many other places around the world. In conjunction with social acceptance, progressive laws have also made it possible for lesbian women to consider adoption and fostering and with increasing access to artificial reproductive technology, they are also having their own biological children with the use of donor sperm. In addition, lesbian women continue to mother children from their previous heterosexual relationships and their partners are mothering non-biological children from their partner's previous heterosexual relationship/s. Subsequently, there has been a significant increase in the number of lesbian women choosing motherhood (Australian Bureau of Statistics [ABS], 2009; Hequembourg, 2009) and partnered lesbian women creating their own *de novo* families. A *de novo* family is a constellation of kin that is headed by two, partnered lesbian women who planned, conceived, birthed and are parenting their children in the context of their same-sex relationship (McNair, 2004). Since *de novo* families in Australia and around the world are increasing, social recognition, acceptance and visibility of lesbian women as mothers is also increasing (Goldberg & Perry-Jenkins, 2007; Renaud, 2007).

Much of the earlier literature on lesbian motherhood (see Golombok & Tasker, 1996; Green, 1978; Huggins, 1989; O'Connell, 1993; Patterson, 1994; Steckel, 1987) focused on the children of (solo and/or partnered) lesbian mothers. Continuing into the subsequent decades, this focus narrowed to specifically examine the effects on children, of being parented by a mother with a lesbian identity (Bos, van Balen, van den Boom & Sandfort, 2004; McNair, Dempsey, Wise & Perlesz, 2002). The majority of these findings overwhelmingly indicated that there were no developmental, social or intellectual disadvantages to children who were parented by a lesbian mother (Adams & Light, 2015; Baiocco *et al.*, 2015; Crouch, Waters, McNair, Power & Davis, 2014).

While these studies have demonstrated that children of lesbian mothers do as well as children raised in heterosexual-parented families, lesbian mothers continue to worry that society will judge the quality of their mothering more harshly because of their lesbian identity (Bos & van Balen, 2010; Braeways, Ponjaert, Van Hall & Golombok, 1997; Hayman, Wilkes, Halcomb & Jackson, 2013; Ryan & Berkowitz, 2009). More recently, the focus of the literature has shifted towards an emphasis on homophobic experiences (see Bos & Gartrell, 2010; Hayman *et al.*, 2013; Hertzmann, 2011; Willis, 2012), the various methods of conception utilised by lesbian women choosing motherhood (see Hayman *et al.* 2015; Nordqvist, 2011; Wojnar & Katzenmeyer, 2014) and their experiences of healthcare (see Cherguit, Burns, Pettle & Tasker, 2013; Hayman *et al.*, 2013; Lee, Taylor & Raitt, 2011; O'Neill, Hamer & Dixon, 2012; Smith, 2015; Weber, 2010). While the journey to motherhood presents significant challenges and adjustments for all women, partnered lesbian women choosing biological motherhood are exposed to additional challenges, purely because of their lesbian identity (Ben-Ari & Livni, 2006). These challenges will be explored in the following sections with a focus on the consequences of stigmatisation, discrimination and homophobia (Goldberg & Smith, 2008; Weber, 2010) and how they work to overcome these challenges. Specifically, justifying the role and position of the non-birth mother in *de novo* families and important decision-making.

Becoming mothers

Following a chronological pathway, this chapter will now explore conception, pregnancy, birth and parenting experiences of lesbian women creating *de novo* families, and the ways that lesbian mothers manage some of the personal, societal and healthcare challenges faced. A brief case study has been included to provide the reader with an opportunity to consider the insights in a real-life context. Additional readings have also been offered at the end of the chapter on specific topics that you may wish to study in more depth.

Planning and conceiving

As more and more lesbian women choose motherhood, the terms *mother* and *lesbian* are no longer mutually exclusive identities (Reed, Miller, Valenti & Timm, 2011). Creating a *de novo* family involves a great deal of planning and numerous decisions that are unique to partnered lesbian women (Chabot & Ames, 2004; Kranz & Daniluk, 2006; Renaud, 2007). Planning typically involves charting the cycle of the woman who will try to conceive, discussing employment and other financial decisions and conversations about healthcare and service providers. Many of the decisions are based on information gained from researching via the internet and conversations with other lesbian mothers, both online (via blogs for example) and face-to-face with their peers and healthcare providers; a process that one woman referred to as researching 'within an inch of her sanity' (Lilly) (Hayman *et al.*, 2015, p. 400). Initially the women need to decide which one of them will try to conceive. Generally, this decision is based on factors like age, health status and individual desire. For example, in some partnerships, one woman might be at an age where conception is impossible or unlikely, or one woman might have health issues that would make it difficult to conceive, or where conception would worsen her health. In our study, Lilly stated she thought she would be best, 'because of my age' and Gemma added that her partner would try to conceive because she 'didn't have a strong desire to carry a child' (Hayman *et al.*, 2015, p. 399).

In some lesbian couples, one woman might identify as *butch* and as such, being pregnant would be incongruent with her gender identity. Where both women desire to conceive, they have the option of taking turns. Sometimes the decision is made based on which woman is able to conceive, for example after several unsuccessful attempts, the couple could decide that the other partner would try to conceive.

With the increasing availability of Assisted Reproductive Technology (ART) it is sometimes the case in *de novo* families that the birth mother is not the biological mother of the child. Some partnered lesbian women choose to use one mother's egg and her partner's body to conceive, carry and deliver the baby. This option is perceived to equalise the relationship between each mother and the child, or may be chosen if the pregnant partner is older and there are concerns about the health of her eggs. Once these decisions are made, then they will need to negotiate more complex decisions around how they will go about conceiving and whether they want to use sperm from a known or an unknown donor.

More recently, increased access to ART has meant lesbian women have far more options for conceiving. Historically, lesbian women needed to identify a male friend who was comfortable donating sperm and go about self-inseminating to achieve a pregnancy. Assuming she had no health issues that would make conception more difficult, together with a regular cycle, this method of conception is fairly successful. Notably, there are some lesbian women who choose to engage in heterosexual intercourse as a means to an end of achieving a pregnancy, although this is very unusual as it is not congruent with lesbian identity (Baetens & Brewaeys, 2001). Today with more options available to lesbian women wishing to conceive, they can choose to use known or unknown donor sperm for various methods of conception including: vaginal insemination (VI), intrauterine insemination (IUI), or in-vitro fertilisation (IVF) (Yager, Brennan, Steele, Epstein & Ross, 2010).

Vaginal insemination (VI) is generally undertaken as self-insemination in a home environment, and has been a practice used by lesbian women since the 1970s (Luce, 2010), but can also be conducted in a clinical setting that is medically supervised. Women choosing VI will have chosen to use sperm from a known donor (discussed in more depth below). Most women choose to self-inseminate at home with known donor sperm and the usual process is that the couple will make contact with the donor just prior to ovulation to arrange a collection. The sperm will be collected in a sterile container and transferred to the vagina via a 3ml syringe. Typically, women engage in activities like placing pillows under their buttocks, positioning legs in the air and/or staying still for extended periods of time, believing that the sperm will find their way to the egg more easily. Some women choose to inseminate more than once during ovulation, to increase chances of achieving a pregnancy. Vaginal insemination can also take place in a clinic and in this case, sperm from an unknown *or* known donor can be used. IUI and IVF take place in a clinical environment. Generally, both women attend the clinic together for all procedures including insemination; Kristie (non-birth mother) stated that, 'We were together, so it was nice. It felt kind of like a joint thing we were doing' (Hayman *et al.*, 2013, p. 280). Each of the non-birth mothers in our study expressed the importance of being as involved as possible in the insemination process, and indeed all aspect of planning, conceiving, pregnancy, birth and beyond.

Decisions around known or unknown sperm donor identity can be a choice that is interdependent with the decision about method of conception. For example, as discussed above a woman choosing VI – sometimes referred to as alternate (or artificial) insemination (AI) outside of the clinical environment – means that she *must* also choose to use known donor sperm. When insemination takes place in a clinical environment, sperm from an unknown or known donor can be used. This sperm is quarantined for six months to reduce the risk of the transmission of infections.

Besides choosing a known donor because the women prefer VI at home, they choose known sperm donation for a variety of other reasons. Some lesbian women choose a known donor because it is important for them to have an ongoing relationship with him in the future, and anticipate that the donor will have a role in the child's life – either from birth or later when (and if) the child chooses to make contact. This was reflected by Ellie who stated that they 'only wanted a registered donor, so when the kids turn 18, they are able to contact him' (Hayman et al., 2013, p. 279). Other women choose an unknown donor because they want to make sure that he does not lay parental claim to the child in the future – Jane confirmed this stating, 'We wanted to make sure that he knew it was going to be our child, not part of – like not his child' (Hayman et al., 2015, p. 402). They want to protect their parental roles and in particular, the role of the non-birth mother.

In addition to choosing a known or unknown sperm donor, the women also need to make other donor-related decisions. Especially when choosing an unknown donor, the women want to make the choice based on some, what they deem to be, important characteristics. For example, they want to know his health status and history, what he looks like (for example his eye and hair colour) as well as his age, ethnicity, job, hobbies and level of education. Some of these characteristics are important for obvious reasons, for example his age and health status might indicate his (perceived) level of fertility. Other characteristics like his hair and eye colour and ethnicity might be important to the women because they will sometimes try and match the physical features of the donor to the non-birth mother. This is done to increase the possibility of the child looking like the non-birth mother. Non-birth mothers in de novo families often have to continually justify their parental role and position – choosing physical characteristics of the sperm donor that match hers, is a way of demonstrating familial connection to the outside world. Connection between the non-birth mother and the child are very important and some couples choose to use sperm from the non-birth mother's relative (usually her brother) to further create an authentic connection. Rosie and Kelly used the sperm of Kelly's (non-birth mother) brother to try and create a stronger biological tie between Kelly and her child (Hayman et al., 2015, p. 401).

Finally, choosing an unknown donor meant that conception would occur in a clinical environment, and with this comes increased health safety. Women choosing self-insemination assume some risk of contracting sexually transmitted infections, while couples using IUI or IVF are afforded the peace of mind that the semen has been tested and quarantined for six months prior to use, thus significantly reducing the risk of disease transmission.

Once all of these important decisions have been made, the couple begins their journey of trying to conceive. Like heterosexual couples and single women, conceiving can be a difficult time for lesbian women also, who describe this period as 'living in fortnightly cycles' – either waiting to test or waiting to ovulate (Hayman et al., 2015). Despite the challenges, lesbian women are fairly successful at conceiving and generally conceive within a year (Hayman et al., 2015).

Pregnancy and birth

Sharing the news of a pregnancy can be a point of difference for lesbian women, when compared to partnered, heterosexual women planning a pregnancy. Often lesbian women do not share the news of their pregnancies with their biological families. This occurs for a number of reasons, but a primary one is that they do not have any/regular contact with their families, who have disowned them due to their lesbian orientation. This can lead to a lack of support received by the couple and in addition can reduce access to mothering role-models. Some families of origin (biological families) are of the opinion that lesbian women should not have children in the context of their same-sex relationship, and that children (especially boys) need a male-gendered father to grow and develop properly (Clarke & Kitzinger, 2005; MacCallum & Golombok, 2004). For this reason, they might reject the pregnant lesbian daughter or at best, ignore the pregnancy. These circumstances exclude some lesbian women from the usual mother-stories traditionally handed down from mother to daughter. Further, some lesbian women choosing motherhood might be ostracised by some segments of the lesbian community who do not perceive motherhood as congruent with a true lesbian identity (Donovan & Wilson, 2008). For these reasons, lesbian women choosing motherhood will often surround themselves strategically with other lesbian mothers and people who support their decision to create a family (O'Neill *et al.*, 2012).

The excitement of a (planned) positive pregnancy test, arranging an ultrasound, wondering if it's a boy or a girl (or both), designing the nursery are experiences familiar to any parents who find they are expecting. In terms of pregnancy and preparing for birth, the experiences of lesbian women are likely similar to those of heterosexual women celebrating a planned pregnancy.

One area of contention highlighted in the research I have conducted with my colleagues is the exclusionary and judgemental attitudes of healthcare providers towards lesbian couples. For example the non-birth mothers are sometimes excluded and their role as a legitimate mother is not always recognised (Hayman *et al.*, 2013). I now present a case study which illuminates some of the issues mentioned so far, and which highlights the potential stigmatising and discriminatory behaviours that non-birth mothers, and *de novo* families can face by midwifery professionals (other examples of discriminatory behaviours by professionals are discussed in Chapter 6).

Case study: Jemima and Angela

Jemima knew she was a lesbian at the age of 14 years. She hid this information from her friends and family fearing she would be disliked, made fun of or worse, kicked out of home. Despite these worries, at the age of 18 years Jemima told her parents about her sexual orientation; that she was a lesbian. Her mother cried and her father left the room – he has not spoken to her since that day. Her relationship with her mother was very strained and Jemima left home at 19 years of age.

Soon after leaving home, Jemima met Angela. Jemima and Angela have been partnered for eight years and decided to have a baby. Both aged in their mid 20s, they decided that Jemima would try to conceive because Angela had experienced polycystic ovary syndrome since her teens, and they believed it would be more difficult for her to become pregnant.

They went about finding information and eventually decided to use a known sperm donor and try vaginal insemination at home. Angela's brother agreed to donate sperm and soon Jemima was pregnant. The pregnancy went well, and Angela's family (who accepted Angela's orientation) were very excited for the couple. Unfortunately, they lived in another state, so the level of support they could offer was minimal. Both Angela and Jemima felt quite alone during the pregnancy. Some of their friends had not spent as much time with them because they were of the opinion that child-bearing was for heterosexual people, and against the true, authentic lesbian identity.

Toward the end of the pregnancy, Jemima and Angela attended an antenatal class at their local hospital, where they were booked-in to give birth to their baby. The midwife running the class was taken aback when she first saw the same-sex couple, and stated she did not know what to call Angela – 'she isn't the father is she?' she asked. Further, the midwife asked, 'Where's the father?' This left Angela and Jemima feeling excluded and embarrassed, and also a little angry. They did not go to any future classes.

Jemima was admitted to the hospital and scheduled for an induction. On admission, Angela and Jemima found it difficult to complete the admission forms – there was nowhere for Angela to put her name, so she ended up drawing a line through the word 'father' and replacing it with the words 'other mother' and putting her name beside it. During admission a midwife asked Jemima many questions, one of which was, 'Was this a planned pregnancy?' Jemima and Angela felt like the midwife was not really thinking about them as an individual family, and they again felt embarrassed. Once the admission process had been completed, they were shown to Jemima's room. On more than one occasion, Angela had to explain who she was – what her relationship was to Jemima and the baby.

After the induction of labour, Jemima was not progressing and because the baby was becoming distressed, it was decided the baby should be delivered by caesarean section. After a complicated caesarean delivery, Jemima needed to stay in the operating theatre, and so Angela decided to go with the baby to the neonatal intensive care unit (NICU). As she arrived at the doorway to the NICU, a nurse approached her and asked her who she was and stated that only family were allowed to enter the NICU. Angela explained that she was the baby's mother and the nurse stated that she knew the baby's mother was still in the operating theatre. Angela tried to explain that she was also the mother, but she was refused entry.

Finally, when a nurse who knew the family arrived, Angela was permitted in to the NICU. An inquisitive nurse who was looking after the baby giggled and asked Angela if they 'used a turkey baster'. While Angela was embarrassed, she went ahead and explained how they had conceived.

This case study is based on several stories shared by participants in our study (Hayman *et al.*, 2015). While these incidents are the exception rather than the rule, and most of the participants shared very positive stories of maternity care – there is much to be learned about systemic/institutional homophobia heteronormative assumptions, and the need for inclusive language/forms in healthcare settings.

Parenting

As alluded to earlier, society does not expect lesbian women to be mothers and in addition, sometimes their families and the lesbian community do not tolerate their decision to become mothers either. Lesbian mothers can be harshly judged stating that it is selfish for lesbian women to have children because they will be bullied because of their mothers' sexual orientation (Clarke, Kitzinger & Potter, 2004) and because all children (but especially boys) require a father role model in order to grow and develop properly (Clarke & Kitzinger, 2005; MacCallum & Golombok, 2004). In addition, some people continue to believe that children raised by lesbian women will grow up to be homosexual (Golombok & Tasker, 1996; Patterson, 2006). The research, as detailed previously, demonstrates that these assertions are not accurate and that children raised by lesbian women do just as well on all measures as children raised in two-parent, heterosexual-parented families and that any bullying experienced by children of lesbian mothers was largely countered by well-developed resilience, nurtured by strong familial relationships (Bos & Gartrell, 2010; Rosenfeld, 2010).

In relation to parenting, partnered lesbian women choosing motherhood experience several complex challenges. Justifying the role of the non-birth mother in their family can be a significant challenge, particularly as she tries to negotiate healthcare and schooling for her children. The role and parental position of the non-birth mother in *de novo* families can be precarious at best and establishing the non-birth mother as a legitimate mother, and equalising each mother-child relationship are very important aspects of creating a *de novo* family.

Often non-birth mothers find that society does not recognise their position and role in their family as a legitimate parent and mother (Hayman *et al.*, 2013). In addition, some non-birth mothers find it difficult to negotiate their role within their family (Paldron, 2014). Because she did not carry nor give birth to a child, the non-birth mother may find herself feeling excluded, especially by members of their family, and particularly by in-laws. Despite biological and non-birth mothers anticipating equal maternal roles (because both parents are the mother), Pelka (2009) found that roles between each of the mothers differed significantly in relation to division of labour, mother-roles and interaction with the child. The birth mother is more likely to be the parent the child goes to for nurturing, feeding, or when they are scared or sad (Goldberg & Perry-Jenkins, 2007), while the child is more likely to seek out their non-birth mother for play activities. Another method of establishing equitable mother-roles is to induce lactation by the non-birth mother and both breastfeed the baby (Wahler & Feister, 2013).

Finally, lesbian mothers justified the role and position of the non-birth mother with the use of strategically chosen names and by engaging in ceremonies (like naming days and commitment ceremonies) that, for them, represented 'marriage' (in the absence of laws that permit legal marriage in Australia). In relation to names, the mothers generally choose special names for the non-birth mother like Ma, Mummy X (X = initial of the woman's first name, like Mummy B for example), Daddy, a first name, or a culturally significant word for Mummy or Daddy (for example, in the study by the author, one non-biological mother is German and she is called 'Mutti' which is German for mother). In addition, most often the baby was given the non-birth mother's surname, and in this case the whole family generally took the non-birth mother's surname (Hayman *et al.*, 2013).

Some lesbian mothers feel the need to act as community educators and teach people about their *de novo* families. In particular, lesbian mothers teach the community about their families and about the methods of conception. Many people will ask questions about how the children are conceived for example. Lesbian mothers take opportunities to debunk myths associated with lesbian motherhood and to educate people about how they go about conceiving their children and make their families work.

Implications for practice

Reflecting on the case study above, the first issue raised is the potential lack of familial and community support for some lesbian women choosing motherhood. Nurses/midwives and other healthcare providers need to be aware that some lesbian women choosing motherhood do not have the support from their families and communities. This may expose them to additional stress and feelings of isolation. It will be important for healthcare professionals to ask lesbian women about their supports, relationships with family and their community. Keeping in mind that some lesbian women even experience ongoing homophobia from their family of origin, they often feel unsupported and maybe even very alone. For this reason, 'family of choice' become a very important source of support for some lesbian women. This is something that the healthcare service, and the professionals, might need to consider in relation to rules related to who is (and is not) permitted to visit new mothers and their babies. Finally, it will be beneficial to keep in mind that ongoing exposure to stress because of exclusion (familial and/or social) and homophobia can affect self-esteem, which may impact on mental health, the likelihood of developing post-natal depression and her capacity to mother – real or perceived.

Second, healthcare professionals need to consider the language they are using – it is inclusive? The forms as an extension of the language used by healthcare professionals also need consideration and re-developing, so that they are flexible enough to capture diverse family constellations and individuals who may fall outside the binary male/female gender system. Midwives and nurses caring for *de novo* families should always ask about the terms used to signify each member of the family, in particular the non-birth mother. This will help the family to feel comfortable and accepted within the health service setting. The use of inclusive language on admission and intake forms will also be helpful. In addition, displaying of posters, pamphlets and other health promotional materials that demonstrate diverse family constellations will also help *de novo* families to feel accepted and acknowledged.

Finally, individual healthcare professionals need to engage in self-examination and reflection about their own attitudes and recognise that heteronormativity can be as harmful as homophobia. Heteronormativity is the assumption that everyone is straight and that being opposite-sex attracted is more acceptable than being same-sex attracted. It can affect the relationship between the lesbian woman seeking healthcare and the healthcare provider. Assuming that a lesbian woman is heterosexual can immediately create a barrier between the woman and her healthcare professional, and subsequently affect the quality of their relationship. For example, if the healthcare professional were to ask about the woman's husband, the woman has to make a decision about letting the professional continue with the incorrect assumption or whether to correct the assumption. Correcting the assumption can be dangerous and may be met with an indignant response to simply being corrected, or even a homophobic reaction. The fact that the healthcare professional has assumed heterosexual orientation can indicate that he/she privileges opposite-sex attracted relationships, and can create fear and feelings of distrust in the patient.

Homophobia can be subtle, like inappropriate questions or refusing to acknowledge the non-birth mother in a same-sex partnership. On occasions, non-birth mothers have been referred to as aunties or sisters, so the healthcare professional feels more comfortable. In addition, making assumptions about a person's sexual orientation can be fraught with dangers. Healthcare providers should ask a person about their orientation instead of making heteronormative assumptions. More importantly, being forced to *come out* over and over again is extremely stressful. Professionals need to consider their personal attitudes and how any assumptions might affect the healthcare experiences of lesbian women. Any notion that the healthcare staff does not approve or devalues their relationship is going to undermine the therapeutic relationship required to deliver quality health care.

Reflection questions

- Consider how the forms or documentation you currently use in your service might include/exclude some/minority members of the community?
- How can the forms be improved? Consider your local policy and procedures.
- What are the benefits of improving forms?
- What are the (health) risks of using forms that exclude some people in our communities?

Conclusion

With the increase in ART and the favourable changes to societal attitudes that are becoming more accepting of partnered lesbian women having children, there has been a significant increase in the number of *de novo* families. While acceptance of lesbian mothering has certainly expanded, unfortunately there still remains significant, attitudinal challenges, specifically homophobia and heteronormativity.

As a natural progression from negative individual/societal attitudes, there remains, in Australia at least, legal inequality in relation to same-sex marriage and the privileges it brings to individuals, families and communities. For these reasons, choosing motherhood can present significant challenges to lesbian women and midwives need to be aware of their specific needs. Homophobia, heteronormativity, use of inappropriate language, lack of knowledge and a lack of consideration of the unique experiences of lesbian women can create barriers to the delivery of quality health care.

Most people feel some level of vulnerability when they are a patient, and for lesbian women this vulnerability is magnified. Any strategies that the healthcare professional can implement to increase a sense of safety and subsequently promote a therapeutic relationship will inevitably improve the overall quality of health care delivered.

References

Adams, J. & Light, R. (2015). Scientific consensus, the law, and same sex parenting outcomes. *Social Science Research, 53*, 300–310.

Australian Bureau of Statistics (2009). *Australian social trends*. Available from: www.abs.gov.au/ausstats/abs@.nsf/mf/4102.0 [Accessed 17 November 2016].

Baetens, P. & Brewaeys, A. (2001). Lesbian couples requesting donor insemination: An update of the knowledge with regard to lesbian mother families. *Human Reproduction Update, 7*(5), 512–519.

Baiocco, R., Santamaria, F., Ioverno, S., Fontanesi, L., Baumgartner, E., Laghi, F. & Lingiardi, V. (2015). Lesbian mother families and gay father families in Italy: Family functioning, dyadic satisfaction, and child well-being. *Sexuality Research and Social Policy, 12*(3), 202–212.

Ben-Ari, A. & Livni, T. (2006). Motherhood is not a given thing: Experiences and constructed meanings of biological and non-birth lesbian mothers. *Sex Roles, 54*, 521–531.

Bos, H. & van Balen, F. (2010). Children of the new reproductive technologies: Social and genetic parenthood. *Patient Education and Counseling, 81*(3), 429–439.

Bos, H. & Gartrell, N. (2010). Adolescents of the USA national longitudinal lesbian family study: Can family characteristics counteract the negative effects of stigmatisation? *Family Process, 49*(4), 559–572.

Bos, H., van Balen, F., van den Boom, D.C. & Sandfort, Th.G.M. (2004). Minority stress, experiences of parenthood and child adjustment in lesbian families. *Journal of Reproductive and Infant Psychology, 22*(4), 291–304.

Braeways, A., Ponjaert, I., Van Hall, E.V. & Golombok, S. (1997). Donor insemination: Child development and family functioning in lesbian mother families. *Human Reproduction, 12*, 1349–1359.

Chabot, J.M. & Ames, B.D. (2004). It wasn't 'let's get pregnant and go do it': Decision making in lesbian couples planning motherhood via donor insemination. *Family Relations, 53*(4), 348–356.

Cherguit, J., Burns, J., Pettle, S. & Tasker, F. (2013). Lesbian co-mother's experiences of maternity healthcare experiences. *Journal of Advanced Nursing, 69*(6), 1269–1278.

Clarke, V. & Kitzinger, C. (2005). We're not living on planet lesbian: Constructions of male role models in debates about lesbian families. *Sexualities, 8*(2), 137–152.

Clarke, V., Kitzinger, C. & Potter, J. (2004). 'Kids are just cruel anyway': Lesbian and gay parents' talk about homophobic bullying. *British Journal of Social Psychology, 43*(4), 531–550.

Crouch, S.R., Waters, E., McNair, R., Power, J. & Davis, E. (2014). Parent-reported measures of child health and wellbeing in same-sex parent families: A cross-sectional survey. *BMC Public Health, 14*(635). doi:10.1186/1471-2458-14-635.

Donovan, C. & Wilson, A.R. (2008). Imagination and integrity: Decision-making among lesbian couples to use medically provided donor insemination. *Culture, Health and Sexuality, 10*(7), 649–665.

Goldberg, A.E. & Perry-Jenkins, M. (2007). The division of labor and perceptions of parental roles: Lesbian couples across the transition to parenthood. *Journal of Social and Personal Relationships, 24*(2), 297–318.

Goldberg, A.E. & Smith, J.Z. (2008). Social support and well-being in lesbian and heterosexual preadoptive parents. *Family Relations, 57*, 281–294.

Golombok, S. & Tasker, F. (1996). Do parents influence the sexual orientation of their children? Findings from a longitudinal study of lesbian families. *Developmental Psychology, 32*(1), 3–11.

Green, R. (1978). Sexual identity of 37 children raised by homosexual or transsexual parents. *American Journal of Psychiatry, 135*, 692–697.

Hayman, B., Wilkes, L., Halcomb, E. & Jackson, D. (2013). Marginalised mothers: Lesbian women negotiating heteronormative healthcare services. *Contemporary Nurse, 44*(1), 120–127.

Hayman, B., Wilkes, L., Halcomb, E. & Jackson, D. (2015). Lesbian women choosing motherhood: The journey to conception. *Journal of GLBT Family Studies, 121*(4), 395–409.

Hayman, B., Wilkes, L., Jackson, D. & Halcomb, E. (2013). De novo lesbian families: Legitimising the other mother, *Journal of GLBT Family Studies, 9*(3), 273–287.

Hequembourg, A. (2009). An exploration of sexual minority across the lines of gender and sexual identity. *Journal of Homosexuality, 56*(3), 273–298.

Hertzmann, L. (2011). Lesbian and gay couple relationships: When internalised homophobia gets in the way of couple creativity. *Psychoanalytic Psychotherapy, 25*(4), 346–360.

Huggins, S.L. (1989). A comparative study of self-esteem of adolescent children of divorced lesbian mothers and divorced heterosexual mothers. *Journal of Homosexuality, 18*(1–2), 123–135.

Kranz, K.C. & Daniluk, J.C. (2006). Living outside the box: Lesbian families created through the use of anonymous donor insemination. *Journal of Feminist Family Therapy, 18*(1–2), 1–33.

Lee, E., Taylor, J. & Raitt, F. (2011). 'It's not me, it's them': How lesbian women make sense of negative experiences of maternity care. A hermeneutic study. *Journal of Advanced Nursing, 67*, 982–990.

Luce, J. (2010). *Beyond expectations: Lesbian/bi/queer women and assisted conception.* Toronto: University of Toronto Press.

MacCallum, F. & Golombok, S. (2004). Children raised in fatherless families from infancy: A follow-up of children of lesbian and heterosexual mothers at early adolescence. *The Journal of Child Psychology and Psychiatry, 45*(8), 1407–1419.

McNair, R. (2004). *Outcomes for children born of A.R.T. in a diverse range of families* (Occasional Paper). Melbourne, VIC: Law Reform Commission.

McNair, R.P., Dempsey, D., Wise, S. & Perlesz, A. (2002). Lesbian parenting: Issues, strengths and challenges. *Family Matters*, 63, 40–49.

Nordqvist, P. (2011). Choreographies of sperm donations: Dilemmas of intimacy in lesbian couple donor conception. *Social Science and Medicine*, 73, 1661–1668.

O'Connell, A. (1993). Voices from the heart: Developmental impact of a mother's lesbianism on her adolescent children. *Smith College Studies in Social Work*, 63, 281–299.

O'Neill, K.R., Hamer, H.P. & Dixon, R. (2012). 'A lesbian family in a straight world': The impact of the transition to parenthood on couple relationships in planned lesbian families. *Women's Studies Journal*, 26(2), 39–53.

Paldron, M.F. (2014). The other mother: An exploration of non-biological lesbian mothers' unique parenting experience. PhD thesis, University of Minnesota. Available from: http://conservancy.umn.edu/handle/11299/167423 [Accessed 10 January 2016].

Patterson, C.J. (1994). Lesbian and gay couples considering parenthood: An agenda for research, service and advocacy. *Journal of Gay and Lesbian Social Services*, 1, 33–55.

Patterson, C.J. (2006). Children of lesbian and gay parents. *Current Directions in Psychological Science*, 5(5), 241–244.

Pelka, S. (2009). Sharing motherhood: Maternal jealousy among lesbian co-mothers. *Journal of Homosexuality*, 56(2), 195–217.

Reed, S.J., Miller, R.L., Valenti, M.T. & Timm, T.M. (2011). Good gay females and babies' daddies: Black lesbian community norms and the acceptability of pregnancy. *Culture, Health and Sexuality: An International Journal for Research, Intervention and Care*, 13(7), 751–765.

Renaud, M.T. (2007). We are mothers too: Childbearing experiences of lesbian families. *Journal of Obstetric, Gynecologic and Neonatal Nursing*, 36(2), 190–199.

Rosenfeld, M.J. (2010). Non-traditional families and childhood progress through school. *Demography*, 47(3), 755–775.

Ryan, M. & Berkowitz, D. (2009). Constructing gay and lesbian parent families 'Beyond the closet'. *Qualitative Sociology*, 32(2), 153–172.

Smith, R. (2015). Healthcare experiences of lesbian and bisexual women in Cape Town, South Africa. *Culture, Health and Sexuality*, 17(2), 180–193.

Steckel, A. (1987). Psychosocial development of children of lesbian mothers. In F.W. Bozett (Ed.), *Gay and lesbian parents* (pp. 75–85). New York: Praeger Publishers.

Wahler, L. & Fiester, A. (2013). Induced lactation for the non gestation mother in a lesbian couple (Commentary). *AMA Journal of Ethics*, 15(9), 753–756.

Weber, S. (2010). A stigma identification framework for family nurses working with parents who are lesbian, gay, bisexual, or transgendered and their families. *Journal of Family Nursing*, 16(4), 378–393.

Willis, P. (2012). Constructions of lesbian, gay, bisexual and queer identities among young people in contemporary Australia. *Culture, Health and Sexuality*, 14(10), 1213–1227. doi :10.1080/13691058.2012.724087.

Wojnar, D.M. & Katzenmeyer, A. (2014). Experiences of preconception, pregnancy, and new motherhood for lesbian nonbiological mothers. *Journal of Obstetric, Gynaecological and Neonatal Nursing*, 43(1), 50–60. doi:10.1111/1552-6909.12270.

Yager, C., Brennan, D., Steele, L.S., Epstein, R. & Ross, L.E. (2010). Challenges and mental health experiences of lesbian and bisexual women who are trying to conceive. *Health and Social Work*, 35(3), 191–200.

Additional reading

Dahl, B., Fylkesnes, A.M., Sørlie, V. & Malterud, K. (2013). Lesbian women's experiences with healthcare providers in the birthing context: A meta-ethnography. *Midwifery, 29*(6), 674–681.

Farr, R.H. & Patterson, C.J. (2013). Coparenting among lesbian, gay, and heterosexual couples: Associations with adopted children's outcomes. *Child Development, 84*(4), 1226–1240.

Gartrell, N.K., Banks, A., Hamilton, J., Reed, N., Bishop, H. & Rodas, C. (1999). The national lesbian family study: 2. Interviews with mothers of toddlers. *Journal of Orthopsychiatry, 69*, 362–369.

Gartrell, N.K., Bos, H.M.W., Peyser, H., Deck, A. & Rodas, C. (2012). Adolescents with lesbian mothers describe their own lives. *Journal of Homosexuality, 59*(9), 1211–1229.

Larsson, A.K. & Dykes, A.K. (2009). Care during childbirth and pregnancy in Sweden: Perspectives of lesbian women. *Midwifery, 25*(6), 682–690.

Spidsberg, B.D. (2007). Vulnerable and strong – lesbian women encountering maternity care. *Journal of Advanced Nursing, 60*(5), 478–486.

Spidsberg, B.D. & Sørlie, V. (2011). An expression of love – midwives' experiences in the encounter with lesbian women and their partners. *Journal of Advanced Nursing, 68*(4), 796–805.

van Rijn-van Gelderen, L., Bos, H.M.W. & Gartrell, N. (2015). Dutch adolescents from lesbian-parent families: How do they compare to peers with heterosexual parents and what is the impact of homophobic stigmatisation? *Journal of Adolescence, 40*, 65–73.

6

WOMEN WITH A DISABILITY, TRANSITION TO MOTHERHOOD AND THE SELF

Denise Lawler

Introduction

People with a disability can experience discriminatory and ostracising societal practices. They are often subjected to negative stereotyping and cast as incompetent and dependent (Scotch & Schriner, 1997). Such stereotyping augments the sense of difference people with a disability feel and may limit the individual's ability to participate fully in society as an autonomous agent (Allen & Allen, 1995; Hahn, 1988). Historically, paternalistic societies controlled the reproductive rights of women with a disability through practices such as segregation and sterilisation, essentially curtailing women's rights to a family. In contemporary society, women are exposed to a range of maternal constructions, including; celebrity mothers, working mothers, teenage mothers or older mothers but missing from this catalogue are mothers with a disability. The chapter begins with an examination of the theoretical underpinnings that inform societal perceptions of women with a disability. It details how two paradigms shape and inform disability in contemporary society, it explores the impact the transition to motherhood has on women with a disability and presents approaches to care that clinicians and practitioners can incorporate to enhance the care provided to women with a disability when becoming mothers. It also details the resilience women with disability demonstrate when negotiating the transition to motherhood and the profound impact the transition has on the woman's understanding, sense and assumptions of self.

Models of disability

Disability is a relative concept defined within the context of how it is used (Raman & Levi, 2002). Traditionally, disability was defined within a physiological, functionalist perspective and was classified according to individual pathology and associated deficits, abnormalities and functional limitations. Currently there are two models of disability, the medical model and social model, which frame and inform society's views and perceptions of people with disability. The models primarily conceptualise disability in two distinctive and divergent ways; (i) the functionalist, biomedical or individual perspective that focuses primarily on how an individual's impairment results in the person feeling inadequate and different or (ii) the bio-psycho-social perspective that is concerned with identifying and decreasing the social and physical barriers an individual encounters when trying to participate in mainstream society.

The notion of a perfect individual, free from chronic illness or disease or a functional limitation emanates from the eugenic movement and throughout history there are well documented examples of where this philosophy was taken to extremes, such as the Swedish policy of conducting hysterectomies on women with a disability (Abberley, 1987; Roy, Roy & Roy, 2012). The medical model defines a person with a disability as an individual who, because of their disability are 'less than whole' (Dartington, Miller & Gwynne, 1981, p. 126), an individual perceived to be unable to function and/or fulfil social roles and responsibilities, such as being a mother and doing mothering (Barnes & Mercer, 2007; Myers, 1965). Almost five decades later people with a disability continue to be perceived as being unable to function and perform socially constructed roles and responsibilities. They are considered different and dysfunctional, someone to be pitied and someone requiring intervention(s) to ameliorate the deficit related to their disability (Barnes & Mercer, 2007, 2010; Brandt & Pope, 1997; McMillan Boyles, Bailey & Mossey, 2008; Sheerin, Keenan & Lawler, 2014). The medical model does not consider people with a disability to be autonomous, independent individuals, rather it beholds that clinicians are responsible for fixing, curing and caring for people and, where possible, returning them to full functional ability. The individual, in turn, is required to cooperate with clinicians and comply with interventions in order to gain some degree of normality (Barnes & Mercer, 2007; Safilios-Rothschild, 1990).

Over the last 50 years people with a disability have refuted the functionalist conceptualisation. With challenges to the medical model intensifying, an alternative approach to disability emerged; namely the social model. This model challenges the assumption that disability equates to infirmity or ill health, rather it considers disability as an aspect of the individual's life and rejects the contention that people with a disability are inherently imperfect. It aims to emancipate people with a disability from social oppression and exclusion (Oliver, 1990) and to some degree has been successful in politicising the social and physical challenges people with a disability experience while attempting to conform to the dominant, non-disabled values and practices of modern society (Barnes & Mercer, 2007, 2010; Lutz & Bowers, 2003; McMillan

Boyles *et al.*, 2008). This approach suggests that there is no causal relationship between impairment and disability rather disability is conceptualised as a construct of society (McClimens, 2005; Tighe, 2001). The actions and attitudes of society and its members are integral factors that encumber people with a disability (Asch, 1998; Hull, 1998) and inform the creation and obliteration of assumptions of self. It asserts that society constructs challenges that impact on the individual's ability to function and fulfil socially prescribed roles and responsibilities, such as being a mother and mothering. Although people with a disability refute the tenets of the medical model of disability in favour for the social model, arguably the medical model remains the dominant model framing and informing how people with a disability are perceived and treated in contemporary society.

Transition to motherhood for women with a disability and one's sense of self

Life consists of a series of transitions integral to the development and maturation of the individual and one's sense of self. Becoming a mother is a significant and intricate transition, that encompasses physical and psychological changes as women adapt, re-orientate and incorporate motherhood in their life (Lawler, Begley & Lalor, 2015; Redwood, 2007). The change and adaptation involves a conscious and unconscious reorganisation of the self (Kralik, Visentin & Van Loon, 2006; Lawler *et al.*, 2015; Oakley, 1980). The process of becoming a mother can be different for women with a disability (Thomson, Kehily, Hadfield & Sharpe, 2011). These women are often depicted as unfit, incompetent and irresponsible mothers (Begley *et al.*, 2010; Walsh-Gallagher, Sinclair & McConkey, 2012) (similar issues of discrimination in relation to lesbian parents is discussed in Chapter 5). Extant theories regarding the transition to motherhood have evolved from the perspective and experiences of non-disabled women, although there is some diversity in population (for example, women over 35 years (Carolan, 2005), lesbian mothers (DiLapi, 1989; Spidsberg, 2007; Wilton & Kaufmann, 2001), adoptive mothers (Fontenot, 2007), teenage mothers (Arthur, Unwin & Mitchell, 2007), imprisoned mothers (Shamai & Kochal, 2008), African American women (Sawyer, 1999), few studies have included women with a disability. The studies that include women with a disability are mainly qualitative, originating from Canada, Australia, America, United Kingdom and Ireland. They tend to focus on the issue of accessibility, profiling the challenges that women with a disability encounter while accessing maternity services and care (Begley *et al.*, 2010; McKay-Moffat & Cunningham, 2006; Prilleltensky, 2003; Smeltzer, Sharts-Hopko, Ott, Zimmerman & Duffin, 2007) and few have investigated the women's transition to motherhood and impact this may have on one's self.

Meeting and adhering to the tenets associated with mothering can be challenging for any woman, but even more for women with a disability because these women engage in mothering with fewer resources and greater challenges than non-disabled mothers. The decision to become a mother is often met with scepticism from non-disabled persons (Begley *et al.*, 2010; Lawler *et al.*, 2015) and when they become mothers their ability to be a good, competent and responsible mother is scrutinised (Kallianes & Rubenfeld, 1997; McKeever, Angus, Lee-Miller & Reid, 2003). The following exemplar demonstrates how women with a disability go to great lengths to present themselves as capable, competent, confident and responsible mothers while simultaneously harbouring a persistent fear that if they do not meet societal norms and expectations of a mother they would lose custody of their child(ren):

> I was referred to the medical social worker because I had a disability ... you cannot do that to any other group in society, you cannot do that to black people, to travellers, to Muslims, to any other section of society, you cannot just block them all and say 'all those people have to be sent to a social worker', it's not acceptable, and yet it is acceptable if you have a disability ... it knocks your confidence, that feeling of being scrutinised and knowing that all it takes is one person to say that 'I am not able to look after her [baby]' and she would be taken away.
>
> (Lawler, 2013, p. 204)

While the transition to motherhood can be challenging for women with a disability, their disability can enhance their mothering abilities and practices (Malacrida, 2009). Women draw on their experiences of having a disability, incorporating the coping and adaptive strategies developed when negotiating an identity and sense of self pre and post-motherhood in a society where disability is perceived as different. These strategies, used creatively and effectively to assist women as they negotiate the normative practices associated with being and the doing of mothering, are informed and shaped by the symbolic relationships created with others.

Factors that influence how women with a disability transition to motherhood

For women with a disability the symbolic relationships created with others, particularly significant others, created during pregnancy and in early motherhood and their appraisal, can be empowering or disempowering, accepting or renouncing of the woman (Gelech & Desjardins, 2011; Sedikides & Brewer, 2001). Such relationships facilitate the development of a sense of agency and individuality and the creation of assumptions about the self that provide meaning and a sense of purpose in the woman's life before and after becoming a mother. These assumptions reside at the core of the women's psyche, are hinged on the concept of benevolence, meaningfulness and self-worthiness (Janoff-Bulman, 1992) and, as the following quote illustrates, provide women with the necessary information to autonomously navigate life, serving as a guide and filter for life experiences and the self, pre and post becoming a mother:

> I had a large family, they [parents, siblings] all helped me to become the person I am. I've been very fortunate, I am the person I am because of them.
>
> (Lawler et al., 2015, p. 6)

The mother-daughter relationship is especially meaningful in the creation of an understanding of and assumptions regarding the self before and after becoming a mother. As the following quotation illustrates, women's experiences of being mothered instil a desire to become a mother, generate an expectation that this desire will be realised and create an assumption that one would be a good, competent, responsible mother:

> My mother was always there for us, my dad was out working ... it was my mother who shaped the person I became and the goals I set in my life, including that of being a mother.
>
> (Lawler, 2013, p. 116)

Parents are also instrumental in the creation of a sense of sameness and inclusiveness. When parents treat their daughter similar to non-disabled siblings and when no allowances are made for physical or sensory differences, the women's sense of sameness intensifies. Consequently, women with a disability do not consider their disability as an impediment rather they regard it as a defining or non-defining entity of the self. The following narratives attest to how women with a disability welcome and appreciate the sense of sameness, inclusiveness and equality promoted and evoked by their parents:

> I feel 100% included in my family, equal and involved, it shapes who I am.
>
> (Lawler, 2013, p. 168)

> I would have grown up in a very mainstream type home, the term disability didn't arise and as a result ... I don't see myself as disabled.
>
> (Lawler, 2013, p. 168)

When parents display an unrelenting sense of confidence in their daughters' abilities, never doubting or questioning the women's ability to achieve their anticipated life goals and desires, including that of becoming and being a responsible, competent mother, this belief instils a sense of self-sufficiency. The following quote demonstrates how the sense of sameness and equality, instilled by parents, positively contribute to the: (i) formation and understanding of the self before and after they become mothers, (ii) development of a positive belief in the self as a woman/mother and (iii) formation of a sense of independence, determination and resilience:

The attitude from my parents, from an expectation, a responsibility and independence point of view was well if you don't do it yourself nobody else is going to do it for you.

(Lawler, 2013, p. 169)

Sense of belonging: a human necessity

Women's everyday interactions with significant others are founded on stability and longevity. Affirmative and positive interactions instil a sense of security, protection, acceptance and belonging, which manifest in feeling connected and related and facilitate a sense of place and purpose both before and after becoming a mother. The sense of security, connectedness and purpose enable women with a disability to function at a positive physical, psychological, emotional, cognitive and spiritual level (Ghavami, Fingerhut, Peplau, Grant & Wittig, 2011). While belonging is an element of connectedness, connectedness is a dimension that creates a sense of togetherness and cohesiveness (Hill, 2006; Lawler, *et al.*, 2015). Maslow (1954) conceptualises the need to belong as a human necessity, a powerful and pervasive human motivation present in all individuals, guiding the individual's emotional, cognitive and behavioural actions and motivating them to develop social bonds. The need is so vital that it underlies one's ability to survive, reproduce, defend or protect oneself from external threats (Baumeister & Leary, 1995). When women with a disability feel a sense of belonging, before and after becoming a mother, they feel important, valued, needed and accepted (Hagerty, Lynch-Sauer, Patusky, Bouwsema & Collier, 1992; Hagerty & Patusky, 1995). They form affirming social bonds with others; it connects them to others, places and things and provides them with a sense of security (Andersen & Chen, 2002; Sargent, Williams, Hargerty, Lynch-Sauer & Hoyle, 2002) and status (Beart, Hardy & Buchan, 2004).

While relationships with others can be affirmative, they can be destructive too. Women with a disability are vulnerable to the perceptions, assumptions and judgements of others. They are vulnerable in a society that classifies and labels them as different (Kallianes & Rubenfeld, 1997; McKeever *et al.*, 2003; Walsh-Gallagher *et al.*, 2012). During pregnancy and in early motherhood, a woman's understanding and assumptions of the self can be disturbed by both the life-changing event and the inconsistent information received from others (family, friends, colleagues and caregivers) about them as a mother and their ability to mother. This information can enhance or significantly impact on the woman's perceptions and assumptions of the self as a mother (Pratt, 1998; Sheerin *et al.*, 2014) as reflected in the following quote:

I am vulnerable, trying to please society, trying to fit in, having it [disability] makes me different so people treated me different, they assume I can do nothing.

(Lawler *et al.*, 2015, p. 8)

Women feel different and, as the following exemplars demonstrate, they experience a range of emotional reactions including; (i) a diminution of their self-worth and self-esteem, (ii) self-doubt about her ability to mother, (iii) anger and (iv) frustration:

> I had difficulty with patronising attitudes ... it's just subtle attitudes from people, you hear people saying this pregnant woman with a disability, there's almost a kind of horror and it kind of makes you feel kind of grotesque and unhuman.
>
> (Lawler, 2013, p. 189)

> I felt that they [caregivers] looked at me like as if I was incapable of making decisions ... an attitude of we're going to talk about you in front of you, not with you.
>
> (Lawler et al., 2015, p. 7)

The process of becoming a mother and the relentless need to prove one's abilities to others significantly undermines the woman's sense of agency and autonomy and may cause some to question their ability to be a good, competent, responsible mother (Janoff-Bulman, 1992; Lawler et al., 2015):

> There is a lot of questions on 'how are you going to manage, how are you going to look after the baby and are you going to be able to do things.
>
> (Lawler, 2013, p. 204)

> Caregivers are very judging ... going around to all the other mothers in the ward saying 'how is she going to cope with the baby?' Then other mothers would say 'they [women with a disability] shouldn't be having babies', if I was a person with no disability I would be respected more.
>
> (Lawler, et al., 2015, p. 7)

This need to prove one's ability to mother unhinges the woman's understanding and expectation of self and induces a psychological and emotional crisis of varying intensity (Stroebe & Schut, 2010). Women with a disability need to respond to the disruption and do so by reorienting the self, recognising what is happening, restructuring their world and establishing new understanding of self as a mother. They substitute assumptions created before they became a mother with new, modified assumptions generated after they become a mother. Research has identified how motherhood for women with a disability can provide a focus; it affirms their sense of femininity and instils a state of maturity. As reflected in the following quotes, being a mother can enhance women's self-confidence, assertiveness and confidence:

> It's a transformation, it's not like a change overnight, it's a process, it happens over time, I became a much calmer person, I learned more about

communication after I became a mother. I was more vulnerable before [pre-motherhood], I'm so much stronger now; I have more faith in myself. I'm much more confident now. I don't feel like I have to please society.

(Lawler et al., 2015, p. 8)

I think it [motherhood] has made me a better person because I'm more grounded, more grown-up, it [motherhood] makes you cop on. It's [being a mother] an amazing special thing to do in your life and I feel my life wouldn't be complete without it.

(Lawler, 2013, p. 234)

Coping with the disruption to one's understanding and assumptions of the self

When interactions with others disrupt women's assumptions and understanding of the self as a mother they initiate a variety of coping strategies (Lazarus & Folkman, 1984). Evidence of this can be seen where the woman sources familial and extra familial support and advice to help overcome the physical or sensory challenges encountered when mothering:

When you have a disability you have to think outside the box, there's ways and means around everything, you have to re-skill; you have to do things differently, because at the end of the day I wanted to do as much for her [daughter] as I could.

(Lawler, 2013, p. 13)

Other measures include employing someone to help with the physical activities of mothering and/or accessing aids that can assist women in the doing of mothering, like an alarming mattress, which may be helpful for women with a visual impairment.

When interacting with others, especially those in a caring capacity like clinicians and practitioners, before and after becoming a mother, some women with a disability may assume a state of helplessness, a state induced by the many constraints encountered when accessing care and services, which impacts on the woman's sense of agency and autonomy (Peterson, Maier & Seligman, 1995). Paradoxically, what appears to be helplessness is in fact the woman's attempt to gain control over a specific situation. Interactions with clinicians and practitioners are often associated with negative connotations, like stigma and discrimination and so, as women continually interact with these persons they assume a passive state. This state helps women deal with and manage the non-affirming interactions while preparing for, becoming a mother and doing mothering. This is exemplified when women, during their interactions with clinicians and practitioners, detach themselves from any meaningful interaction and dialogue choosing instead to follow instruction rather than seek alternative ways of doing things:

> I felt that others [caregivers] looked at me like as if I was incapable of caring for my baby and being a mother … so I just didn't interact or engage with them.
>
> (Lawler, 2013, p. 189)

Critical to the establishments of new understanding and assumptions of the self is the relinquishment/letting go of roles and aspects of the pre-motherhood self that the woman considers incompatible with mothering and their role as a mother. This is discernible in the woman's behaviour and actions, including the; (i) modification of one's social behaviour, (ii) alteration of one's physical appearance, (iii) reprioritising of one's life and personal goals, and (iv) reconfiguration of one's interpersonal relationships (Lawler *et al.*, 2015). Through the cognitive process of letting go and by engaging with and doing mothering, and gaining mastery over activities that others felt they were unable to do, the woman gains a sense of confidence and becomes more aware of what is worthwhile in life. Life takes on new meaning and as the following quote illustrates the process of letting go for women with a disability, collates with an abating of the sense of vulnerability felt by the women:

> I just let go of trying to make people understand, let go of what I think other's perceptions of me are and of trying to fight against those perceptions. When I let go, it's a lot easier; I don't have to prove myself to others anymore.
>
> (Lawler *et al.*, 2015, p. 8)

The impact of motherhood on women with a disability

Motherhood affords women with a disability a sense of (i) purpose and being, (ii) normality and sameness where being a mother and not their physical or sensory disability becomes their defining attribute. Being a mother engenders a sense of pride, purpose, self-worth and value, and reinstates the sense of belonging and place imbued by significant others during childhood. Motherhood represents a gain for women with a disability, promoting a sense of achievement, enhancing the women's self-esteem and engenders a positive understanding and sense of self. With motherhood, women engage in a process of affirming the attributes of the self that they value while recognising other elements that need changing or modifying. They identify their strengths and limitations, establish more supportive and fulfilling relationships, rethink and reprioritise their life goals and plans, and relinquish entities of the self considered incompatible with the maternal self. Their child(ren) and their role as a mother take precedence over other aspects of their life, including their career:

> My children are my priority, they come before me, it's my children that come first above everything else; they're at the forefront of my mind all the time.
>
> (Lawler, 2013, p. 224)

Thinking ahead and planning for the future becomes a priority. Financial security and an increased awareness of one's own mortality, inspire women with a disability to adopt a healthier lifestyle. More importantly, the reform of the self is not eclipsed by the woman's disability. This is in contrast to others who have explored the transition to motherhood from the perspective of non-disabled women and theorised that becoming a mother equates with a loss of self or self-identity but this sense of loss does not resonate with the experiences of women with a disability (Barclay, Everitt, Rogan, Schmied & Wyllie, 1997; Darvill, Skirton & Farrand, 2008; Flakowicz, 2007; Lawler et al., 2015; Oakley, 1980). Rather, as this chapter illustrates through the biological act of becoming a mother, women with a disability experience a reconstruction of the self. While pre-motherhood some may consider motherhood as all-encompassing and consuming, subsequent personal experiences of motherhood and the emotional rewards accompanying it change perceptions. Motherhood is, for women with a disability, a life-changing psychosocial event representing a meaningful gain, a gain created from a disruptive experience. Moving from being a non-mother to a mother has an immense impact on all aspects of life. New information that evolves from becoming a mother, being a mother and doing mothering provides a sense of what is worthwhile in their life, life takes on new meaning, plans are reprioritised and a new appreciation of the self is gained. Motherhood is a new chapter in the woman's life story, one that incorporates new understanding and assumptions of the self, established from their lived experience of becoming a mother, being a mother and doing mothering, a life with new direction and purpose (Lawler et al., 2015).

Implications for practice

During pregnancy and motherhood clinicians and practitioners have a responsibility to provide quality of care to all women including women with a disability. To aid in this process, a number of recommendations are suggested as follows:

1   All relevant staff be provided with disability and diversity training and awareness.
2   All women's needs are assessed at first point of contact with the maternity services, clinicians and practitioners, and an individualised plan of care be devised, implemented and evaluated in partnership with each woman.
3   A post-registration programme (continuous development programme) be developed for all staff involved in the provision of care for women with a disability.
4   Issues relating to equality, diversity, and disability be included in all curricular guidelines and standards in midwifery, nursing, medical and allied health professional undergraduate and postgraduate education programmes.
5   Specialist posts be created and developed in each maternity unit to support women with a disability during the continuum of pregnancy, childbirth and early motherhood. An example of such practice initiative is the lead for

Perinatal Health and Disability located in Liverpool Women's Hospital (UK) (see www.liverpoolwomens.nhs.uk/Library/health_professionals/Health_talk/ LWH_HealthTalk_Iss1_AW.pdf).

6   Collaborate with and develop a mechanism of referral to appropriate voluntary and non-voluntary disability agencies like Disabled Parents Network (UK) to identify, source and enhance support and resources for parents with a disability.

Conclusion

This chapter provided a different perspective on the transition to motherhood, one from the perspective and experiences of women with a disability. It detailed how significant others, more specifically the woman's own mother, significantly inform the construction and creation of assumptions of self. These assumptions reside at the core of the woman's psyche, informing the self, the woman's life and actions therein, and serve as a guide and filter for life experiences. The support and affirming actions of significant others motivate women's resolve to pursue their life goals, including that of becoming a mother. The chapter exemplified how becoming a mother, being a mother and doing mothering is, for women with a disability, a redefining event, one that causes women to realise their abilities rather than disabilities. Being a mother bestows a status and a sense of value and purpose that pre-motherhood eludes such women. Motherhood provides women with a disability with a sense of purpose and being, affords them a sense of normality and sameness where their ability to mother and not their differences become their defining attribute. Being a mother engenders a sense of pride, purpose, self-worth and value, and reinstates the sense of belonging and place imbued in childhood by significant others.

References

Abberley, P. (1987). The concept of oppression and the development of social theory of disability. *Disability, Handicap and Society, 2*(1), 5–19.

Allen, B. & Allen, S. (1995). The process of social construction of mental retardation: Towards value based interaction. *The Journal of the Association for Persons with Severe Handicaps, 20,* 158–160.

Andersen, S.M. & Chen, S. (2002). The relational self: An interpersonal social-cognitive theory. *Psychological Review, 109*(4), 619–645.

Arthur, A., Unwin, S. & Mitchell, T. (2007). Teenage mothers' experience of maternity services: A qualitative study. *British Journal of Midwifery, 15*(11), 672–677.

Asch, A. (1998). Distracted by disability. *Cambridge Quarterly of Healthcare Ethics, 7,* 77–87.

Barclay, L., Everitt, L., Rogan, F., Schmied, V. & Wyllie, A. (1997). 'Becoming a mother' – an analysis of women's experience of early motherhood. *Journal of Advanced Nursing, 25,* 719–728.

Barnes, C. & Mercer, G. (2007). *Disability.* Cambridge: Polity Press.

Baumeister, R.F. & Leary, M.R. (1995). The need to belong: desire for interpersonal attachments as a fundamental motivation. *Psychological Bulletin, 117*(3), 497–529.

Beart, S., Hardy, G. & Buchan, L. (2004). Changing selves: A grounded theory account of belonging to a self-advocacy group for people with intellecutal disabilities. *Journal of Applied Research in Intellectual Disabilities, 17*(2), 91–100.

Begley, C., Lalor, J., Lawler, D., Higgins, A., Sheerin, F., Alexander, J., Nicholl, H., Lawler, D., Keenan, P., Tuohy, T. & Kavanagh, R. (2010). *The strengths and weakness of the publicly-funded Irish health services provided to women with disabilities in relation to pregnancy, childbirth and early motherhood.* Dublin: National Disability Authority.

Brandt, E.N. & Pope, A.M. (1997). *Enabling America: Assessing the role of rehabilitation science and engineering.* Washington, DC: National Academy Press.

Carolan, M. (2005). 'Doing it properly': The experience of first mothering over 35 years. *Health Care for Women International, 26,* 764–787.

Dartington, T., Miller, E.J. & Gwynne, G. (1981). *A life together.* London: Tavistock.

Darvill, R., Skirton, H. & Farrand, P. (2008). Psychological factors that impact on women's experiences of first time motherhood: A qualitative study of the transition. *Midwifery, 26*(3), 357–366.

DiLapi, E.M. (1989). Lesbian mothers and motherhood hierarchy. *Journal of Homosexuality, 18*(1–2), 101–121.

Flakowicz, M. (2007). Daughter, mother, wife: transitions from ideals to the real family. *Infant Observation, 10*(3), 295–306.

Fontenot, H.B. (2007). Transition and adaptation to adoptive motherhood. *JOGNN: Journal of Obstetric, Gynecology and Neonatal Nursing, 36,* 175–182.

Gelech, J.M. & Desjardins, M. (2011). I am many: The reconstruction of self following acquired brain injury. *Qualitative Health Research, 21*(1), 62–74.

Ghavami, N., Fingerhut, A., Peplau, L., Grant, S.K. & Wittig, M.A. (2011). Testing a model of minority identity achievement, identity affirmation and psychological wellbeing among ethnic minority and sexual minority individuals. *Cultural Diversity and Ethnic Minority Psychology, 17*(1), 79–88.

Hagerty, B., Lynch-Sauer, J., Patusky, K., Bouwsema, M., & Collier, P. (1992). Sense of belonging: a vital mental concept. *Archives of Psychiatric Nursing, 6*(3), 172–177.

Hagerty, B., & Patusky, K. (1995). Developing a measure of sense of belonging. *Nursing Research, 44*(1), 9–13.

Hahn, H. (1988). The politics of physical differences: disability and discrimination. In M. Nagler (Ed.), *Perspectives on disability.* 2nd edition. (pp. 37–42). Palo Alto, CA: Health Markets Research.

Hill, D.L. (2006). Sense of belonging as connectedness, American Indian worldview and mental health. *Archives of Psychiatric Nursing, 20*(5), 210–216.

Hull, R. (1998). Defining disability: A philosophical approach. *Res Publica, 4*(2), 199–210.

Janoff-Bulman, R. (1992). *Shattered assumptions: Towards a new psychology of trauma.* New York: Free Press.

Kallianes, V. & Rubenfeld, P. (1997). Disability, women and reproductive rights. *Disability and Society, 12*(2), 203–222.

Kralik, D., Visentin, K. & Van Loon, A. (2006). Transition: A literature review. *Journal of Advanced Nursing, 55*(3), 320–329.

Lawler, D. (2013). Reconstructing myself: The transition to motherhood for women with a disability. PhD, Trinity College Dublin, Dublin.

Lawler, D., Begley, C. & Lalor, J. (2015). (Re)constructing myself: The process of transition to motherhood for women with a disability. *Journal of Advanced Nursing, 71*(7), 1672–1683.

Lazarus, R. & Folkman, S. (1984). *Stress, appraisal and coping.* New York: Springer Publishing.

Lutz, B.J. & Bowers, B.J. (2003). Understanding how disability is defined and conceptualised in the literature. *Rehabilitation Nursing, 28*(3), 74–78.

McClimens, A. (2005). From vagabonds to Victorian values: A social construction of a disability identity. In G. Grant, P. Goward, D. Richardson & P. Ramcharan (Eds.), *A life cycle approach to valuing people* (pp. 28–46). Maidenhead: Open University Press.

McKay-Moffat, S. & Cunningham, C. (2006). Services for women with disabilities: Mothers' and midwives' experiences. *British Journal of Midwifery, 14*(8), 472–477.

McKeever, P., Angus, J., Lee-Miller, K. & Reid, D. (2003). It's more of a production: Accomplishing mothering using a mobility device. *Disability and Society, 18*(2), 179–197.

McMillan Boyles, C., Bailey, P.H. & Mossey, S. (2008). Representation of disability in nursing and healthcare literature: An integrative review. *Journal of Advanced Nursing, 62*(4), 428–437.

Malacrida, C. (2009). Pereforming motherhood in a disablist world: Dilemmas of motherhood, feminity and disability. *International Journal of Qualitative Studies in Education, 22*(1), 99–117.

Maslow, A. (1954) *Motivation and personality*. New York: Harper.

Myers, J.K. (1965). Consequences and prognoses of disability. In M.B. Sussman (Ed.), *Sociology and rehabilitation* (pp. 35–53). Washington DC: American Sociological Association.

Oakley, A. (1980). *Women confined: Towards a sociology of childbirth*. Oxford: Martin Robertson.

Oliver, M. (1990). *The politics of disablement: A sociological approach*. Basingstoke: Palgrave Macmillan.

Peterson, C., Maier, S.F. & Seligman, M.E.P. (1995). *Learned helplessness: A theory for the age of personal control*. New York: Oxford University Press.

Pratt, D.D. (1998). *Five perspectives on teaching in adult and higher education*. Malabar, FL: Krieger Publishing.

Prilleltensky, O. (2003). A ramp to motherhood: The experience of mothers with physical disabilities. *Sexuality and Disability, 12*(1), 21–47.

Raman, S. & Levi, S.J. (2002). Concepts of disablement in documents guiding physical therapy. *Disability and Rehabilitation, 24*(15), 790–797.

Redwood, T. (2007). Becoming a mother: A phenomological exploration of transition to motherhood, its impact and implications for the professional lives of nurses, midwives and health visitors. Unpublished Doctoral dissertation, University of East Anglia.

Roy, A., Roy, A. & Roy, M. (2012). The human rights of women with intellectual disability. *Journal of the Royal Society of Medicine, 105*(9), 384–389.

Safilios-Rothschild, C. (1990). *The sociology and social psychology of disability and rehabilitation*. New York: Random House.

Sargent, J., Williams, R., Hagerty, B., Lynch-Sauer, J. & Hoyle, K. (2002). Sense of belonging as a buffer against depressive symptoms. *Journal of American Psychiatric Nurses Association, 8*(4), 120–129.

Sawyer, L.M. (1999). Engaged mothering: The transition to motherhood for a group of African American women. *Journal of Transcultural Nursing, 10*, 14–21.

Scotch, R.K. & Schriner, K. (1997). Disability as human variation: implications for policy. *The Annals of the American Academy of Political and Social Science, 549*(1), 148–159.

Sedikides, C. & Brewer, M.B. (2001). Individual self, relational self, and collective self: Partners, opponents or strangers? In C. Sedikides & M.B. Brewer (Eds.), *Individual self, relational self, collective self* (pp. 1–3). Philadelphia, PA: Psychology Press.

Shamai, M. & Kochal, R.B. (2008). Motherhood starts in prison: The experience of motherhood among women in prison. *Family Process, 47*(3), 323–340.

Sheerin, F., Keenan, P. & Lawler, D. (2014). Mothers with intellectual disabilities: Interactions with children and family services in Ireland. *British Journal of Learning Disabilities, 41*, 189–196.

Smeltzer, S., Sharts-Hopko, N.C., Ott, B.B., Zimmerman, V. & Duffin, J. (2007). Perspectives of women with disabilities on reaching those who are hard of hearing. *The Journal of Neuroscience Nursing: The Journal of the American Association of Neuroscience Nurses, 39*(3), 163–171.

Spidsberg, B.D. (2007). Vulnerable and strong – lesbian women encountering maternity care. *Journal of Advanced Nursing, 60*(5), 478–486.

Stroebe, M.S. & Schut, H. (2010). Meaning making in the dual process model of coping with bereavement. In R.A. Neimeyer (Ed.), *Meaning reconstruction and the experience of Loss.* 4th edition (pp. 55–73). Washington, DC: American Psychological Association.

Thomson, R., Kehily, M.J., Hadfield, L. & Sharpe, S. (2011). *Making modern mothers.* Bristol: Policy Press.

Tighe, C. (2001). Working at disability: A qualitative study of the meaning of health and disability for women with physical impairments. *Disability and Society, 16*(4), 511–529.

Walsh-Gallagher, D., Sinclair, M. & McConkey, R. (2012). The ambiguity of disabled women's experiences of pregnancy, childbirth and motherhood: A phenomenological understanding. *Midwifery, 28*(2), 156–162.

Wilton, T. & Kaufmann, T. (2001). Lesbian mothers' experiences of maternity care in the UK. *Midwifery, 17*, 203–211.

7

DOMESTIC AND FAMILY VIOLENCE

Angela Taft and Leesa Hooker

Introduction

Pregnancy and early family formation is a profound and life-changing event for a woman and her intimate partner. Frequently it encompasses her family and community as well. It can be bound by and celebrated with cultural practices. It is a time when a woman can expect those around to care for and nurture her and the coming child. It therefore comes as a shock to everyone, including health care professionals, that those closest to her, her intimate partner and perhaps the extended family can inflict harm and cause intentional injury to her and/or the developing fetus.

Domestic and family violence (DFV) is a globally prevalent 'wicked' public health problem, causing profound harm to women and their families, especially during the reproductive period (World Health Organisation [WHO], 2013a). Women experiencing violence and abuse can have more unplanned and unwanted pregnancies; induced abortions; adverse pregnancy outcomes; and more children and at a younger age than women who are not abused (Taft, Watson & Lee, 2004). They are also more likely to experience postnatal depression and have early parenting difficulties (Hooker, Kaspiew & Taft, 2016a; Howard, Oram, Galley, Trevillion & Feder, 2013). Health care professionals who see women in the perinatal period are in a unique position to identify and support those experiencing DFV early and if women are ready – to help them gain access to needed services. While professionals can and should play a vital role in preventing and reducing this problem, solutions to DFV are complex and multi-level, and involve collaborations among governments and service providers across society to deal with the underlying causes.

This chapter discusses how health care professionals can understand the violence that women in the perinatal period may experience, and what is current best practice to support them. It reviews the prevalence and health impact of DFV in the perinatal period and describes women's experience and stages of women's pathways to safety. It also provides evidence to date for what health care professionals should look for, how to respond effectively and when, where and to what interventions to refer to if they are available. In this chapter DFV will refer to any incident or pattern of incidents of controlling, coercive threatening behaviour, violence or abuse between those aged 16 or over who are, or have been, intimate partners or family members regardless of gender or sexuality. It includes intimate partner violence and child abuse.

Prevalence and incidence of intimate partner violence

In 2013, the WHO published global estimates of the prevalence of intimate partner (physical and sexual) violence and its impact on women, including their reproductive health (WHO, 2013a). These ranged from the lowest prevalence of one in every five or six ever-partnered women (16.3 per cent) experiencing violence in their lifetime in the East Asia region, to one in every two women suffering violence in Central Sub-Saharan Africa. High-income regions like Western Europe (19.3 per cent) and North America (21.3 per cent) had rates similar to East Asia.

Women can be vulnerable not only to physical, sexual or psychological abuse, but also to being killed. Globally, 38 per cent of all murders of women are committed by intimate partners (WHO, 2013a). A recent systematic review found that the femicide rates are highest in high-income countries (Stöckl *et al.*, 2013).

Domestic and family violence and pregnancy

While pregnancy is a risk factor for the commencement of violence, women who are abused during pregnancy have most commonly been abused beforehand (Bloom, Bullock, Sharps, Laughon & Parker, 2011). In the 2012 population survey of Personal Safety by the Australian Bureau of Statistics, an estimated 186,000 women had experienced violence by a current cohabiting partner. Of those who had been pregnant, one in five (21.7 per cent) reported that violence occurred during the pregnancy and for almost two thirds of women (61.4 per cent) this had been their first experience of violence in their relationship (Australian Bureau of Statistics, 2013).

A recent multi-country study estimated the prevalence of violence during pregnancy to be between four and eight per cent of pregnant women (Devries *et al.*, 2010). A 2012 Canadian population survey (n=6421) studied the prevalence and timing of violence in pregnancy. They found that any abuse in the two years before the interviews was 10.9 per cent (6 per cent before pregnancy only, 1.4 per cent during pregnancy only, 1 per cent postpartum only, and 2.5 per cent in any combination of these times). The prevalence of any abuse was higher among low-income (21.2 per cent), single (35.3 per cent), and (Canadian) Aboriginal mothers (30.6 per cent). In 52 per cent of the cases, abuse was perpetrated by an intimate partner (Berry, Harrison & Ryan, 2009; Daoud, Smylie, Urquia, Allan & O'Campo,

2012). Women can experience many forms of violence during pregnancy, some of which are reflected within the following quotes:

> I was upset really because ... I was pregnant and I went to work for a deposit on a home. That's what we agreed on and he came home and he bought a very expensive motorbike.

> [He] grabbed the chair and smashed it right next to the baby and he did that on purpose to scare me and it hit the baby.

> You're not going to the hospital. You can leave the bloody kid there, I don't want it in my house, I don't want to ever see it again and you can take [him] and throw him out somewhere too. I want some attention for myself.
>
> (Head & Taft, 1995, pp. 30–31)

What are the factors influencing DFV?

DFV is complex and the factors influencing why it occurs can be present at several levels. The ecological model (Figure 7.1) is a useful framework to use when considering the many interrelating factors that influence the perpetration and victimisation of DFV. Factors at any level can intersect to make a woman more susceptible or resilient to DFV, and her partner or family members more or less likely to abuse her (WHO, 2010). No one factor alone is responsible for women's vulnerability to DFV but her gender, race and class, for example, may intersect to render her more or less vulnerable and more or less able to stay safe.

Some of the key factors that can contribute to DFV are discussed as follows.

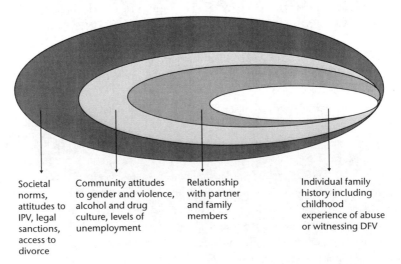

Societal norms, attitudes to IPV, legal sanctions, access to divorce

Community attitudes to gender and violence, alcohol and drug culture, levels of unemployment

Relationship with partner and family members

Individual family history including childhood experience of abuse or witnessing DFV

FIGURE 7.1 Ecological model of impact factors on domestic and family violence
Adapted from Heise, 1998.

Gender inequality

DFV is *gender-based*, and while DFV can be found among men and boys, it is far more prevalent in almost all forms (e.g. physical, sexual, psychological, financial) among women and girls because of gender inequality. It can commence as female feticide, continue as childhood sexual abuse of girls and then intimate partner and sexual violence against women (Flitcraft, 1995). Childhood abuse, including childhood sexual abuse or witnessing family violence is strongly associated with DFV and is a predisposing factor for victimisation in adulthood (WHO, 2013a). Because women are responsible for bearing children, the impact of violence and trauma during pregnancy and thereafter can result in profound and detrimental effects on her own and her children's mental and physical health; on her parenting capacity and through this to her children's healthy development (Hooker *et al.*, 2016a).

Socio-economic factors

While DFV globally is found across all classes and communities, it is disproportionately found among families where there is disadvantage (Abramsky *et al.*, 2011). This can include low levels of education among women or men, unemployment among male partners, among women with disabilities and those on forms of welfare or benefits (Krnjacki, Emerson, Llewellyn & Kavanagh, 2016; Woolhouse, Gartland, Hegarty, Donath & Brown, 2011).

Alcohol

Alcohol misuse by a male partner is strongly associated with DFV and increases the levels of injury severity, but this can be worse if both partners are drinking (Abramsky *et al.*, 2011; Graham, 2011). High rates of DFV are found among Indigenous communities in many high-income countries, which intersects with multiple forms of disadvantage and dispossession, resulting in high levels of trauma (Berry *et al.*, 2009; Daoud, Smylie, Urquia, Allan & O'Campo, 2013; Valpied & Hegarty, 2015).

Migrant and refugee women

Migrant and refugee women may be more likely than others to experience DFV (Stockman, 2015). In some countries, generally those where women's human and reproductive rights are abused, gender-based violence is common – for example, those with dowry traditions, under-age marriage and considerable gender inequality (Morash, Bui, Zhang & Holtfreter, 2007). There is some evidence that diaspora (migrant) communities bring with them the same rates of DFV as those found in countries of origin, but that victims are doubly disadvantaged as they are often unaware of their rights, of the laws and resources to help them and are isolated by both their abuse, and by migrant status and cultural distance (Raj, Silverman,

McCleary-Sills & Liu, 2005; Taft, Small & Hoang, 2008) (also refer to Chapter 3 for further insights faced by asylum seeking and refugee women).

Health and other impacts of DFV on parents, infants and communities

The WHO reviewed the evidence for and summarised the pathways through which intimate partner violence can affect a woman's health (refer to Figure 7.2). These symptoms should inform a health professional's index of suspicion to ask a woman about DFV.

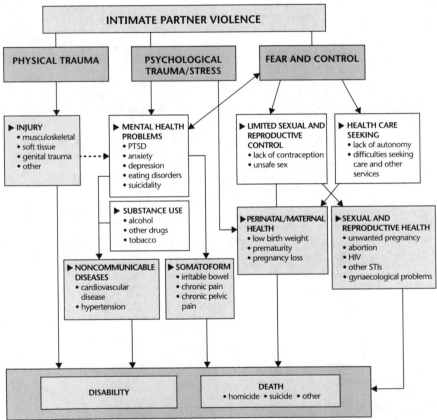

There are multiple pathways through which intimate partner violence can lead to adverse health outcomes. This figure highlights three key mechanisms and pathways that can explain many of these outcomes. Mental health problems and substance use might result directly from any of the three mechanisms, which might, in turn, increase health risks. However, mental health problems and substance use are not necessarily a precondition for subsequent health effects, and will not always lie in the pathway to adverse health.

FIGURE 7.2 Pathways and health effects on intimate partner violence

World Health Organisation, 2013a – reprinted with permission.

What is clear from this diagram is that major health damage results from violence and abuse. This can include the cumulative effects of stress and trauma, depending on the length of time a woman experiences fear and controlling behaviours.

Impact on women's mental health

The experience of abuse, fear and stress can result in high levels of anxiety, depression and post-traumatic stress (Woolhouse et al., 2011) that can be even worse four years after the birth (Woolhouse, Gartland, Mensah & Brown, 2014). A meta-analysis found that women experiencing partner violence during pregnancy have a threefold likelihood of experiencing postnatal depression and a greater prevalence of anxiety and post-traumatic stress disorder symptoms in the ante- and the postnatal period (Howard et al., 2013). Women experiencing violence are also more likely to have suicidal ideation and commit suicide (Devries et al., 2011).

Reproductive health

Women experiencing partner violence may also be subject to sexual abuse. This may mean they are not able to influence when or what kind of sex they have, whether contraception is used and how frequently to space any children. This can result in more frequent sexually transmitted infections, rates of HIV/AIDS in low and middle-income countries, and the high prevalence of unwanted pregnancies and induced abortions (WHO, 2013a).

Self-medication to deal with stress can result in women experiencing violence being more likely to smoke, drink alcohol or use other drugs (also refer to Chapter 8 for further insights into substance misuse in a perinatal population). Substance use, smoking and eating disorders, in addition to stress and cortisol levels, may explain the higher rates of low birthweight, growth restricted babies and other adverse birthing outcomes, including stillbirth found among women experiencing violence (WHO, 2013a).

The impact of abuse on parenting and infants

Hooker et al. (2016a, p. 14) highlight how:

> The traditional stereotype of the 'ideal mother' and the reality of motherhood is often very different, especially for women who are abused. These ideals have found abused women frequently being blamed for not parenting well, being labelled 'bad mothers' who fail to protect and care for their children.

Unsurprisingly, a recent Australian study found that women who have experienced DFV have a worse experience of motherhood than women who have not experienced violence (Hooker, Samaraweera, Agius & Taft, 2016b). Effective parenting requires warm loving relationships and a secure attachment with the primary caregiver (most often the mother). This is ideal for the healthy development of children, but DFV can be disruptive to the development of these bonds and damage attachment at this vulnerable time. Personality and brain growth critical to their later abilities is developing in an infant's first three years and is disrupted in environments of fear and chronic anxiety, such as those in a violent family environment.

Evidence points to the mostly negative impact of abuse on women's and men's ability to parent and the largely detrimental effect that DFV has on children (Hooker et al., 2016a). DFV can result in more parenting stress and more aggressive childrearing behaviours by the mother to monitor children's behaviour when the abuser is present. This can involve mothers using punitive parenting methods to control children in order to keep them safe. Impaired emotions and hypervigilance and inconsistent and distant parenting often result. Women's difficulty in regulating their own behaviour in response to abuse can prevent appropriate responses and interactions with infants and children.

Children exposed to violence are at greater risk of behavioural, physical and mental health problems. Mood and anxiety disorders, Attention Deficit Hyperactivity Disorder (ADHD) and oppositional/defiant or conduct problems were all identified from several meta-analyses (Kitzmann, Gaylord, Holt & Kenny, 2003; Sternberg, Baradaran, Abbott, Lamb & Guterman, 2006; Wolfe, Crooks, Lee, McIntyre-Smith & Jaffe, 2003). Male children display more externalising and females more internalising problems. Witnessing violence is as damaging as being directly physically abused.

In a longitudinal study of mothers and children beginning in pregnancy, Bogat et al. (2011) found that mothers with emotionally supportive networks experienced less detrimental effects from DFV. They also found that mothers who were able to leave abusive partners were more likely to have greater attachment to their infants by four years than those still in the relationships. They concluded that this period is an ideal time to intervene to help the mother find safety and target therapeutic work to the mother–child bond (Bogat et al., 2011; Hooker et al., 2016a).

DFV also has economic implications for women in terms of loss of earnings due to ill-health (physical and psychological) and healthcare costs. The many forms of injury and somatoform illnesses, and together with the above health and parenting consequences results in the increased prevalence of women experiencing abuse attending all forms of health care services (Hegarty, Gunn, Chondros & Taft, 2008; Larkins et al., 2015).

Women's experience of DFV, their journeys to safety and what they hope for from health care professionals and system

Women's 'stages of change' refers to transitions in the woman's process of making changes in her life in relation to DFV. The concept is based on the Transtheoretical Model of Change or Stages of Change model (Prochaska & Velicer, 1997), and when adapted to DFV includes five stages: pre-contemplation (no awareness of abuse); contemplation (acknowledging the problem), preparation (planning for safety and/or leaving the relationship), action (implementing plans), maintenance (maintaining the new action) (Reisenhofer & Taft, 2013).

One of the ways in which these stages can be explored and understood is following disclosures to trusted professionals. However, whether women do or do not disclose can also depend on the skills and attitudes of the professional. For the woman, disclosure can commence a long and difficult journey. Many women experience difficulties even after leaving their partner, but eventually reach safety and improved well-being. Support from a health care professional can make a profound difference to her levels of confidence and self-esteem and knowledge of the range of help available in her community (Feder, Hutson, Ramsey & Taket, 2006) and because women in the perinatal period are more frequently permitted to see professionals, this is an ideal opportunity and a repeated one, to reach out to her early and offer her support. This issue is reflected in the following quote:

> I'd never specifically went [to the GP] myself, it was only when I was allowed to go to the doctors when I was pregnant.
>
> (Hegarty & Taft, 2001, p. 435)

Feder *et al.* (2006) undertook a meta-analysis of qualitative studies of over 800 women's experiences with health care professionals. They found that generally women hoped for consistent approaches: non-judgemental, nondirective, and individually tailored, with an appreciation of the complexity of partner violence. Women at later stages of an abusive relationship expressed the hope that professionals would repeatedly ask about partner violence (Feder *et al.*, 2006).

The professional's role

For professionals to become 'effective agents' in ending the cycle of violence in women's lives, they must accept two premises. The first premise is that DFV is a serious public health issue, rather than a private problem, which falls within the purview of health professional care. The second premise is that no woman, under any circumstances, deserves to be physically, sexually or emotionally abused. Professionals must take care to maintain empathy and support for women, refrain from judgement and remember that escaping from violence is a process not an event (Bloom *et al.*, 2011, p. 168). Professionals should never therefore prescribe that women leave an abuser, but support them. When the woman judges she is sufficiently resourced, safe and confident enough to leave, she will herself know best when she can do so. However, professionals need regular ongoing training and support by their organisation to feel confident to overcome their own barriers and offer women the support appropriate to their needs and readiness to act (O'Doherty, Taft, Hegarty, Ramsay, Davidson & Feder, 2014).

Bloom *et al.* (2011) advise that statements by a professional to the abuse survivor that she is a worthwhile person and does not deserve to be hurt, can be extremely empowering to a woman in a vulnerable position. They remind us that she has often been told by her abuser that no one will believe her and that she deserves the abuse and she may have come to believe this herself (Bloom *et al.*, 2011, p. 168). An overview of best practice recommendations in providing care to women experiencing DFV (WHO, 2013b) are provided in Box 7.1.

BOX 7.1. WHO BEST PRACTICE RECOMMENDATIONS RELEVANT TO THE PERINATAL PERIOD (ADAPTED FROM WHO, 2013B)

Women-centred care

- Non-judgemental, supportive and validating
- Careful listening, in private
- Confidentiality, within legal limits
- Practical care and support
- Information on helpful resources
- Safety assessment of the woman and her children

Identification and care

- Use of policy and organisational guidelines
- Regular training about how to ask and respond
- Routine asking of all pregnant women
- Case finding approach for all others
- Written information on DVF provided in private areas
- Supportive psychological/advocacy/empowerment interventions
- Mother–child interventions

Screening and assessment

There is a current debate about the best way to identify women in health care and other settings in universal and in targeted settings (Taket, Wathen & MacMillan, 2004; Wathen, MacGregor, Sibbald & MacMillan, 2013). A recent Cochrane systematic review found no high quality evidence for universal screening (asking all women in every setting) over case finding (looking for women symptomatic of DFV) (O'Doherty *et al.*, 2014). However, both Cochrane and the WHO considered pregnancy a significantly vulnerable period and recommended screening (asking all presenting women, irrespective of symptoms whether they are experiencing DFV) in antenatal settings (O'Doherty *et al.*, 2014; WHO, 2013b). In Australia, national clinical practice guidelines require midwives to explain to all women at the first antenatal visit that asking about domestic violence is a routine part of antenatal care (Australian Health Minister's Advisory Council, 2012). UK guidance suggests trained staff in antenatal, postnatal and other high risk areas (mental health, sexual and reproductive health services) ask all women about DFV exposure, and not just when indicators of abuse are present (National Institute for Health and Care Excellence, 2014).

Screening is not an end in itself, but the first stage of a system-wide health care response. Some organisations have not put sufficient resources aside other than for screening – into training, collaboration, and policy and programme responsibility to support staff who have been mandated to screen. Fully implementing a context for routine enquiry and responsive integrated care for women experiencing DFV needs to be embedded into everyday practice rather than as a separate activity (Humphreys & Campbell, 2011) (also refer to Chapter 14 for insights into integrated service models of care).

How professionals can ask about DFV

There is evidence that women may prefer to be screened indirectly – that is by self-completing either a computer or paper-based screen rather than direct questioning, so that she can decide whether she is ready to disclose today and whether or not to this professional (Hooker, Small & Taft, 2016c; MacMillan et al., 2006). Taft et al., (2015) found use of a self-completion Maternal Health and Well-being Checklist increased screening and disclosure rates threefold in a postpartum trial among mothers attending community-based maternal and child nurse clinics (Hooker et al., 2016c). The Abuse Assessment Screen (McFarlane & Parker, 1994) was designed to be used during pregnancy, but there are useful reviews of screening tools that professionals may consult if deciding what is appropriate for your setting and which is the most rigorous tool (Basile, Hertz & Back, 2007; Feder et al., 2009). The Danger Assessment Scale (Campbell, 2000) is a useful tool to assess women's level of risk of danger.

It is important for professionals to be mindful of their own and woman's barriers to asking and disclosure. Particularly in the perinatal period, the presence of children can be motivation for women to either remain or leave an abusive relationship. In this situation, it can be useful for you to outline the harm that DFV can do to infants and children. Asking women about abuse must always be done in a safe and confidential setting. During the perinatal period, it can be difficult for you to talk to women if their partners or other family members are there. Many midwives or nurse-midwives providing antenatal care use urine testing or other innovative strategies to see the woman alone if they have suspicions that she may be abused (Valpied & Hegarty, 2015).

If a woman discloses to you, you should make a careful assessment of their goals and the 'stage of change' a woman has reached (Reisenhofer & Taft, 2013). Professionals can use the stages of change to provide a means of assessing women's movement toward their own self-identified goals. You will need an understanding of what may affect her decision-making in order to support women in their often stop-start movements in her journey to safety. Bloom et al. (2011) outlined how women in early stages of a relationship struggle to make sense of the mixed messages from the abuser, work on making a loving relationship, overlook the warning signals and shoulder the blame. Later phases can be described as enduring, disengaging and recovering (Bloom *et al.*, 2011, p. 158).

Empowerment – strengthening a woman's sense of self-worth and self-efficacy – is critical in enabling a woman to reach safety for herself and her children. Professionals can support women to identify and implement their personal goals and enhance their self-efficacy to move positively across the change stages. Reisenhofer and Taft (2013) identified three primary objectives that women in differing stages may wish to achieve. These are: 1) minimising harm and promoting well-being within an abusive relationship, 2) achieving safety and well-being within the relationship by halting the abuse, or 3) achieving safety by ending/leaving intimate relationships (Reisenhofer & Taft, 2013).

Interventions to help women in the perinatal period and after

There is only now a developing body of strong evidence about what can help women in any circumstance or what can help specifically in pregnancy. Increasingly nurse home visiting schemes and mentor mothers offer promise for increasing early intervention and social support in the postpartum period (Jack, Jamieson, Wathen & MacMillan, 2008; Taft, Small, Hegarty, Watson & Lumley, 2011). Much more research needs to be done into what can help women suffering different forms of abuse, at differing stages of change and what are the most effective therapeutic interventions to help heal the mother–child dyad after abuse. At present there is a strong emphasis on the benefit of trauma-informed care (Bloom *et al.*, 2011; Reeves, 2015).

While DFV can have a detrimental effect on women's ability to parent, it is possible for mothers to have some resilience to the effects of abuse if they have adequate social support, fewer mental health issues and they have children with an easy temperament. Professionals should seek to build support networks around women if possible and refer women and their children to therapeutic services.

Intensive advocacy/empowerment based interventions may improve short-term quality of life and reduce physical abuse one to two years after the intervention for women from domestic violence shelters or refuges. Brief advocacy (such as counselling and DFV support sessions) may also provide small short-term mental health benefits and reduce abuse, particularly in pregnant women and for less severe abuse (Rivas *et al.*, 2015). In antenatal settings, brief advocacy in a Chinese antenatal clinic (Tiwari *et al.*, 2010) was effective in reducing depression. A multi-strategy psycho-behavioural trial to reduce DFV, smoking and substance use among pregnant low-income black women in a US setting was effective in reducing abuse (Kiely, el-Mohandes, el-Khorazaty & Gantz, 2010).

Hooker *et al.* (2016a) reviewed the effects of DFV on parenting, what may help mothers and children recover after abuse, and what might reduce the post-traumatic stress and renew mother-child attachment. Most effective therapies were combined or dyadic psychotherapeutic interventions based on attachment and trauma theory. While there was little evidence with studies that included control groups, Hooker *et al.* (2016a) described promising (intensive home visiting) studies undertaken in the Australian Aboriginal and Torres Strait Islander community (also refer to Chapter 4). Increasingly behaviour change groups for men who use violence are attempting to combine strategies for DFV reduction, mental illness and substance abuse and parenting. However, there was very little evidence for what works to support enhanced parenting by abusive men (Hooker *et al.*, 2016a).

Conclusion

Women pregnant, giving birth and raising an infant deserve a supportive and loving environment. DFV in the perinatal period violates this promise and is a complex, prevalent problem globally. It is more prevalent and dangerous for women in the perinatal period and a critical time for early intervention and support by professionals. Because the factors impacting on DFV exist at society, community, family and individual level, professionals need a supportive context in which to respond. They require knowledge of legislative support, policing and effective services to which to refer women, regular training and up-to-date resources and to work in partnership with services at a community level. They need the support of the system that surrounds them and from their managers from the top down.

Training needs to inform and upskill professionals to understand the complex context for DFV, about the intersection and levels of factors affecting women's vulnerability to DFV and the process and pathways through which women need to travel before they feel safe to make permanent and beneficial change. Assessing the context of a woman's abuse will help professionals to empower women to set their own goals, at their own pace in order to form a therapeutic alliance helping women to action for beneficial changes and eventually safety, well-being and strength.

References

Abramsky, T., Watts, C.H., Garcia-Moreno, C., Devries, K., Kiss, L., Ellsberg, M., Jansen, H. & Heise, L. (2011). What factors are associated with recent intimate partner violence? Findings from the WHO multi-country study on women's health and domestic violence. *BMC Public Health*, *11*(109). doi:10.1186/1471-2458-11-109.

Australian Bureau of Statistics. (2013). *Personal safety survey, Australia*. Australian Bureau of Statistics. Canberra. Available from: www.abs.gov.au/ausstats/abs@.nsf/mf/4906.0 [Accessed 17 January, 2016].

Australian Health Minister's Advisory Council. (2012). *Clinical practice guidelines: Antenatal care-module 1*. Australian Government Department of Ageing, Canberra. Available from: www.health.gov.au/internet/main/publishing.nsf/content/015FBFDD266795DBCA2 57BF0001A0547/$File/ANC_Guidelines_Mod1_v32.pdf [Accessed 18 November 2015].

Basile, K.C., Hertz, M.F. & Back, S.E. (2007). *Partner violence and sexual violence victimisation assessment instruments for use in healthcare settings: Version 1.* Atlanta, GA: Centers for Disease Control and Prevention, National Center for Injury Prevention and Control.

Berry, J.G., Harrison, J.E. & Ryan, P. (2009). Hospital admissions of indigenous and non-indigenous Australians due to interpersonal violence. *Australian and New Zealand Journal of Public Health, 33*(3), 215–222.

Bloom, T., Bullock, L., Sharps, P., Laughon, K. & Parker, B.J. (2011). Intimate partner violence during pregnancy. In J. Humphreys & J. Campbell (Eds.), *Family violence and nursing practice* (pp. 155–179). New York: Springer Publishing Company.

Bogat, G.A., Levendosky, A.A., von Eye, A. & Davidson II, W.S., (2011). Effects of intimate partner violence on the attachment relationship between mother and child: Data from a longitudinal study beginning during pregnancy. In S.A. Graham-Bermann & A. Levendosky (Eds.), *How intimate partner violence affects children: Developmental research, case studies and evidence-based intervention* (pp. 19–46). Washington DC: American Psychological Association.

Campbell, J.C., Sharps, P. & Glass, N. (2000). Risk assessment for intimate partner homicide. In G.F. Pinard & L. Pagani (Eds.), *Clinical assessment of dangerousness: Empirical contributions* (pp. 136–157). New York: Cambridge University Press.

Daoud, N., Smylie, J., Urquia, M., Allan, B. & O'Campo, P. (2013). The contribution of socio-economic position to the excesses of violence and intimate partner violence among Aboriginal versus non-Aboriginal women in Canada. *Canadian Journal of Public Health, 104*(4), e278–283.

Daoud, N., Urquia, M., O'Campo, P., Heaman, M., Janssen, P.A., Smylie, J. & Theissen, K. (2012). Prevalence of abuse and violence before, during and after pregnancy in a national sample of Canadian women. *American Journal of Public Health, 102*(10), 1893–1901.

Devries, K.M., Kishor, S., Johnson, H., Stöckl, H., Bacchus, L.J., Garcia-Moreno, C. & Watts, C. (2010). Intimate partner violence during pregnancy: Analysis of prevalence data from 19 countries. *Reproductive Health Matters, 18*(36), 158–170.

Devries, K., Watts, C., Yoshihama, M., Kiss, L., Schraiber, L.B., Deyessa, N., Heise, L., Durand, J., Mbwambo, J., Jansen, H., Berhane, Y., Ellsberg, M., Garcia-Moreno, C. & WHO Multi-Country Study Team. (2011). Violence against women is strongly associated with suicide attempts: evidence from the WHO multi-country study on women's health and domestic violence against women. *Social Science & Medicine, 73*(1), 79–86.

Feder, G., Hutson, M., Ramsey, J. & Taket, A.R. (2006). Women exposed to intimate partner violence: Expectations and experiences when they encounter health care professionals: A meta-analysis of qualitative studies. *Archives of Internal Medicine, 166*(1), 22–37.

Feder, G., Ramsay, J., Dunne, D., Rose, M., Arsene, C., Norman, R., Kuntze, S., Spencer, A., Bacchus, L., Hague, G., Warburton, A. & Taket, A. (2009). How far does screening women for domestic (partner) violence in different health-care settings meet criteria for a screening programme? Systematic reviews of nine UK National Screening Committee critieria. *Health Technology Assessment, 13*(16), 1–113. doi:10.3310/hta13160.

Flitcraft, A. (1995). From public health to personal health: Violence against women across the life span. *Annals of Internal Medicine, 123*(10), 800–802.

Graham, K., Bernards, S., Wilsnack, S.C. & Gmel, G. (2011). Alcohol may not cause partner violence but it seems to make it worse: A cross national comparison of the relationship between alcohol and severity of partner violence. *Journal of Interpersonal Violence, 26*(8), 1503–1523.

Head, C. & Taft, A. (1995). *Improving general practitioner management of women experiencing domestic violence: A study of the beliefs and experiences of women victim/survivors and of GPs.* Canberra: General Practitioner Evaluation Program, GP Branch, Commonwealth Department of Health, Housing and Community Services.

Hegarty, K., Gunn, J., Chondros, P. & Taft, A. (2008). Physical and social predictors of partner abuse in women attending general practice. *British Journal of General Practice, 58,* 484–487.

Hegarty, K.L. & Taft, A.J. (2001). Overcoming the barriers to disclosure and inquiry of partner abuse for women attending general practice. *Australian & New Zealand Journal of Public Health, 25*(5), 433–437.

Heise, L. (1998). Violence against women: An integrated ecological model. *Violence Against Women,* 4(262), 262–290.

Hooker, L., Kaspiew, R. & Taft, A. (2016a). Domestic and family violence and parenting: Mixed methods insights into impact and support needs. *ANROWS Landscapes series* (01/16). Sydney: Australia's National Research Organisation for Women's Safety.

Hooker, L., Samaraweera, N., Agius, P., & Taft, A. (2016b). Intimate partner violence and the experience of motherhood: A cross-sectional analysis of factors associated with a poor experience of motherhood. *Midwifery, 34,* 88–94.

Hooker, L., Small, R. & Taft, A.J. (2016c). Understanding sustained domestic violence identification in maternal and child health nurse care: Process evaluation from a two year follow-up of the MOVE trial. *Journal of Advanced Nursing, 72*(3), 534–544.

Howard, L., Oram, S., Galley, H., Trevillion, K. & Feder, G. (2013). Domestic violence and perinatal mental disorders: A systematic review and meta-analysis. *PLoS Med, 10*(5), e1001452. doi:10.1371/journal.pmed.1001452.

Humphreys J, & Campbell J. (Ed.). (2011). *Family violence and nursing practice.* 2nd edn. New York: Springer Publishing.

Jack, S.M., Jamieson, E., Wathen, C.N. & MacMillan, H.L. (2008). The feasibility of screening for intimate partner violence during postpartum home visits. *Canadian Journal of Nursing Research, 40*(2), 150–170.

Kiely, M., el-Mohandes, A., el-Khorazaty, M.N. & Gantz, M.G. (2010). An integrated intervention to reduce intimate partner violence in pregnancy: A randomised controlled trial. *Obstetrics and Gynaecology, 115*(2), 273–283.

Kitzmann, K.M., Gaylord, N.K., Holt, A.R. & Kenny, E.D. (2003). Child witnesses to domestic violence: A meta-analytic review. *Journal of Consulting and Clinical Psychology,* 71(2), 339. doi:10.1037/0022-006X.71.2.339.

Krnjacki, L., Emerson, E., Llewellyn, G. & Kavanagh, A. (2016). Prevalence and risk of violence against people with disabilities: Findings from an Australian population-based study. *Australian and New Zealand Journal or Public Health, 40*(1), 16–21.

Larkins, C., Drinkwater, J., Hester, M., Stanley, N., Szilassy, E. & Feder, G. (2015). General practice clinicians' perspectives on involving and supporting children and adult perpetrators in families experiencing domestic violence and abuse. *Family Practitioner, 32*(6), 701–705.

McFarlane, J. & Parker, B. (1994). *Abuse during pregnancy: A protocol for prevention and intervention.* New York: National March of Dimes Birth Defects Foundation.

MacMillan, H.L., Wathen, C.N., Jamieson, E., Boyle, M., McNutt, L-A., Worster, A., Lent, B., Webb, M &: McMaster Violence Against Women Research Group. (2006).

Approaches to screening for intimate partner violence in health care settings: A randomized trial. *Journal of American Medicine Association, 296*(5), 530–536.

Morash, M., Bui, H.N., Zhang, Y. & Holtfreter, K. (2007). Risk factors for abusive relationships: A study of Vietnamese American immigrant women. *Violence Against Women, 13*(7), 653–675.

National Institute for Health and Care Excellence. (2014). *Domestic violence and abuse: Multi-agency working. NICE guideline (PH 50)*. London: National Institute for Health and Care Excellence.

O'Doherty, L., Taft, A., Hegarty, K., Ramsay, J., Davidson, L.L. & Feder, G. (2014). Screening women for intimate partner violence in health care settings: Abridged Cochrane systematic review and meta-analysis. *British Medical Journal, 348*. doi:10.1136/bmj.g2913.

Prochaska, J. & Velicer, W.F. (1997). The transtheoretical model of health behavior change. *American Journal of Health Promotion, 12*(1), 38–48.

Raj, A., Silverman, J.G., McCleary-Sills, J. & Liu, R. (2005). Immigration policies increase south Asian immigrant women's vulnerability to intimate partner violence. *Journal of the American Medical Women's Association, 60*(1), 26–32.

Reeves, E. (2015). A synthesis of the literature on trauma-informed care. *Issues in Mental Health Nursing, 36*(9), 698–709.

Reisenhofer, S. & Taft, A.J. (2013). Women's journey to safety: The transtheoretical model in clinical practice when working with women experiencing IPV: A scientific review and clinical guidance. *Patient Education and Counselling, 93*(3), 536–548.

Rivas, C., Ramsay, J., Sadowski, L., Davidson, L.L., Dunne, D., Eldridge, S., Hegarty, K., Taft, A. & Feder, G. (2015). Advocacy interventions to reduce or eliminate violence and promote the physical and psychosocial well-being of women who experience intimate partner abuse (Review). *Cochrane Database of Systematic Reviews* (12). doi:10.1002/14651858.CD005043.pub3.

Sternberg, K.J., Baradaran, L.P., Abbott, C.B., Lamb, M.E. & Guterman, E. (2006). Type of violence, age, and gender differences in the effects of family violence on children's behavior problems: A mega-analysis. *Developmental Review, 26*(1), 89–112.

Stöckl, H., Devries, K., Rotstein, A., Abrahams, N., Campbell, J., Watts, C. & Moreno, C.G. (2013). The global prevalence of intimate partner homicide: A systematic review. *Lancet, 382*(9895), 859–865.

Stockman, J.K., Hayashi, H. & Campbell, J.C. (2015). Intimate partner violence and its health impact on ethnic minority women. *Journal of Women's Health, 24*(1), 64–79.

Taft, A., Hooker, L., Humphreys, C., Hegarty, K., Walter, R., Adams, C., Agius, P. & Small, R. (2015). Maternal and child health nurse screening and care for mothers experiencing domestic violence (MOVE): A cluster randomised trial. *BMC Medicine, 13*(150). doi:10.1186/s12916-015-0375-7.

Taft, A., Small, R., Hegarty, K., Watson, L., Gold, L. & Lumley, J. (2011). Mothers' AdvocateS In the Community (MOSAIC) – non-professional support to reduce intimate partner violence and depression in mothers: A cluster randomised trial in primary care. *BMC Public Health, 11*(178). doi:10.1186/1471-2458-11-178.

Taft, A., Small, R. & Hoang, K. (2008). Intimate partner violence in Vietnam and among diaspora communities in western societies: A comprehensive review. *Journal of Family Studies, 14*(2–3), 167–182.

Taft, A.J., Watson, L. & Lee, C. (2004). Violence against young Australian women and associated reproductive events: A cross sectional analysis. *Australian and New Zealand Journal of Public Health, 28*(4), 324–329.

Taket, A., Wathen, N. & MacMillan, H. (2004). Should health professionals screen all women for domestic violence? *PLoS Medicine, 1*(1), 7–10.

Tiwari, A., Fong, D.Y.T., Yuen, K.H., Yuk, H., Pang, P., Humphreys, J. & Bullock, L. (2010). Effect of an advocacy intervention on mental health in Chinese women survivors of intimate partner violence: A randomised controlled trial. *Journal of the American Medical Association, 304*(5), 536–543.

Valpied, J. & Hegarty, K. (2015). Intimate partner abuse: Identifying, caring for and helping women in healthcare settings. Review. *Women's Health, 11*(1), 51–63.

Wathen, C.N., MacGregor, J.C.D., Sibbald, S.L. & MacMillan, H.L. (2013). Exploring the uptake and framing of research evidence on universal screening for intimate partner violence against women: A knowledge translation case study. *Health Research Policy and Systems, 11*(13). doi:10.1186/1478-4505-11-13.

Wolfe, D.A., Crooks, C.V., Lee, V., McIntyre-Smith, A. & Jaffe, P.G. (2003). The effects of children's exposure to domestic violence: A meta-analysis and critique. *Clinical Child and Family Psychology Review, 6*(3), 171–187.

Woolhouse, H., Gartland, D., Hegarty, K., Donath, S. & Brown, S.J. (2011). Depressive symptoms and intimate partner violence in the 12 months after childbirth: A prospective pregnancy cohort study. *British Journal of Obstetrics and Gynaecology, 119*(3), 315–323.

Woolhouse, H., Gartland, D., Mensah, F.K. & Brown, S.J. (2014). Maternal depression from early pregnancy to 4 years postpartum in a prospective pregnancy cohort study: Implications for primary health care. *British Journal of Obstetrics and Gynaecology, 122*(3), 312–321.

World Health Organisation. (2013a). *Global and regional estimates of violence against women: Prevalence and health effects of intimate partner violence and non-partner sexual violence.* Geneva: World Health Organisation.

World Health Organisation. (2013b). *Responding to intimate partner violence and sexual violence against women – WHO clinical and policy guidelines.* Geneva: World Health Organisation.

World Health Organisation & London School of Hygeine and Tropical Medicine. (2010). *Preventing intimate partner and sexual violence against women: Taking action and generating evidence.* Geneva: World Health Organisation.

8

MATERNAL SUBSTANCE USE IN THE PERINATAL PERIOD

Lucinda Burns, Victoria Coleman-Cowger and Courtney Breen

Introduction

The *Diagnostic and statistical manual of mental disorders* (5th Edition) is the American Psychiatric Association's (APA) official manual of mental disorders. The DSM-5 definition of a substance use disorder (SUD) is a problematic pattern of use leading to clinically significant impairment or distress as manifested by the presence of two or more symptoms such as tolerance, craving, and withdrawal (APA, 2013). The adverse effects of substance use disorders on fetal development are well known. Given this, women who use substances and are pregnant or may become pregnant are a high priority for treatment and support. However, mothers often feel a substantial amount of guilt and remorse about their substance use and fear that admission of use may lead to loss of custody of their child (Stengel, 2013; Stone, 2015). Consequently, only a small proportion of pregnant women with substance use problems disclose their use and receive treatment (Center for Behavioral Health Statistics and Quality [CBHSQ], 2013). In this chapter we examine the nature, patterns, outcomes and treatments for the most commonly used substances in pregnancy in Australia and the United States (US); tobacco, alcohol, marijuana, opioids and methamphetamine. We conclude with the implications of substance use in the perinatal period for clinical practice.

Alcohol

Prevalence

Recent Australian population data (Australian Institute of Health and Welfare, 2014) show that since 2007, alcohol consumption in pregnancy has reduced and the proportion abstaining risen, although other research suggests the proportion of pregnant women drinking at very high levels has not changed (Cameron, Davey,

Kendall, Wilson & McClure, 2013). In the US the Centers for Disease Control and Prevention (CDC) assesses alcohol use among pregnant women with the Behavioral Risk Factor Surveillance System (BRFSS) (CBHSQ, 2015). According to aggregated data from 2011 to 2013, 1 in 10 pregnant women reported any alcohol use and 1 in 33 reported binge drinking in the past 30 days.

Predictors and outcomes

A systematic review of 14 studies from a range of countries found the most consistently reported predictors of alcohol use in pregnancy were pre-pregnancy alcohol use (quantity and frequency), smoking, and maternal exposure to violence and abuse (Skagerström, Chang, & Nilsen, 2011). A number of other factors are less consistently predictive: age, unemployment, marital status and education level (O'Keeffe *et al.*, 2015; Skagerström, Chang, & Nilsen, 2011). This lack of consistency may be due to different patterns of alcohol use in subgroups, for example, older women have a longer history of drinking, but the amount consumed may be less, where younger women may be more likely to binge drink.

Alcohol is a well-known teratogen (i.e. causes birth defects). The first descriptions of prenatal alcohol effects in children of mothers with an alcohol-use disorder appeared in the late 1960s (Lemoine, Harousseau, Borteyru & Menuet, 1968) and early 1970s (Jones & Smith, 1973). Heavy maternal alcohol consumption during pregnancy is associated with birth defects, growth impairment, developmental disabilities and neurodevelopmental dysfunction (ARND Consensus Statement, 2011; Burns, Mattick & Cooke, 2006; Stratton, Howe & Battaglia, 1996). These indicators of brain dysfunction extend across a continuum that ranges from mild to severe impairment (Stratton *et al.*, 1996) and can result in ongoing disability (Streissguth, Bookstein, Barr, Sampson, O'Malley & Young, 2004). The continuum of harm is called Fetal Alcohol Spectrum Disorder with Fetal Alcohol Syndrome (FAS) the severe end of the spectrum. A diagnosis of FAS relies on a triad of features: characteristic facial dysmorphology; impaired growth prenatally and/or postnatally; and structural and/or functional abnormalities of the central nervous system (Stratton *et al.*, 1996).

Tobacco

Prevalence

In Australia, whilst a significant proportion of women will cease smoking once their pregnancy has been confirmed, smoking persists in a subgroup of heavy smokers. Of women who gave birth in Australia in 2012, 12 per cent reported smoking during the first 20 weeks of pregnancy and 9 per cent reported smoking after 20 weeks (Li, Zeki, Hilder & Sullivan, 2013). There has also been a trend towards fewer cigarettes smoked per day (Centre for Epidemiology and Evidence, 2014). In the US the annual average rate of past month cigarette use in 2012 and

2013 among pregnant women aged 15 to 44 was 15 per cent (CBHSQ, 2015). This rate was lower than women who were not pregnant, confirming a significant proportion of women spontaneously quit smoking prior to giving birth.

Predictors and outcomes

Smoking during pregnancy is more common among younger women, single women, women who are socioeconomically disadvantaged, those with lower rates of education, Indigenous women (also refer to Chapter 4) and women in rural areas. These inequities appear to be increasing over time (Coleman-Cowger, Rosenberry & Terplan, 2016; Mohsin, Bauman & Forero, 2011). The harm caused by tobacco smoking during pregnancy are well established, in particular low birth weight for gestational age and associated poor health outcomes in later life (Agrawal *et al.*, 2010). The emergence of electronic cigarettes presents a new public health issue (England *et al.*, 2014). One recent US study suggests that e-cigarettes are perceived by pregnant women as being less harmful than traditional cigarettes, and this may lead to increased use (Mark, Farquhar, Chisolm & Coleman-Cowger, 2015).

Cannabis

Prevalence

Recent US survey data found 5.5 per cent of pregnant women self-reported past month cannabis use (SAMHSA, 2014). Population data on cannabis use in pregnancy is not available in Australia but an analysis of cohorts in Australia, the United Kingdom (UK) and Ireland, showed the overall proportion of women reporting the use of marijuana before or during pregnancy was 5.6 per cent, with Australia having the highest rate (11.6 per cent), followed by New Zealand (4.5 per cent), Ireland (3.8 per cent), and UK (3.7 per cent) (Garg *et al.*, 2016; Leemaqz *et al.*, 2016).

Predictors and outcomes

A number of studies have found that women who were younger, less educated, single, unemployed, socioeconomically disadvantaged, or belonged to a racial or ethnic minority group were more likely to use cannabis and tobacco during pregnancy (Brown *et al.*, 2016; el-Marroun *et al.*, 2008; Ko, Farr, Tong, Creanga & Callaghan, 2015) as were multigravida women and women with unplanned pregnancies (el-Marroun *et al.*, 2008). Cannabis has been associated with adverse pregnancy outcomes, including preterm birth (PTB), small for gestational age (SGA), placental abruption and antepartum haemorrhage (el-Marroun *et al.*, 2008). Given cannabis is often mixed with tobacco, the harms associated with nicotine in pregnancy are also present. Cannabis use during pregnancy is related to subtle but consistent deficits in neuro-behavioural and cognitive outcomes, although these may be mediated by genetic, environmental and social factors (Ross, Graham, Money & Stanwood, 2015), and recent reviews suggest further research in this area is required (Hall, 2015; Volkow *et al.*, 2016).

Opioids

Prevalence

Estimates of the use of heroin by pregnant women are currently not available from population surveys. The most recent Australian population survey conducted every three years estimated less than one per cent of the population had recently used heroin and this was a significant decrease from the previous survey (Australian Institute of Health and Welfare, 2014). The US 2013 National Survey on Drug Use and Health (NSDUH) (SAMHSA, 2014) found heroin use by pregnant women to be 0.4 per cent.

Predictors and outcomes

In a recent Australian study of women who were in treatment for heroin dependence, the majority were receiving government benefits and reported recent financial problems (Taplin & Mattick, 2015). Only 24 per cent had completed school. Half the women had a criminal history (also refer to Chapter 9) and 18 per cent had current domestic violence problems (also refer to Chapter 7). They also had significant mental health problems: 54.2 per cent reported recent psychiatric illness and 38.5 per cent were on a psychiatric medication (further insights into women with perinatal mental health problems are discussed in Chapter 2). Two-thirds (64.5 per cent) had been physically and/or sexually abused in childhood.

Observational studies have found that heroin use in pregnancy is associated with intrauterine growth restriction (IUGR), low birth weight, neonatal death and Neonatal abstinence syndrome (NAS) (Greig, Ash & Douiri, 2012). NAS occurs where the fetus is exposed to heroin (or other opioids) in pregnancy and then shows signs of opioid withdrawal after birth (Beckwith & Burke, 2015; Healy, English, Daniels & Ryan, 2014).

Methamphetamine

Prevalence

A chart review of 879 known perinatal drug users birthing in metropolitan hospitals in New South Wales (NSW) showed that the proportion of amphetamine use increased from 21.4 per cent in 2004 to 25.8 per cent in 2007, despite a decrease in general-population amphetamine use over that time (Abdel-Latif, Oei, Craig, Lui, 2013). In the US NSDUH in 2014, 569,000 people were current methamphetamine users although there was no specific information on methamphetamine use in pregnancy (SAMHSA, 2014).

Predictors and outcomes

Available research points to increased rates of premature delivery, placental abruption, small size, lethargy, and heart and brain abnormalities (DellaGrotta *et al.*, 2010). Women who use methamphetamine in pregnancy are at risk of developing anaemia or other nutritional deficiencies (Wright, Schuetter, Fombonne, Stephenson & Haning, 2012). Other pregnancy complications include pregnancy-induced hypertension and preterm birth (also refer to Chapter 10 for insights into mothers with premature infants), meconium stained amniotic fluid, premature rupture of membranes and precipitate labour (Oei *et al.*, 2009). A study funded by the US National Institute on Drug Abuse examining developmental outcomes in children born to mothers who used methamphetamine in pregnancy have found neurobehavioral problems such as decreased arousal and increased stress and subtle but significant attention impairments in these children (LaGasse *et al.*, 2012; Smith *et al.*, 2008). Similar findings have been found in a cohort study undertaken in South Africa (Dyk, Ramanjam, Church, Koren & Donald, 2014). Poorer inhibitory control was also found in children exposed to a heavy dose in utero placing them at high risk for impaired executive function and its consequences (Smith *et al.*, 2008).

Screening for substance use

Principles of screening

There are a number of general principles that guide screening for drug and alcohol use in pregnancy. Questions should be posed in a non-judgemental manner, avoiding expressions that may be interpreted as negative or pejorative (NSW Department of Health, 2014). In a study by Harvey and colleagues, women on an opioid replacement programme (methadone) described how they felt judged by staff in the maternity unit, believing labels such as 'junkie', 'drug addict' and bad mother were applied to them (Harvey, Dahlen, Nicholls & Schmied, 2015). These women stated they were 'scared', 'terrified' about opening up about their drug use as they had heard 'horror stories' of children being removed into care (Harvey *et al.*, 2015, p. 291).

Questions are best embedded in the usual antenatal history at initial assessment and repeated at each re-assessment. Simple questions about quantity and frequency of drug use should be initially asked as it is important to establish whether each substance is used occasionally, on a regular recreational or non-dependent basis, or whether there is ongoing problematic use. Answers to these questions will indicate when referral to specialist services is warranted or, if a brief intervention, incorporating techniques such as motivational interviewing (see below) may be appropriate. In some US clinics urine drug testing is undertaken to validate substance use or non-use.

Substances specific screening tools

Alcohol

There are numerous screening tools available to clinicians to assess alcohol problems (Babor, Higgins-Biddle, Saunders & Monteiro, 2001; National Institute on Alcohol Abuse and Alcoholism (NIAAA), 2003). A systematic review of brief screening tools for alcohol use in pregnancy (Burns, Gray & Smith, 2010) concluded that the T-ACE (an acronym based on questions included), the TWEAK (acronym also based on screener questions), and the AUDIT-C (a three item version of the Alcohol Use Disorders Identification Test – AUDIT) show promise for screening for risk drinking, and AUDIT-C may also be useful for identifying alcohol dependency or abuse.

In Australia, the most recent guidelines for treatment of substance use in pregnancy suggest the AUDIT- C (see Box 8.1), that ask about quantity and frequency will suffice for assessment in pregnancy (NSW Department of Health, 2014).

BOX 8.1 AUDIT-C

Q1: How often did you have a drink containing alcohol in the past year?

Never	(0 points)
Monthly or less	(1 point)
Two to four times a month	(2 points)
Two to three times per week	(3 points)
Four or more times a week	(4 points)

Q2: How many drinks did you have on a typical day when you were drinking in the past year?

1 or 2	(0 points)
3 or 4	(1 point)
5 or 6	(2 points)
7 to 9	(3 points)
10 or more	(4 points)

Q3: How often did you have six or more drinks on one occasion in the past year?

Never	(0 points)
Less than monthly	(1 point)
Monthly	(2 points)
Weekly	(3 points)
Daily or almost daily	(4 points)

The T-ACE is the screening tool recommended for pregnant women in the US by the American College of Obstetricians and Gynecologists (ACOG) and the NIAAA. It is reported to have acceptable validity with women of different ethnicities in the US (Jones, Bailey & Sokol, 2013). The T-ACE is an adaption of the CAGE that adds a tolerance question (T) and removes the guilt question (G) (Russell, 1994) (see Box 8.2)

BOX 8.2 T-ACE

T Tolerance: How many drinks does it take to make you feel high?

A Have people **annoyed** you by criticising your drinking?

C Have you ever felt you ought to **cut down** on your drinking?

E Eye-opener: Have you ever had a drink first thing in the morning to steady your nerves or get rid of a hangover?

The T-ACE is based on the CAGE. A score of two or more is considered positive. Affirmative answers to questions A, C, or E = 1 point each. Reporting tolerance to more than two drinks (the T question) = 2 points.

Tobacco

The revised Fagerström Test for Nicotine Dependence (FTND) is a simple six-question tool for assessing level of nicotine dependence and is useful as an indication of whether pharmacotherapy may be required to support a quit attempt (Heatherton, Kozlowski, Frecker & Fagerström, 1991) (see Box 8.3)

BOX 8.3 FAGERSTRÖM TEST FOR NICOTINE DEPENDENCE

1   How soon after you wake up do you smoke your first cigarette?
    After 60 minutes   *(0)*
    31–60 minutes   *(1)*
    6–30 minutes   *(2)*
    Within 5 minutes   *(3)*

2   Do you find it difficult to refrain from smoking in places where it is forbidden?
    No   *(0)*
    Yes   *(1)*

3   Which cigarette would you hate most to give up?
    The first in the morning   *(1)*
    Any other   *(0)*

---

4   How many cigarettes per day do you smoke?

10 or less	*(0)*
11–20	*(1)*
21–30	*(2)*
31 or more	*(3)*

5   Do you smoke more frequently during the first hours after awakening than during the rest of the day?

No	*(0)*
Yes	*(1)*

6   Do you smoke even if you are so ill that you are in bed most of the day?

No	*(0)*
Yes	*(1)*

Score

Your score was_____

Your level of dependence on nicotine is:

0–2	Very low dependence
3–4	Low dependence
5	Medium dependence
6–7	High dependence
8–10	Very high dependence

Other substances

For substances that do not have specific screening instruments, dependence can be measured by the Severity of Dependence Scale. Each of the five items is scored on a four-point scale (0–3). The total score is obtained through the addition of the five-item ratings. The higher the score, the higher the level of dependence (Gossop *et al.*, 1995) (see Box 8.4)

BOX 8.4 SEVERITY OF DEPENDENCE SCALE

Circle the answer that best applies to how you have felt about your use of .... over the last month.

1   Did you ever think your use of ....(drug) was out of control?

Never or almost never	*(0)*
Sometimes	*(1)*
Often	*(2)*
Always	*(3)*

2   Did the prospect of missing a fix/dose make you very anxious or worried?

Never or almost never   (0)

Sometimes   (1)

Often   (2)

Always   (3)

3   How much did you worry about your use of the drug?

Not at all   (0)

A little   (1)

Often   (2)

Always or nearly always   (3)

4   Did you wish you could stop?

Never or almost never   (0)

Sometimes   (1)

Often   (2)

Always   (3)

5   How difficult would you find it to stop or go without ....(drug)?

Not difficult at all   (0)

Quite difficult   (1)

Very difficult   (2)

Impossible   (3)

SCORE_____

Readiness and confidence to change scales

In addition to the substance specific screening tools it is important to assess the readiness of the woman to change her substance use. This is very important as if she is not ready, little will be achieved through treatment. A number of readiness to change questions are available. Examples are included in Box 8.5 below (Alcohol and Drugs Training Research Unit, 1992).

BOX 8.5 READINESS AND CONFIDENCE TO CHANGE QUESTIONS

Readiness to change

Do you want to change your use of (drug) right now?

No   (0)

Probably not   (1)

Unsure   (2)

Possibly   (3)

Definitely   (4)

Confidence to change

Do you think you could change your use of (drug) now if you wanted to?

Definitely could not	*(0)*
Probably could not	*(1)*
Unsure	*(2)*
Probably could	*(3)*
Definitely could	*(4)*

For some women pregnancy can be an important motivator for change. Women in the study by Harvey *et al.* (2015) discussed their hope for a better future and to achieve their goal of being a 'good mother' – Kristy stated:

> I have to sort of take that [child protection involvement] because I have to work with that if I want to have my children. That's my biggest goal is to keep the children and not only to keep them but to do the right thing by them. It's no good me having them if I am abusing them or I am going out doing stuff. I'm not giving them the life that they could have. It's a vicious cycle that keeps going around and around unless you put your foot into it and go 'no more'. I'm not, you know, I'm going to change this and make it because you pass it down to them.
>
> (Harvey *et al.*, 2015, p. 288)

Treatment

Motivational interviewing

Motivational interviewing (MI) is a technique that accepts that clients who need to make changes in their lives are at different levels of readiness to do so. The MI approach seeks to help clients think differently about their behaviour and ultimately to consider what might be gained through change. This happens through asking open-ended questions, making affirmations, using reflections and summarising what has been discussed. It is non-judgemental, non-confrontational and non-adversarial and the health professional is viewed more as a facilitator than a clinician.

The 5 As

The United States Preventive Services Task Force, ACOG and Australian guidelines (Breen, Awbery & Burns, 2014; NSW Department of Health, 2014) currently recommend asking all pregnant women about tobacco use and providing them with assistance to quit utilising the 5As manual behavioural framework (see Box 8.6). The five 'A's referred to are: Ask, Advise, Assess, Assist, Arrange. This approach and can be used to encourage women to decrease/cease use of all different forms of substances.

BOX 8.6 THE 5As FRAMEWORK

1   ASK: All pregnant women should be asked about their tobacco use.

2   ADVISE: This involves strong direct personal advice by the provider to the pregnant woman to cease smoking. Education about the impact on the fetus and mother should be provided.

3   ASSESS: Determine how willing the woman is to change her behaviour after hearing the provider's advice. Stress the importance of understanding the reasons for smoking and wanting to make changes. Prompt the client to identify 'pros' and 'cons' of smoking and to rate them on a scale of 0 to 10. Work through the same process for the 'pros' and 'cons' of change.

4   ASSIST: This refers to helping the patient make a change if she appears ready. Explain what triggers are (i.e. specific feelings or events which prompt strong thoughts about wanting to smoke). Ask the client if she has attempted to stop previously and if so ask what she found helpful. Explain why high-risk situations need to be avoided and suggest they develop a relapse prevention plan. Stress the normality of urges/cravings and that they rarely last more than 30 minutes. Give examples of some techniques that may be of assistance for withdrawal and/or cravings (e.g. distraction, delay, de-catastrophising, distressing).

5   ARRANGE: Refer the patient for further assessment and treatment, and set up follow-up appointments. Interventions including counselling, relapse prevention and support are.

Supported referrals to specialist treatment and antenatal care should be provided where appropriate.

Substance specific treatments

It is important to note that abstinence will not be immediately possible for some women and substitution treatment or harm minimisation approaches will be the most appropriate. Substance use disorders are characterised by periods of remission and relapse; thus treatment must be tailored to address this variable course. Given substance dependence is a chronic relapsing disorder, and a high proportion of pregnancies are reported to be unplanned (Frezza, di Padova, Pozzato, Terpin, Baraona & Lieber, 1990; Muggli et al., 2016; Naimi, Lipscomb, Brewer & Gilbert, 2003), the focus of treatment should be one of assertive long-term follow-up to support the woman and prevent additional unplanned pregnancies. Appropriate treatment will also depend on factors including: other mental and physical health problems, access to services including transport and severity of the problem.

A stepped and individualised approach is recommended, where the least intensive treatment is implemented first, and if not successful, followed by more intense treatment (Kay-Lambkin, Baker, McKetin & Lee, 2010). In addition to psychosocial treatments, if consumption is problematic and/or the woman is substance dependent it may be necessary to provide a supervised detoxification. Depending on the substance and severity of the dependence this may be as an inpatient.

Alcohol

Given concerns for the health of the fetus, pharmacotherapies available to treat alcohol dependence are contraindicated in pregnancy, other than standard nutritional support. Importantly, alcohol withdrawal may precipitate fetal distress and possible demise and inpatient admission is advised where possible (Bhat & Hadley, 2015; NSW Department of Health, 2014). Ongoing home visiting to support parenting skill development is recommended both during and after pregnancy. Treatment should be specific to the woman and her situation and may include integrated treatment if other problems such as post-traumatic stress disorder (PTSD) or other comorbid disorders are also present (further insights into PTSD onset following childbirth are presented in Chapter 11).

Smoking

Guidelines suggest interventions for smokers should be based on their willingness to quit; those who are willing to quit (smoking cessation), those unwilling to quit (motivational interviewing) and former smokers who have recently quit (relapse prevention). A stepped care approach to smoking cessation is advocated, including nicotine replacement therapy (NRT) when a pregnant woman is otherwise unable to quit, and when the likelihood and benefits of cessation outweigh the risks of NRT and potential continued smoking (Haddad & Davis, 2016). It is recommended that pregnant women who smoke use intermittent (gum, lozenge, inhaler, tablet) rather than continuous (patches) NRT preparations, and use the lowest dose possible (NSW Department of Health, 2014).

Opioids & Methamphetamine

Withdrawal from heroin (and other opioids) during pregnancy is not routinely encouraged as evidence of safety and effectiveness is sparse and relapse to illicit heroin use is more likely to pose a significant risk to the mother and infant alike (Jones *et al.*, 2014; Krans, Cochran & Bogen, 2015). Stabilisation and maintenance on methadone or buprenorphine is recommended (Minozzi, Amato, Vecchi, & Davoli, 2013). Both these treatments are associated with improved fetal development and infant birth weight and reduction in neonatal mortality. A recent study confirmed the safety profile for both treatments in pregnancy (Jones, Finnegan & Kaltenbach, 2012). However, it should be noted that further research is required as the impact of opioids on the developing brain remain unknown. Pregnant women may already be prescribed opioids (e.g. morphine or oxycodone) for significant pain problems before they become pregnant. The advantages and disadvantages of continuing prescription opioids during pregnancy or a structured withdrawal off opioids is suggested in consultation with a pain specialist (NSW Department of Health, 2014).

There are no pharmacological treatments for methamphetamine. Current guidelines highlight the importance of early engagement in antenatal care and psychosocial interventions to address comorbid physical and mental health problems (NSW Department of Health, 2014). The majority of these infants require only minimal supportive treatment, for example, gavage feeding for about a week. Few have been shown to need pharmacological treatment

Policy and guidelines

Given the complex interplay between the dose, timing and frequency of substance use together with cultural differences, it is unlikely that a universal cut off for safe use of any substance will ever be established. Given the legal status and substantial evidence base for alcohol use, the Australian National Health and Medical Research Council, the body that determines national health guidelines has most recently stated that 'For women who are pregnant or planning a pregnancy, not drinking is the safest option'. The Australian guidelines note women who have consumed alcohol should be reassured that the risk to the fetus from low-level drinking (such as one or two drinks per week) during pregnancy are likely to be low (National Health and Medical Research Council, 2009). The UK National Institute for Health and Clinical Excellence (NICE) guidelines also recommends abstinence (NICE, 2010). The ACOG has also long-supported this stance (ACOG and the American Academy of Pediatrics, 2007).

Implications for practice

Initiatives aimed at reducing maternal and fetal harm should be embedded in a broad framework of care that includes the provision of information about the impact of substance use in pregnancy to all women of childbearing age. Early provision of antenatal care and increased number of visits is associated with improved pregnancy and birth outcomes (Wright et al., 2012). Care of women who are substance dependent and pregnant should include referral to specialist care, appointment of a case manager, continuity of care and assertive follow-up (refer to Chapter 14 for the benefits of integrated care for women with substance misuse in pregnancy). The provision of contraceptive advice is critical in reducing the rates of future unplanned pregnancies. Women with substance use disorders are also likely to have a range of comorbid mental health disorders. Poor mental health can be exacerbated by substance use and pregnant women who use substances may be more likely to have panic attacks, anxiety, or depression which in turn have their own deleterious health effects.

The framework of care should be grounded in a model of social justice and the ethical provision of services. Confidentiality is a fundamental right of people using health care services, and all services should be guided by relevant privacy legislation. Women who are substance dependent and pregnant need to be treated in a respectful and non-judgemental manner, as emphasised here by Emma (a woman on a methadone programme):

> Treat people the way they [staff] treated me, with a bit of respect. Just to not look down on anyone and treat them like they're a normal person and not like they're on Methadone ... I wasn't scared to ask questions, I would have been worried to ask if they were rude.
>
> (Harvey *et al.*, 2015, p. 295)

Issues of child protection are, however, paramount. In Australia substance use alone is not an indicator for a child protection notification, although child welfare should be a consideration in all treatments for women who are substance dependent and notifications made accordingly. In the US, there remains one state (Tennessee) that criminalises drug use during pregnancy; 18 states consider substance abuse during pregnancy to be child abuse under civil child-welfare statutes; and three states consider it grounds for civil commitment.

The majority of women will cease or reduce substance use during pregnancy, although a minority will continue to use and to use heavily and this group requires increased support. Treatment for this group is complex and requires individual case management given the reasons for use are a complex interplay between the environment, physiology and individual characteristics. It is recommended that all preventive and treatment approaches be grounded in a collaborative framework to ensure follow through of comprehensive treatment that takes cultural and environmental factors into account. This should include flexibility in access including outreach and assertive follow-up. All health services for pregnant women who are substance dependent should be non-judgemental and provided in a holistic framework that is centred around the woman's current priorities and needs, and grounded in evidence based policies and procedures.

Conclusion

Substance use in pregnancy is of international concern. Whilst use has decreased for the population overall, it has not changed for women whose use is heavy and chronic, the group most likely to develop poor maternal and fetal outcomes. It is therefore critical that a no 'wrong door approach' be taken, where women are able to access services through any care facility, whether this is through direct care or referral. Most importantly, early engagement in antenatal care is required with long-term follow-up and an empathetic approach that engenders trust, ensuring delivery of the best possible treatments for mother and fetus/infant alike.

References

Abdel-Latif, M.E., Oei, J., Craig, F., Lui, K. & NSW and ACT NAS Epidemiology Group. (2013). Profile of infants born to drug-using mothers: A state-wide audit. *Journal of Paediatrics and Child Health*, *49*(1), E80-E86.

Agrawal, A., Balasubramanian, S., Smith, E.K., Madden, P.A.F., Bucholz, K.K., Heath, A.C. & Lynskey, M.T. (2010). Peer substance involvement modifies genetic influences on regular substance involvement in young women. *Addiction*, *105*(10), 1844–1853.

American College of Obstetricians and Gynecologists and the American Academy of Pediatrics. (2007). *Guidelines for perinatal care*. 6th edition. Elk Grove Village, IL: AAP; Washington, DC: ACOG; p. 103, 284–286, 323–325, 352.

American Psychiatric Association. (2013). *Diagnostic and statistical manual of mental disorders*. 5th edition. Arlington, VA: American Psychiatric Association.

ARND Consensus Statement. (2011). Consensus statement on recognising Alcohol-Related Neurodevelopmental Disorder (ARND) in primary health care of children. Available from: www.niaaa.nih.gov/sites/default/files/ARNDConferenceConsensusStatement Booklet_Complete.pdf [Accessed 20 October 2016].

Australian Institute of Health and Welfare. (2014). *National drug strategy household survey report 2013*. Canberra: Australian Institute of Health and Welfare.

Babor, T., Higgins-Biddle, J., Saunders, J. & Monteiro, M. (2001). *The alcohol use disorders identification test: Guidelines for use in primary care*. 2nd edition. Available from: http://apps. who.int/iris/bitstream/10665/67205/1/WHO_MSD_MSB_01.6a.pdf [Accessed 23 October 2016].

Beckwith, A.M. & Burke, S.A. (2015). Identification of early developmental deficits in infants with prenatal heroin, methadone, and other opioid exposure. *Clinical Pediatrics*, *54*(4), 328–335.

Bhat, A. & Hadley, A. (2015). The management of alcohol withdrawal in pregnancy – case report, literature review and preliminary recommendations. *General Hospital Psychiatry*, *37*(3), 273.e271–273.e273.

Breen, C., Awbery, E. & Burns, L. (2014). *Supporting pregnant women who use alcohol or other drugs: A review of the evidence*. Sydney: National Drug and Alcohol Research Centre, UNSW Australia. Available from https://ndarc.med.unsw.edu.au/sites/default/files/ ndarc/resources/Supporting%20Pregnant%20Women%20who%20use%20Alcohol%20 or%20Other%20Drugs%20-%20A%20review%20of%20the%20evidence.pdf [Accessed 20 October 2016].

Brown, S.J., Mensah, F.K., Ah Kit, J., Stuart-Butler, D., Glover, K., Leane, C., Weetra, D., Gartland, D., Newbury, J. & Yelland, J. (2016). Use of cannabis during pregnancy and birth outcomes in an Aboriginal birth cohort: A cross-sectional, population-based study. *BMJ Open*, *6*(2). doi:10.1136/bmjopen-2015-010286.

Burns, E., Gray, R. & Smith, L. (2010). Brief screening questionnaires to identify problem drinking during pregnancy: A systematic review. *Addiction*, *105*, 601–614.

Burns, L., Mattick, R. & Cooke, M. (2006). The use of record linkage to examine alcohol use in pregnancy. *Alcoholism: Clinical and Experimental Research*, *30*(4), 642–648.

Cameron, C., Davey, T., Kendall, E., Wilson, A. & McClure, R.J. (2013). Changes in alcohol consumption in pregnant Australian women between 2007 and 2011. *Medical Journal of Australia*, *199*(5), 355–357.

Center for Behavioral Health Statistics and Quality (CBHSQ). (2013). *Trends in substances of abuse among pregnant women and women in treatment of childbearing age in treatment.* Available from: www.samhsa.gov/data/sites/default/files/spot110-trends-pregnant-women-2013.pdf [Accessed 4 October 2016].

Center for Behavioral Health Statistics and Quality (CBHSQ). (2015). *Behavioral health trends in the United States: Results from the 2014 national survey on drug use and health.* Available from: www.samhsa.gov/data/sites/default/files/NSDUH-FRR1-2014/NSDUH-FRR1-2014.pdf [Accessed 20 September 2016].

Centre for Epidemiology and Evidence. (2014). *New South Wales mothers and babies 2012.* Available from: www.health.nsw.gov.au/hsnsw/Publications/mothers-and-babies-2012.pdf [Accessed 15 July 2016].

Coleman-Cowger, V.H, Koszowski, B., Rosenberry, Z.R. & Terplan, M. (2016). Factors associated with early pregnancy smoking status among low-income smokers. *Maternal and Child Health Journal, 20*(5), 1054–1060.

DellaGrotta, S., LaGasse, L.L., Arria, A.M., Derauf, C., Grant, P., Smith, L.M., Shah, R., Huestis, M., Liu, J. & Lester, B.M. (2010). Patterns of methamphetamine use during pregnancy: Results from the infant development, environment, and lifestyle (IDEAL) study. *Maternal and Child Health Journal, 14*(4), 519–527.

Dyk, J., Ramanjam, V., Church, P., Koren, G. & Donald, K. (2014). Maternal methamphetamine use in pregnancy and long-term neurodevelopmental and behavioral deficits in children. *Journal of Population Therapeutics and Clinical Pharmacology, 21*(2), e185–196.

el-Marroun, H., Tiemeier, H., Jaddoe, V.W.V., Hofman, A., Mackenbach, J.P., Steegers, E.A.P, Verhulst, F.C., van den Brink, W. & Huizink, A.C. (2008). Demographic, emotional and social determinants of cannabis use in early pregnancy: The Generation R study. *Drug and Alcohol Dependence, 98*(3), 218–226.

England, L.J., Anderson, B.L., Tong, V.T.K., Mahoney, J., Coleman-Cowger, V.H., Melstrom, P. & Schulkin, J. (2014). Screening practices and attitudes of obstetricians-gynecologists toward new and emerging tobacco products. *American Journal of Obstetrics & Gynecology, 211*(6), 695.e1–695.e7.

Frezza, M., di Padova, C., Pozzato, G., Terpin, M., Baraona, E. & Lieber, C.S. (1990). High blood alcohol levels in women. *New England Journal of Medicine, 322*(2), 95–99.

Garg, M., Garrison, L., Leeman, L., Hamidovic, A., Borrego, M., Rayburn, W.F. & Bakhireva, L. (2016). Validity of self-reported drug use information among pregnant women. *Maternal and Child Health Journal, 20*(1), 41–47.

Gossop, M., Darke, S., Griffiths, P., Hando, J., Powis, B., Hall, W. & Strang, J. (1995). The severity of dependence scale (SDS): Psychometric properties of the SDS in English and Australian samples of heroin, cocaine and amphetamine users. *Addiction, 90*(5), 607–614.

Greig, E., Ash, A. & Douiri, A. (2012). Maternal and neonatal outcomes following methadone substitution during pregnancy. *Archives of Gynecology and Obstetrics, 286*(4), 843–851.

Haddad, A. & Davis, A.M. (2016). Tobacco smoking cessation in adults and pregnant women: Behavioral and pharmacotherapy interventions. *JAMA 315*(18), 2011–2012.

Hall, W. (2015). What has research over the past two decades revealed about the adverse health effects of recreational cannabis use? *Addiction, 110*(1), 19–35.

Harvey, S., Schmied, V., Nicholls, D. & Dahlen, H. (2015). Hope amidst judgement: The meaning mothers accessing opioid treatment programmes ascribe to interactions with health services in the perinatal period. *Journal of Family Studies, 21*(3), 282–304.

Healy, D., English, F., Daniels, A. & Ryan, C. (2014). Emergence of opiate-induced neonatal abstinence syndrome. *Irish Medical Journal*, *107*(2), 46.

Heatherton, T.F., Kozlowski, L.T., Frecker, R.C. & Fagerström, K.-O. (1991). The Fagerström test for nicotine dependence: A revision of the Fagerström tolerance questionnaire. *British Journal of Addiction*, *86*(9), 1119–1127.

Jones, H., Finnegan, L. & Kaltenbach, K. (2012). Methadone and buprenorphine for the management of opioid dependence in pregnancy. *Drugs*, *72*(6), 747–757.

Jones, H.E., Deppen, K., Hudak, M.L., Leffert, L., McClelland, C., Sahin, L., Starer, J., Terplan, M., Thorp, J.M., Walsh, J. & Creanga, A.A. (2014). Clinical care for opioid-using pregnant and postpartum women: The role of obstetric providers. *American Journal of Obstetrics and Gynecology*, *210*(4), 302–310.

Jones, K. & Smith, D. (1973). Recognition of the fetal alcohol syndrome in early infancy. *The Lancet*, *302*(7836), 999–1001.

Jones, T.B., Bailey, B.A. & Sokol, R.J. (2013). Alcohol use in pregnancy: Insights in screening and intervention for the clinician. *Clinical Obstetrics & Gynecology*, *56*(1), 114–123.

Kay-Lambkin, F., Baker, A., McKetin, R. & Lee, N. (2010). Stepping through treatment: Reflections on an adaptive treatment strategy among methamphetamine users with depression.. *Drug and Alcohol Review*, *29*, 475–482.

Ko, J.Y., Farr, S.L., Tong, V.T., Creanga, A.A. & Callaghan, W.M. (2015). Prevalence and patterns of marijuana use among pregnant and nonpregnant women of reproductive age. *American Journal of Obstetrics and Gynecology*, *213*(2), 201.e201–210.e210. http://dx.doi.org/10.1016/j.ajog.2015.03.021.

Krans, E.E., Cochran, G. & Bogen, D.L. (2015). Caring for opioid dependent pregnant women: Prenatal and postpartum care considerations. *Clinical obstetrics and gynecology*, *58*(2), 370–379.

LaGasse, L.L., Derauf, C., Smith, L.M., Newman, E., Shah, R., Neal, C., Arria, A., Huestis, M.A., Della Grotta, S., Lin, H., Dansereau, L.M. & Lester, B.M. (2012). Prenatal methamphetamine exposure and childhood behavior problems at 3 and 5 years of age. *Pediatrics*, *129*(4), 681–688.

Leemaqz, S.Y., Dekker, G.A., McCowan, L.M., Kenny, L.C., Myers, J.E., Simpson, N.A., Poston, L. & Roberts, C.T.; SCOPE Consortium. (2016). Maternal marijuana use has independent effects on risk for spontaneous preterm birth but not other common late pregnancy complications. *Reproductive Toxicology*, *62*, 77–86.

Lemoine, P., Harousseau, H., Borteyru, J.P. & Menuet, J.C. (1968). Les enfants des parents alcooliques: Anomalies observées à propos de 127 cas (The children of alcoholic parents: anomalies observed in 127 cases). *Quest Medical*, *25*, 476–482.

Li, Z., Zeki, R., Hilder, L., & Sullivan, E. (2013). *Australia's mothers and babies 2011*. Canberra: Australian Institute of Health and Welfare.

Mark, K., Farquhar, B., Chisolm, M. & Coleman-Cowger, V.H. (2015). Knowledge, attitudes, and practice of electronic cigarettes use among pregnant women. *Journal of Addiction Medicine*, *9*, 266–272.

Minozzi, S., Amato, L., Vecchi, S. & Davoli, M. (2013). Maintenance agonist treatments for opiate dependent pregnant women. *Cochrane Database of Systematic Reviews* (12). http://onlinelibrary.wiley.com/doi/10.1002/14651858.CD006318.pub2/abstract doi:10.1002/14651858.CD006318.pub2.

Mohsin, M., Bauman, A.E. & Forero, R. (2011). Socioeconomic correlates and trends in smoking in pregnancy in New South Wales, Australia. *Journal of Epidemiology and Community Health*, *65*(8), 727–732.

Muggli, E., O'Leary, C., Donath, S., Orsini, F., Forster, D., Anderson, P.J., Lewis, S., Nagle, C., Craig, J.M., Elliott, E. & Halliday, J. (2016). 'Did you ever drink more?' A detailed description of pregnant women's drinking patterns. *BMC Public Health*, *16*(1), 683. doi:10.1186/s12889-016-3354-9.

Naimi, T., Lipscomb, L., Brewer, R. & Gilbert, B. (2003). Binge drinking in the preconception period and the risk of unintended pregnancy: Implications for women and their children. *Pediatrics*, *111*(5 part 2), 1136–1141.

National Health and Medical Research Council. (2009). *Australian guidelines to reduce health risks from drinking alcohol*. Available from: www.nhmrc.gov.au/guidelines-publications/ds10 [Accessed 23 October, 2016].

National Institute for Health and Clinical Excellence (NICE). (2010). *Pregnancy and complex social factors: A model for service provision for pregnant women with complex social factors*. Available from: www.nice.org.uk/guidance/cg110 [Accessed 23 October 2016].

National Institute on Alcohol Abuse and Alcoholism (NIAAA). (2003). *Assessing alcohol problems: A guide for clinicians and Researchers*. 2nd edition. Available from: http://pubs.niaaa.nih.gov/publications/AssessingAlcohol/index.pdf [Accessed 23 October 2016].

NSW Department of Health. (2014). *NSW clinical guidelines for the management of substance use during pregnancy, birth and the postnatal period*. North Sydney: NSW Department of Health.

Oei, J.L., Abdel-Latif, M.E., Craig, F., Kee, A., Austin, M.-P. & Lui, K. on behalf of the NWS and ACT NAS Epidemiology Group. (2009). Short-term outcomes of mothers and newborn Infants with comorbid psychiatric disorders and drug dependency. *Australian and New Zealand Journal of Psychiatry*, *43*(4), 323–331.

O'Keeffe, L.M., Kearney, P.M., McCarthy, F.P., Khashan, A.S., Greene, R.A., North, R., Poston, L., McCowan, L.M.E., Baker, P.N., Dekker, G.A., Walker, J.J., Taylor, R. & Kenny, L.C. (2015). Prevalence and predictors of alcohol use during pregnancy: Findings from international multicentre cohort studies. *BMJ Open*, *5*(7). doi:10.1136/bmjopen-2014-006323.

Ross, E.J., Graham, D.L., Money, K.M. & Stanwood, G.D. (2015). Developmental consequences of fetal exposure to drugs: What we know and what we still must learn. *Neuropsychopharmacology*, *40*(1), 61–87.

Russell, M. (1994). New assessment tools for drinking in pregnancy: T-ACE, TWEAK, and others. *Alcohol Health and Research World*, *18*(1), 55–61.

Skagerström, J., Chang, G. & Nilsen, P. (2011). Predictors of drinking during pregnancy: A systematic review. *Journal of Womens Health*, *20*(6), 901–913.

Smith, L.M., LaGasse, L.L., Derauf, C., Grant, P., Shah, R., Arria, A., Huestis, M., Haning, W., Strauss, A., DellaGrotta, S., Fallone, M., Liu, J. & Lester, B.M. (2008). Prenatal methamphetamine use and neonatal neurobehavioral outcome. *Neurotoxicology and Teratology*, *30*(1), 20–28.

Stengel, C. (2013). The risk of being 'too honest': Drug use, stigma and pregnancy. *Health, Risk & Society*, *16*(1), 36–50.

Stone, R. (2015). Pregnant women and substance use: Fear, stigma, and barriers to care. *Health & Justice*, *3*(2), 1–15 doi:10.1186/s40352-015-0015-5.

Stratton, K., Howe, C. & Battaglia, F. (Eds.). (1996). *Fetal alcohol syndrome*. Washington, DC: Institute of Medicine National Academy Press.

Streissguth, A.P., Bookstein, F.L., Barr, H.M., Sampson, P.D., O'Malley, K. & Young, J.K. (2004). Risk factors for adverse life outcomes in fetal alcohol syndrome and fetal alcohol effects. *Journal of Developmental & Behavioral Pediatrics*, *25*(4), 228–238.

Substance Abuse and Mental Health Services Administration (SAMHSA). (2014). Results from the 2013 national survey on drug use and health: Summary of national findings.

Available from: www.samhsa.gov/data/sites/default/files/NSDUHresultsPDFWHTML 2013/Web/NSDUHresults2013.pdf [Accessed 23 October, 2016].

Taplin, S. & Mattick, R. (2015). The nature and extent of child protection involvement among heroin-using mothers in treatment: High rates of reports, removals at birth and children in care. *Drug and Alcohol Review, 34*(1), 31–37.

Volkow, N.D., Swanson, J.M., Evins, A.E., DeLisi, L.E., Meier, M.H., Gonzalez, R., Bloomfield, M.A.P., Curran, H.V. & Baler, R. (2016). Effects of cannabis use on human behavior, including cognition, motivation, and Psychosis: A review. *JAMA Psychiatry, 73*(3), 292–297.

Wright, T.E., Schuetter, R., Fombonne, E., Stephenson, J. & Haning, W.F. (2012). Implementation and evaluation of a harm-reduction model for clinical care of substance using pregnant women. *Harm Reduction Journal, 9*(1), 5. doi:10.1186/1477-7517-9-5.

9

WOMEN WHO ARE INCARCERATED

Cathrine Fowler and Chris Rossiter

Introduction

A loud bang on the door in the middle of the night. Darkness – then bright lights. Loud noises and shouting. Strange people in the house. Furniture and possessions upended. Sleeping children waking suddenly, frightened and crying out for their mothers ...

For a small but growing number of women, terror such as this marks the beginning of a traumatic journey as they and/or their partners are arrested. Many incarcerated mothers report a common story of separation, not knowing where their children have been taken or whether they are safe, and an ongoing struggle to maintain contact with their children. For some, this story does not end when they are released, as their incarceration may result in long-term or permanent loss of custody of their children.

Although women make up a relatively small proportion of the prison population in countries such as Australia and the United Kingdom (UK), their imprisonment rate is increasing faster than men (Prison Reform Trust, 2015; Corrective Services New South Wales, 2014). In Australia over the last ten years, whereas the number of male prisoners increased by 29 per cent, the number of female prisoners increased by 39.7 per cent (Australian Bureau of Statistics, 2016). While in the UK the number of women in prison nearly trebled (Prison Reform Trust, 2015).

Many female prisoners are mothers of infants or young children. The number of children with a mother in prison in the UK is estimated to be more than 17,000 (Prison Reform Trust, 2015). In New South Wales (NSW), Australia, nearly two-thirds of Indigenous women in prison have children up to the age of 18, as do 57.8 per cent of non-Indigenous women (Corrective Services NSW, 2014). In addition, around 4.6 per cent of women are pregnant on entry to prison (Australian Institute of Health and Welfare (AIHW), 2015). In the United States of America (USA) the pregnancy rate of incarcerated women is between six per cent and ten per cent (American College of Obstetricians and Gynecologists, 2011). Around nine per cent of incarcerated parents have at least four dependent children (AIHW, 2015); others have stepchildren and grandchildren.

Within corrective facilities, there are constant tensions between maintaining security and safety, achieving rehabilitation requirements, and ensuring the emotional and physical needs of correctional staff and of incarcerated pregnant women, mothers and their children. Clearly, imprisonment poses multiple challenges to a woman in sustaining her maternal role (Celinska & Siegal, 2010). For many women and their children, the outcome of incarceration is major disruption to their emerging relationship, due to prolonged periods of separation. This often reinforces an intergenerational cycle of incarceration, poverty, trauma and violence. Yet, crucially, governments, services and professionals can assist incarcerated women who are pregnant or have infants to make significant changes in their parenting beliefs and behaviour. Implementing interventions with a parenting focus for women in prison can potentially improve the life outcomes for their infants.

This chapter aims to provide an overview of the challenges encountered by incarcerated mothers, their infants and families. It illustrates the complexity of the issues experienced by mothers in custody and discusses the potential for programmes within the prison system to support them.

Background

Women's journeys to incarceration are complex and varied. Crucially, many women arrive in prison with co-morbidities of addiction, mental illness and significant trauma histories of family violence, and physical, emotional and sexual abuse in childhood (AIHW, 2015). This is often compounded by smoking and alcohol consumption (also refer to Chapter 8), inadequate access to legal assistance, limited capacity to speak or understand English or a lack of family support.

Indigenous people are frequently over-represented within the prison population in many countries. In Australia, Indigenous people are 12 times more likely to be incarcerated than non-indigenous Australians (Australian Institute of Criminology, 2016), exacerbating the impact of colonisation and the forced removal of children (Human Rights and Equal Opportunities Commission, 1997) (also refer to Chapter 4 for further insights into issues faced by Indigenous women). While Aboriginal people represent 3 per cent of the population in Canada, they account for 24 per cent of admissions to provincial or territorial correctional services; for Aboriginal Canadian women, the rate was 36 per cent (Statistics Canada, 2015).

In the USA people from minority groups are also at high risk of incarceration due to reduced family resources, further compounding these families' disadvantage and vulnerability (Wildeman & Western, 2010). A similar situation exists in the UK with disproportionately high rates of incarceration of people from minority groups (Institute of Race Relations, 2016). As mothers usually take the major responsibility for the daily care of children the impact of incarceration is often amplified. If the mother is incarcerated she is in most instances separated from her children, and the father frequently does not take any responsibility for the children. If the father is incarcerated the mother is required to care for the children with minimal financial or emotional support. Geller, Garfinkel, Cooper and Mincy (2009) found that families with an incarcerated parent experienced severe hardship that often included unemployment and poor health. Women prisoners are more likely to come from situations of poverty, eat unhealthy diets and have lower levels of education than the population overall (AIHW, 2015; Sutherland, 2013).

A significant issue is the intergenerational cycle of offending and imprisonment evident amongst some families with a parent who has been incarcerated (Farrington, Ttofi, Crago & Coid, 2015). This is often related to impaired parenting behaviours (Raudino, Fergusson, Woodward & Horwood, 2013). Children observe their parents' criminal acts and violent behaviour. They learn antisocial behaviour rather than the pro-social behaviour that is required to support the development of self-regulation and an enduring secure relationship between parent and child (Bowlby, 1988; Raudino et al., 2013). While not all incarcerated women lack self-regulation (self-control), those that do experience self-regulatory difficulties have a reduced ability to provide sensitive, appropriate and timely parenting to their infants, placing children at risk of abuse. These mothers lack the skills to use strategies to reduce conflict and risk-taking (Magar, Phillips & Hosie, 2008). Instead conflict may escalate into impulsive, explosive and frequently dangerous behaviours that result in incarceration (deWall, Baumeister, Stillman & Gailliot, 2007). The potential for a trajectory of antisocial and criminal behaviour often starts early for children with incarcerated parents, and may be exacerbated by low family incomes, mental health problems, and irregular or poor schooling experiences. It is important to understand that incarcerated mothers have often had limited exposure to supportive or appropriate parenting themselves. Over 17 per cent of women in NSW prisons had experienced their own parents' incarceration and nearly one-third had been placed in care before the age of 16 (Indig et al., 2010).

The following sections focus on the issues experienced by incarcerated mothers during pregnancy and the postnatal period, and the impact on the mother and her infant and young children. Parenting programmes are discussed and implications for practice and research explored. Examples aim to aid reflection on the multiple and complex issues faced by incarcerated mothers.

Pregnancy

Pregnancy brings an added dimension to the lives of incarcerated women as they anticipate the birth of their babies. Incarceration during pregnancy induces significant stress and places this group of women at high risk of adverse maternal and fetal outcomes (Mukherjee, Pierre-Victor, Bahelah & Madhivanan, 2014; Shaw, Downe & Kingdon, 2015). Many of these women continue to engage in risky health behaviours such as smoking, drug and alcohol use and may not have accessed antenatal care prior to incarceration (Mukherjee *et al.*, 2014; Sutherland, 2013; Walker, Hilder, Levy & Sullivan, 2014).

Pregnant incarcerated women are likely to have high levels of depression and anxiety (AIHW, 2015). While imprisonment provides opportunities for health interventions, perinatal outcomes are often poorer given their existing disadvantages and the impact of mental health issues, substance use disorders and smoking during pregnancy (AIHW, 2015; Mukherjee *et al.*, 2014; Shaw *et al.*, 2015). An Australian retrospective cohort study using linked health data found that incarcerated pregnant women had poor pregnancy or neonatal outcomes. Their babies were more likely to be born prematurely, have low birth weight and require hospitalisation compared to community controls, consistent with data from the UK and USA (Walker *et al.*, 2014).

In most developed countries, incarcerated women have ready access to midwives and other psychological and medical care to monitor the pregnancy, and their mental and physical health. The relationship with a midwife is important as it provides professional support and advocacy for the mother and infant. Some pregnant women are transferred to prisons with adjacent hospitals prior to labour. While beneficial for maternity care, this may mean they are removed from being in close proximity to other children or family members, making visits expensive and difficult. Labour and birth can be an isolating and frightening experience. Women are not always allowed to have a support person or prison midwife present, increasing their stress and resulting in higher levels of pain. In some countries this is changing. For example, in the UK, a local charity Birth Companions provides support for incarcerated women during pregnancy, birth and the postnatal period (Marshall, 2010).

For many incarcerated pregnant women, a major stressor is the issue of who will care for their new-born infant and how soon they will be separated following birth, causing additional emotional distress (Eloff & Moen, 2003; Huang, Atlas & Parvez, 2012). Some infants are placed into the care of members of the mother's family; others are placed in temporary foster care. A small number of infants are permanently removed from their mothers' care. Permanent removal of a child into out-of-home care does not usually occur simply because the woman is in prison. Loss of permanent custody of the infant is usually due to this infant or other children being identified as abused or at high risk of abuse or neglect. Children are often removed due to continued use of illegal substances resulting in the mother's inability to safely care for them (Doab, Fowler & Dawson, 2015) (see Chapter 8 for further insights into substance misuse amongst perinatal women).

Some incarcerated women are required to make very difficult decisions about their pregnancy and their baby. For example, in the following story Mae had to make a decision about keeping her baby or relinquishing her child for adoption. As you read the following story think about the care and information you would provide Mae if you were a healthcare professional working in the prison system:

- How would you assist her manage this situation?

- What information would you provide Mae to prepare for the birth of her child and the early post-partum period? Consider both her emotional and physical needs.

Case study: Mae

Mae was born in Vietnam and obtained a short-term visa to study at an Australian university. Her boyfriend encouraged her to supplement her finances by helping him sell drugs within the local Vietnamese community. Mae and her boyfriend were arrested. She was sentenced to four years in an Australian prison, then deportation to Vietnam after her sentence. When arrested Mae was four months pregnant.

After consultations with a prison psychologist, Mae decides to have her baby adopted. Mae is reluctant to contact her parents about the pregnancy and imprisonment, as she fears they will disown her when she returns to Vietnam. She will not be able to financially care for her baby in Vietnam as a single mother.

The midwife provides Mae with regular antenatal care, monitoring her pregnancy and mental health. The midwife is concerned about Mae's mental health state and refers Mae to the prison psychiatrist who prescribes medication for depression. The mental health nurse provides ongoing counselling and monitors Mae's medication.

Postnatal period

Many incarcerated mothers are separated from their babies within hours of birth if they gave birth in a local hospital, as they are returned to prison to continue their sentence. Most infants are released to family or foster carers in the community, although some require admission to a neonatal intensive care unit to treat neonatal abstinence syndrome (Kanwaljeet & Campbell-Yeo, 2015) before being released to their carers.

This separation is extremely traumatic, especially if women have not received appropriate emotional support during the pregnancy, labour and birth (Andersen, Melvaer, Videbech & Lamont, 2012; Hodnett, Gates, Hofmeyr & Sakala, 2013). The provision of psychological support can vary in both availability and quality between prisons and countries. Crucially, this separation from her infant can exacerbate the woman's existing mental illness and distress (Celinska & Siegal, 2010). Mothers who were able to have some control over who cared for their children were found to experience less role strain than mothers who were not given the same opportunity (Celinska & Siegal, 2010).

Enabling incarcerated mothers to be with their infants during the first hours and days after birth is essential to strengthen the maternal bond. They can get to know the smell and movement of the baby and ideally learn to breastfeed (Bowlby, 1988; Eloff & Moen, 2003; Huang, Atlas & Parvez, 2012). Breastfeeding can help incarcerated women make the transition to motherhood (Huang *et al.*, 2012) through developing the mother–infant bond and a responsive relationship (Oxford & Findlay, 2015). In the occasions when breastfeeding may not be possible, it is crucial for mothers to have early and extended contact and to feed the infant.

One option for mothers with new-born infants is residence in a mother baby unit, or prison nursery, available to women with a low security risk. Infants and babies can live with their mothers up to school age and, thereafter, can come to stay for weekends and school holidays. However, access to these units in Australia as in many countries is often limited – if appropriate facilities even exist. For instance in NSW, a committee reviews the feasibility of the baby staying with the mother, considering the child's safety, vacancies within the unit and the mother's security category (Hyslop, 2009).

In the following story, Julie is provided with an opportunity to care for her new-born. While reading the story reflect on:

- your beliefs and feelings about allowing infants to stay with their incarcerated mothers;
- whether all incarcerated mothers should be provided with the opportunity to care for their infants while incarcerated;
- the experience of the infant while with their incarcerated mother.

Case study: Julie

Julie has four children with two different fathers, ranging from 16 years to 6 months. Julie was sentenced for four and a half years for 'aggravated assault with intent to rob'. Her 6-month-old daughter Susie was with foster carers who brought her to visit once a month. The other children have been permanently removed from Julie's care because of her drug addiction and violent behaviour. Julie has not had any contact with the older children for several years.

There is a mother baby unit at the prison where Julie is located and she requested to be housed there with her baby once a vacancy occurred. Since entering prison Julie has been compliant with the prison rules and she has willingly attended anger and addiction management programmes. The unit committee agreed for her to move to the unit, on condition that she continues to attend the anger and addiction management programmes and a parenting programme. Julie's interaction with her baby is closely monitored and she has regular review meetings with the child protection workers responsible for Susie's safety. The child and family health nurse (similar to health visitors in UK) monitors Susie's growth and development during her monthly child health check visits.

Impact of incarceration on mothers and children

Incarceration causes a loss of control and power to make everyday decisions that women are used to making about their daily activities and their children. In prison, the day's activities are governed by the need to maintain control and security within the prison community. Decisions about what the prisoners wear, how they structure their day, and who they can associate with are restricted and closely monitored.

Crucially, this control of their lives includes whether or not women are able to have access to their children. Their access is often limited for numerous reasons beyond their control, as illustrated in the following story about Sally.

Case study: Sally

Sally has two young children who are being cared for by their paternal grandmother. Sally's partner is also in prison for drug offences. The children are living in a small country town five hours' drive from the prison where Sally is incarcerated. The grandmother is reluctant to bring the children to visit, as she does not always have enough money for the train and accommodation in the city. The children can be difficult to manage as they become upset and overwhelmed by the visit to such an alien environment. Grandma finds having to be searched prior to entering the prison confronting and upsetting. She also feels a greater need to visit the children's father, her son. On occasions she has brought the children to visit Sally, but visiting has been cancelled without notice due to a prison security concern. The children are disappointed and return home without seeing their mother.

Sally's experience is common for many incarcerated mothers, causing disappointment and distress. The story illustrates the complex difficulties faced by prisoners and their families.

Mothers sometimes limit or restrict visits by their children and other family members in an attempt to reduce the distress that can be experienced (Celinska & Siegal, 2010). Other mothers make a decision to not tell their young children where they are, to avoid the child experiencing stigma about having a parent in prison. A study of incarcerated mothers found that one-quarter reported that none of their children knew that they were in prison and another 15 per cent had not told all their children (Fowler, Rossiter, Power, Dawson & Roche, 2016). The children are told 'Mummy is sick and in hospital' or 'Mummy has to go away to work'. While this avoidance may work while children are very young, they are likely to feel deceived by their mothers as they grow and become more aware. Children can become extremely angry, further damaging the relationship.

Some mothers have little contact with their children while they are incarcerated. One Australian study found that 41.5 per cent of incarcerated mothers received no visits from their children and less than a quarter (23.1 per cent) had regular visits from all their children. Over one-third rarely or never speak to their children by phone. This compares with incarcerated fathers of whom 32.8 per cent receive no visits (Fowler et al., 2016). This illustrates the particular difficulties that mothers face in keeping in contact with their children. Whereas many incarcerated fathers have a partner (or ex-partner) who can care for their children and potentially arrange visits, this is much less common for incarcerated mothers, whose children are more likely to be placed in foster care or with more distant relatives.

Regardless of the crime or length of sentence, women want to be 'good' mothers (Celinska & Siegal, 2010). This often requires them to be defensive about their use of drugs, alcohol and their parenting style. Yet this is often the behaviour that has been the underlying reason for the separation from their children (Celinska & Siegal, 2010). The reasons women give for being separated from their children often demonstrate limited reflective functioning (also discussed in Chapter 2) as they do not appear to understand the impact their behaviour or lifestyle choices will have on their children. Reflective functioning refers to a parent's capacity to understand their own and others' behaviour in regard to underlying mental states and intentions (Slade, 2005). However, reflective functioning is essential for insightful and sensitive parenting; its absence can disrupt parent–infant communication (Grienenberger, Kell & Slade, 2005) and impact on the ability to develop productive social relationships (Slade, 2005). For example, South African research into mother–child interaction patterns in prison identified that the mothers did not demonstrate insight into how their infants might find certain experiences stressful (Eloff & Moen, 2003).

Impact on the children

There is a growing body of literature about the impact of parental incarceration on children and the importance of maintaining contact between child and parent (Poehlmann, Dallaire, Looper & Shear, 2010). Infants and children can be exposed to discrimination, violence and abuse as an outcome of parental incarceration (Dawson, Jackson & Nyamathi, 2012). They frequently experience unmet material needs and residential instability that often result in behavioural problems (Geller et al., 2009).

The implications and impact of having an incarcerated parent are multiple and complex. Children are at risk of negative academic and social outcomes that frequently include internal and external behavioural problems, substance abuse, truancy, school failure, criminal behaviour and incarceration (Poehlmann et al., 2010). However, there is a lack of rigorous and innovative evidence-based studies of interventions to address the many risk factors facing the children of inmates (Dawson et al., 2012).

For some children, maternal incarceration results in minimal change or disruption as others have cared for them for much of their lives. For other children the incarceration of one or both parents can result in major upheaval, requiring a sudden removal from the familiar surrounds of their home and receiving care from unfamiliar people. Non-kinship or 'looked after' care occurs when no extended family members are willing to take an infant or child for long-term care. The arrangement may lack stability if the children experience numerous changes to their placement during their mother's incarceration. Multiple moves result in disruption, confusion and potential risk of abuse. The separation of infants or young children from their mothers can be compounded by the need to accommodate siblings with different families in geographically distant locations.

Parenting programmes

In recent years, correctional agencies have developed and offered parenting programmes and activities for inmates, acknowledging the impact of incarceration in undermining the critical mother–child relationship (Rossiter, Power, Fowler, Jackson, Hyslop & Dawson, 2015). These parenting programmes increasingly use a relational rather than a behavioural approach. Relational parenting programmes are based on attachment theory and aim to enhance the mother's knowledge of child development. They focus on developing maternal sensitivity and recognition of children's needs. There is no clear evidence that engaging in parenting programmes assists to reduce the recidivism rate. However, it is anticipated that raising mothers' awareness of their parenting behaviour can make a difference to the significant impact of incarceration on their children's behaviour, physical and emotional health and future life prospects (Perry, Fowler & Heggie, 2009). One example is the Mothering at a Distance programme offered for the past ten years in women's correctional facilities in NSW. It provides a relationship-based programme that encourages co-production of knowledge (Perry, Fowler, Heggie & Barbara, 2011) (see Box 9.1 below). The mothers who participated in the programme were able to: identify the unique role they played in their children's lives; develop improved self-image and understanding; experience validation as mothers; and crucially, understand their children's world and experiences and how their children needed them to be available (Rossiter et al., 2015).

Many incarcerated women have limited literacy skills and previously found schooling difficult. Many have only ever experienced a deficit model of education, where failure was common. Parenting classes need to overcome barriers that inhibit women's ability to participate in education. They should be carefully developed to engage women and, whenever possible, use a strength-based approach that builds on existing knowledge rather than highlighting the women's deficits as mothers. These relational parenting programmes recognise the limited exposure many mothers have had to sensitive and responsive parenting (Rossiter et al., 2015).

Ideally the mothers are able to practise these new skills with their children. If infants or young children are able to stay with their mothers within the prison, there can be positive outcomes. A study of the intergenerational attachment of 30 mother–infant dyads raised in a prison nursery (Byrne, Goshin & Joestl, 2010) provided evidence that infants can be raised with secure attachment to their mothers, even though the mother's internal attachment was categorised as insecure, as determined by standard measures of attachment. A nurse practitioner provided an intervention, consisting of weekly visits incorporating: anticipatory guidance for infant development, responsive parenting, maternal life goals and issues of re-entry into the community. Mothers received feedback using videotapes of unstructured play with their children as part of the intervention. On re-entry to the community the mothers received biweekly letters and telephone calls from the nurse for 12 months. Of the study group of infants, 60 per cent were tested post-intervention as having secure attachment. These findings were unexpected, as the researchers had anticipated greater numbers of infants with disorganised attachment. While this study had a limited sample, it demonstrated the benefits that could occur from children being placed within a safe environment where the mother felt supported by prison staff and benefited from regular contact with a nurse who assisted in developing maternal sensitivity and enhancing the mother–infant relationship.

BOX 9.1 MOTHERING AT A DISTANCE

A ten-session programme for pregnant women or women with children aged 0–5.

The programme aims to:

- reduce the distress caused by separation due to incarceration for female offenders and their young children;
- reduce the trauma for young children caused by separation and visiting their mothers in a correctional setting;
- enable women during the short contact period with their young children to develop strategies to:
    - enhance the mother–child relationship;
    - increase maternal sensitivity and appropriate responsiveness to infant's signals;
    - increase ability to reflect on their own and infant's behaviour, thoughts and feelings in regard to attachment – caregiving interactions;
    - build on maternal and infant strengths;
    - increase the mother's knowledge and skills to care for her infant to enhance the positive impact of their current care-giving patterns and behaviours;
    - reduce negative (punitive) parenting interactions;
    - develop pro-social play skills and behavioural management, with the aim of breaking the intergenerational cycle of crime.

The programme uses learning strategies that encourage the women to share their maternal experiences and observations of their children – they co-produce knowledge with the programme facilitators about their children and parenting. The facilitators assist the mothers to reconstruct their understanding of their infant's behaviours from a negative understanding to a more positive developmentally based understanding. Much of the learning occurs while the women do craft activities making presents for their children: jigsaw puzzles, picture frames and books. The programme focuses on asking questions to elicit the women's knowledge within a conversational setting. One mother stated at the end of the programme that she had learnt 'there was more to being a mother than loving your baby' (Perry *et al.*, 2009; Rossiter *et al.*, 2015).

Implications for practice

Incarceration for women can provide improved access to health care. In many developed countries correctional systems' duty of care requires them to provide treatment for drug and alcohol addiction and mental illness, as well as physical health and dental care. Improved nutrition and involvement in physical exercise can contribute to overall improvement in women's health.

Working with incarcerated or recently released mothers requires a delicate balance of supporting the pregnant women, mothers and infants, providing appropriate interventions that are sustainable within a secure environment, and ensuring compliance with security requirements. A broad consensus exists that incarcerated mothers and their infants should not be separated (Albertson, O'Keefe, Lessing-Turner, Burke & Renfrew, 2012). However, there is a lack of adequate mother baby facilities (Albertson et al., 2012). Many correctional systems are already overcrowded and cannot find appropriate safe spaces to accommodate mothers with babies or young children.

Mother baby units also require staff that understand and can support the needs of new mothers and infants, including breastfeeding support. These units require strategies to ensure that young children have regular contact with the outside world, including opportunities that further enrich their lives, for example, experiencing playgroups, preschool, interaction with family members, visits to the park, and access to pets.

Using incarceration as an opportunity to provide interventions that aim to significantly improve maternal behaviour can make a difference in the lives of mothers and their infants (Geller et al., 2009). This is particularly true of parenting programmes that focus on child development, mother–infant relationships and development of maternal sensitivity.

Mothers who have been separated from their infants require regular and sustained opportunities to interact and be with their children. Mothers who have had their children removed to out-of-home care require structured reunification support, staged to ensure that mothers have the capacity to care for their babies. It is especially important to ensure a woman is able to manage her infant or young child's behaviour using sensitive and developmentally appropriate rather than punitive parenting approaches. Where the mother and child have had limited or no contact, reunification plans must foreground the risk of further traumatising the child. The child may have developed strong bonds with existing carers and be distressed by this new separation.

Strength- and relationship-based approaches to work with mothers and their children will enhance the women's maternal and other strengths. However, identifying a woman's strengths is not enough; she will usually require support and encouragement to develop these strengths and put them into action (Feeley & Gottlieb, 2000).

A key strategy is to model the sensitive, appropriate and timely behaviour that provides a style of mothering that most incarcerated women have not experienced as children. This parallel process enables mothers to start forming a new model of parenting (Fowler & McGarry, 2011). Using co-productive approaches to generating parenting knowledge can assist mothers develop confidence and problem-solving capacity (Fowler, Lee, Dunston, Chiarella & Rossiter, 2012). This requires a switch from an expert model of clinical practice to a more exploratory and joint problem-solving approach to working with mothers.

Implications for research

It is important to note that undertaking research within a correctional facility is often extremely difficult due to the constant tension between the need for access to research participants and the need for security. Despite these limitations, research about incarcerated women has increased during the past decade. This is possibly due to the growing interest in early intervention and potential improvements in the life trajectories of infants and their mothers. However, further research is required on interventions that are effective in supporting incarcerated mothers and their infants (Shaw et al., 2015), moving beyond studies of parenting programmes that are descriptive in nature and limited in size.

A useful methodological approach to consider in this setting is Appreciative Inquiry. This approach focuses on the participants' strengths rather than deficits. It enables the exploration of peak experiences and identifies factors that support success (Cooperrider & Whitney, 2001). It also enables researchers to focus on participants' experiences as parents rather than as inmates or criminals.

Conclusion

Having a criminal record should not preclude women from being mothers and maintaining the care of their infants with adequate supports. This is with the proviso that the child remains safe and able to take advantage of the opportunities most families take for granted, that provide for healthy child growth and development.

Incarceration not only punishes a woman but also her children. The correctional system in most countries provides an important service of keeping the community safe. Yet we also need to provide compassionate care for incarcerated pregnant women, mothers and their infants and other children. Many correctional systems are making significant attempts to introduce these changes to provide compassionate and child-friendly care.

Incarceration provides a potential change point or opportunity to make available parenting interventions for women who would normally not willingly interact with health professionals, educators and other government services. In particular, these women fear the removal of their children and are willing to actively participate in programmes in the hope that it will help ensure that they maintain custody of their children on release from prison.

It is unrealistic to think that you will not work with mothers who have been incarcerated or their families. But unless you have been told or are able to develop a trusting relationship and ask the right questions, you may never know of their experience. Working with incarcerated mothers or mothers who have had this experience requires an ability to look beyond the crime and understand the complex life experiences that have resulted in incarceration.

References

Albertson, K., O'Keefe, C., Lessing-Turner, G., Burke, C. & Renfrew, M. (2012). *Tackling health inequalities through developing evidence based policy and practice with childbearing women in prison: A consultation.* Sheffield: Sheffield Hallam University.

American College of Obstetricians and Gynecologists. (2011). Committee Opinions No. 511: Health care for pregnant and postpartum incarcerated women and adolescent females. *Obstetrics & Gynecology, 118*(5), 1198–1202.

Andersen, L., Melvaer, L., Videbech, P., & Lamont, R. (2012). Risk factors for developing post-traumatic stress disorder following childbirth: A systematic review. *Acta Obstetricia et Gynecologica Scandinavica, 91*(11), 1261–1272.

Australian Bureau of Statistics. (2016). *Prisoners in Australia.* Canberra: ABS.

Australian Institute of Criminology. (2016). *Indigenous justice.* Available from: www.aic.gov.au/crime_types/in_focus/indigenousjustice.html [Accessed 15 March 2016].

Australian Institute of Health and Welfare. (2015). *The health of Australia's prisoners: 2015.* Cat. No. 207. Canberra: AIHW.

Bowlby, J. (1988). *A secure base: Clinical application of attachment theory.* London: Tavistock/Routledge.

Byrne, M., Goshin, L. & Joestl, S. (2010). Intergenerational transmission of attachment for infants raised in a prison nursery. *Attachment & Human Development, 12*(4), 375–393.

Celinska, K. & Siegal, J. (2010). Mothers in trouble: Coping with actual or pending separation from children due to incarceration. *The Prison Journal, 90*(4), 447–474.

Cooperrider, D. & Whitney, D. (2001). A positive revolution in change: Appreciative inquiry. *Public Administration and Public Policy, 87*, 611–630.

Corrective Services NSW. (2014). *Children of parents in custody: Facts and figures June 2014.* Sydney: Corrective Services NSW.

Dawson, A., Jackson, D. & Nyamathi, A. (2012). Children of incarcerated parents: Insights to addressing a growing public health concern in Australia. *Children and Youth Services Review, 34*, 2433–2441.

deWall, C., Baumeister, R., Stillman, T. & Gailliot, M. (2007). Violence restrained: Effects of self-regulation and its depletion on aggression. *Journal of Experimental Social Psychology, 43*, 62–76.

Doab, A., Fowler, C. & Dawson, A. (2015). Factors that influence mother-child reunification for others with a history of substance use: A systematic review of the evidence to inform policy and practice in Australia. *International Journal of Drug Policy, 26*(9), 820–831.

Eloff, I. & Moen, M. (2003). An analysis of mother-child interaction patterns in prison. *Early Child Development and Care, 173*(6), 711–720.

Farrington, D., Ttofi, M., Crago, R. & Coid, J. (2015). Intergenerationa: Similarities in risk factors for offending. *Journal of Developmental and Life Course Criminology, 1*, 48–62.

Feeley, N. & Gottlieb, L. (2000). Nursing approaches for working with family strengths and resources. *Journal of Family Nursing, 6*(1), 9–24.

Fowler, C. & McGarry D. (2011). Praxis: The essential nursing construct. In A. Cashin & R. Cook (Eds.), *Evidence-based practice in nursing informatics: Concepts and applications* (pp. 40–50). Hershey, PA: IGI Global.

Fowler, C., Lee, A., Dunston, R., Chiarella, M. & Rossiter, C. (2012). Co-producing parenting practice: Learning how to do child and family health nursing differently. *Australian Journal of Child and Family Health Nursing, 9*(1), 7–11.

Fowler, C., Rossiter, C., Power, M., Dawson, A. & Roche, M. (2016). *Breaking the cycle for incarcerated parents: Towards pro-social parenting. Final report.* Sydney: University of Technology, Centre for Midwifery, Child & Family Health.

Geller, A., Garfinkel, I., Cooper, C. & Mincy, R. (2009). Parental incarceration and child well-being: Implications for urban families. *Social Science Quarterly, 90*(5), 1186–1202.

Grienenberger, J., Kell, K. & Slade, A. (2005). Maternal reflective functioning, mother-infant affective communication, and infant attachment: Exploring the link between mental states and observed caregiving behavior in the intergenerational transmission of attachment. *Attachment & Human Development, 7*(3), 299–311.

Hodnett, E., Gates, S., Hofmeyr, G., & Sakala, C. (2013). Continuous support for women during childbirth (review). *Cochrane Database of Systematic Reviews* (7), 1–118. doi:10.1002/14651858.CD003766.pub5.

Huang, K., Atlas, R. & Parvez, F. (2012). The significance of breastfeeding to incarcerated pregnant women: An exploratory study. *Birth, 39*(2), 145–155.

Human Rights and Equal Opportunities Commission. (1997). *Bringing them Home: National inquiry into the separation of Aboriginal and Torres Strait Islander children from their families.* Sydney: HREOC.

Hyslop, D. (2009). Parenting programs in NSW Women's Correctional Centres. *Australasian Journal of Correctional Staff Development, 4*, 1–6.

Indig, D., Topp, L., Ross, B., Mamoon, H., Border, B., Kumar, S., & McNamara, M. (2010). *2009 NSW inmate health survey: Key findings report.* Sydney: Justice Health.

Institute of Race Relations. (2016). *Criminal justice system statistics.* Available from: www.irr.org.uk/research/statistics/criminal-justice/ [Accessed 10 April 2016].

Kanwaljeet, J. & Campbell-Yeo, M. (2015). Consequences of prenatal opioid use for newsborns. *Acta Paediatrica, 104*, 1066–1069.

Magar, E., Phillips, L. & Hosie, J. (2008). Self-regulation and risk-taking. *Personality and Individual Differences, 45*, 153–159.

Marshall, D. (2010). Birth companions: Working with women in prison giving birth. *British Journal of Midwifery, 18*(4), 225–228.

Mukherjee, S., Pierre-Victor, D., Bahelah, R. & Madhivanan, P. (2014). Mental health issues among pregant women in correctional facilities: A systematic review. *Women & Health, 54*(8), 816–842.

Oxford, M. & Findlay, D. (Eds.). (2015). *Caregiver/parent-child interaction: Feeding manual.* 2nd edition. Seattle, WA: NCAST.

Perry, V., Fowler, C. & Heggie, K. (2009). *Evaluation of the mothering at a distance program.* Sydney: Corrective Services NSW.

Perry, V., Fowler, C., Heggie, K. & Barbara, K. (2011). The impact of a correctional-based parenting program in strengthening parenting skills of incarcerated mothers. *Current Issues in Criminal Justice, 22*(3), 457–472.

Poehlmann, J., Dallaire, D.H., Looper, A., & Shear, L. (2010). Children's contact with their incarcerated parents: Research findings and recommendations. *American Psychologist, 65*(6), 575–598.

Prison Reform Trust. (2015). *Prison: The facts*. Bromley Briefings. Summer 2015. London: Prison Reform Trust.

Raudino, A., Fergusson, D., Woodward, L. & Horwood, L. (2013). The intergenerational transmission of conduct problems. *Society Psychiatry and Psychiatric Epidemiology, 48*(3), 465–476.

Rossiter, C., Power, T., Fowler, C., Jackson, D., Hyslop, D. & Dawson, A. (2015). Mothering at a distance: What incarcerated mothers value about a parenting programme. *Contemporary Nurse, 50*(2–3), 238–255.

Shaw, J., Downe, S. & Kingdon, C. (2015). Systematic mixed-methods review of interventions, outcomes and experiences for imprisoned pregnant women. *Journal of Advanced Nursing, 71*(7), 1451–1463.

Slade, A. (2005). Parental reflective functioning: An introduction. *Attachment & Human Development, 7*(3), 269–281.

Statistics Canada. (2015). Adult correctional statistics in Canada 2013/2014. Available from: www.statcan.gc.ca/pub/85-002-x/2015001/article/14163-eng.htm#a8 [Accessed 17 April 2016].

Sutherland, M. (2013). Incarceration during pregnancy. *Nursing for Women's Health, 17*(3), 225–230.

Walker, J., Hilder, L., Levy, M. & Sullivan, E. (2014). Pregnancy, prison and perinatal outcomes in New South Wales, Australia: A retrospective cohort study using linked health data. *BMC, Pregnancy and Childbirth, 14*, 214.

Wildeman, C. & Western, B. (2010). Incarceration in fragile families. *The Future of Children, 20*(2), 157–177.

10

GIVING BIRTH EARLIER THAN EXPECTED

Mothers whose new-born requires neonatal intensive care

Nancy Feeley

Introduction

A premature birth is one that occurs before 37 weeks of gestation. In the United Kingdom premature birth accounts for 7 per cent of live births (Office for National Statistics, 2014), and the Canadian rate is comparable at 7.7 per cent (Public Health Agency of Canada, 2013). In the United States, the rate is higher with 11.4 per cent of infants born preterm (Centers for Disease Control and Prevention, 2014). Following birth, preterm neonates are admitted to a Neonatal Intensive Care Unit (NICU) for medical care that supports their adjustment to life and bodily functions.

Although both mothers and fathers experience adversity following a preterm birth, most of the research has studied mothers, and much less is known about fathers. Hence, this chapter focuses on the evidence about mothers. The chapter describes the prevalence of psychological distress that they may experience in the midst of this event and afterwards. Factors that place women at risk or protect them from psychological distress are identified. Intervention programmes that are efficacious in promoting their well-being and parenting, as well as innovative models of care that hold promise to do so, are discussed. Lastly, this chapter ends with implications for practice.

Psychological distress among mothers of infants born preterm

There are many aspects of a NICU hospitalisation that mothers may experience as stressful. Preterm infants require hospitalisation for weeks or months, and mothers often experience early and repeated separation from their new-born. The NICU is a critical care environment that utilises medical technology which can limit mother–infant contact, and can be perceived as frightening. Mothers may observe events (e.g. resuscitation) and procedures that cause psychological distress.

Their infant's appearance and responses can also be disturbing. They may also be concerned about the survival or medical status of their infant as indicated in the following quote:

> There was like acute events when you thought she might die, when she gets a tube blocked and they have problems getting a tube in or … so you think she's not going to be able to breathe, she's not going to survive … and you become obsessed with what her saturations are like and it's very stressful watching that and seeing the alarm going off for long periods and seeing it go up and down, that on a day to day is pretty stressful to watch.
>
> (Watson, 2011, p. 1466)

Although parental presence is encouraged in many NICUs, both quantitative and qualitative studies highlight how women feel their role as a mother is restricted when infant care is primarily in the hands of health care professionals (Montirosso, Provenzi, Calciolari & Borgatti, 2012). Mothers may wish to participate in infant care, but are unable to do so to the extent that they desire.

Feelings of guilt, worries about infant health and uncertainty about the future are common and persist after discharge (Ballantyne, Benzies, Rosenbaum & Lodha, 2015; Kantrowitz-Gordon, Altman & Vandermause, 2016). Mothers with other children need to balance their desire to be with their hospitalised infant with the needs of siblings. Mothers themselves may also have health issues after childbirth. Following discharge they confront challenges including frequent medical appointments and the need to perform medical procedures for their infant (Murdoch & Franck, 2012).

Studies have examined different types of stress mothers may experience using two self-report questionnaires. The Parental Stressor Scale: Neonatal Intensive Care questionnaire (PSS:NICU) (Miles, Funk & Carlson, 1993) examines how stressful a parent finds the NICU environment, the infant's appearance and behaviour and restriction of their parenting role during hospitalisation. A meta-analysis examining NICU-stress measured with the PSS:NICU found that parents whose infant weighed less at birth experience greater stress about the alteration of their parental role (Schappin, Wijnroks, Uniken Venema & Jongmans, 2013). Mothers also had higher NICU-stress than fathers, but the effect size was small. A quote from a qualitative study illustrates how stressful some parents find the environment:

> When I walked into this big room with all the incubators and other critically ill little babies, I couldn't focus on just mine. There were so many machines sending out loud beeps. As I walked closer to the corner where they kept my baby, I nearly collapsed. He had so many lines and tubes attached to his tiny body … it was terrible … I just wanted to run away.
>
> (Lee, Long & Boore, 2009, p. 330)

In contrast, the Parenting Stress Index (PSI) is a measure that captures the stress any parent might experience parenting after the postpartum period. A meta-analysis of studies using the PSI found that compared to parents of children born full-term, parents of children born preterm experienced more stress particularly in regard to child behaviour and temperament; however, the effect size was small (Schappin *et al.*, 2013). Although parents of preterm children scored higher, their average score was below the level reflecting high parenting stress.

A systematic review found that rates of postpartum depression are as high as 40 per cent among mothers of infants born before 38 weeks, and at 8 weeks postpartum their risk is 1.6 times greater compared to mothers of full-term infants (Vigod, Villegas, Dennis & Ross, 2010). Furthermore, mothers of infants born before 33 weeks have higher depressive symptoms for 12 months after birth and symptoms did not decrease after discharge.

Less is known about anxiety disorders. Ross's systematic review revealed a prevalence of 4.4–8.2 per cent for generalised anxiety disorder among postpartum women (Ross & McLean, 2006). Much higher rates from 18 to 43 per cent were evident in mothers of NICU infants (Segre, McCabe, Chuffo-Siewert & O'Hara, 2014). A 2003 study was one of the first to suggest that post-traumatic stress disorder (PTSD) might be experienced following preterm birth (Holditch-Davis, Bartlett, Blickman, & Miles, 2003) (for further insights into PTSD following childbirth refer to Chapter 11). Interviews with mothers revealed they re-experienced events that occurred during hospitalisation, avoided reminders of birth and hospitalisation, and experienced symptoms of arousal long after discharge. For example, one mother continued to vividly recall how her new-born appeared to her while hospitalised:

> Just like that bird that had fallen out of the nest. And just laying there ... He just looked so little and frail ... and I still hear the bells and the clinking.
> (Holditch-Davis *et al.*, 2003, p. 165)

In a systematic review of 31 studies, preterm birth was identified to be a risk factor for PTSD following childbirth (Andersen, Melvaer, Videbech, Lamont & Joergensen, 2012). A meta-analysis found that although the prevalence of postpartum PTSD is estimated at 3.1 per cent, the rate of 15.7 per cent in at-risk samples (i.e. women with a psychiatric history, history of trauma or preterm birth) is considerably higher (Grekin & O'Hara, 2014). Moreover, preterm birth and NICU admission had a strong association with postpartum PTSD. Of note, PTSD and postnatal depression (PND) are frequently co-morbid yet few studies assess these concurrently (Soderquist, Wijma, Thorbert & Wijma, 2009). In the few studies of mothers of preterm infants, correlations of 0.5 to 0.8 have been reported (Lefkowitz, Baxt & Evans, 2010; Shaw, Bernard, Deblois, Ikuta, Ginzburg & Koopman, 2009).

Impact of maternal psychological distress

During hospitalisation greater maternal NICU-stress has been related to less maternal visitation and fewer hours of providing skin-to-skin care (Gonya & Nelin, 2013). It is well-established that mothers' interactive behaviour with their infant plays an important role in shaping later child development. Decades of studies show that maternal psychological distress has adverse effects on mother–infant interactions, and this is evident among mothers of preterm infants. Stress and anxiety are thought to interfere with their ability to notice and respond to infant interaction cues (Hsu & Jeng, 2013), and the cues of preterm infants are more difficult to interpret. A further complication is that preterm children are at increased risk for developmental delays and are more reliant on parent interactive behaviour compared to their full-term peers (Erickson, Duvall, Fuller, Schrader, Maclean & Lowe, 2013).

Mothers who are anxious in the early months after birth interact less effectively with their infant in later infancy, and their child has more behaviour problems and poorer cognitive development in early childhood (Feeley, Gottlieb & Zelkowitz, 2005; Zelkowitz & Papageorgiou, 2005). There is some evidence that PTSD symptoms are also associated with less sensitive maternal interactive behaviour (Feeley, Zelkowitz, Charbonneau, Lacroix & Papageorgiou, 2010), and toddler sleep problems (Pierrehumbert, Nicole, Muller-Nix, Forcada-Guex & Ansermet, 2003).

Mothers of preterm infants with depressive symptoms have poorer affective involvement and less positive communication in interactions with their infants (Korja et al., 2008). Maternal depressive symptoms are associated with greater parenting stress (Gray, Edwards, O'Callaghan, Cuskelly & Gibbons, 2013), and poorer cognitive development (Mulder, Carter, Frampton & Darlow, 2014) and greater behavioural and emotional problems among children born preterm (Huhtala et al., 2012).

Risk factors for psychological distress

As mothers experience different types of psychological distress, a longitudinal study examined several types simultaneously including symptoms of depression, anxiety, PTSD and NICU-stress assessed with the PSS:NICU (Holditch-Davis et al., 2015). Based on mothers' scores on these measures during hospitalisation they identified five sub-groups of mothers who had similar patterns of psychological distress. Two groups remained at risk for distress one year after discharge: mothers who had elevated symptoms on all measures, and those with elevated symptoms of both depression and anxiety. Although both group's symptoms decreased initially, in the second half of the first year symptoms increased. Both groups perceived their infant as vulnerable, and their infants were sicker during hospitalisation (Holditch-Davis et al., 2015). Taken together with the studies cited earlier, this evidence suggests that risk for ongoing psychological distress can be predicted during the NICU stay.

Mothers of sicker or more premature infants appear to be at greater risk and their distress can persist.

Evidence shows that risk factors for PND in mothers of preterm infants are reduced support (Vigod *et al.*, 2010) and not living with the infant's father (Garfield *et al.*, 2015). Circumstances surrounding the birth and hospitalisation, as well as health concerns as the child grows, may affect mother's support. They have difficulty relating to parents of term infants as their parenting concerns seem trivial (Kantrowitz-Gordon *et al.*, 2016). Following health professionals' advice, parents often limit contact with family and friends to protect the infant from infection and this can lead to isolation and lack of support (Whittingham, Boyd, Sanders & Colditz, 2014), as reflected in the following quote:

> We were home for three years. They [the children] were in isolation basically in our house. So they weren't allowed in, you know, play groups or preschool of anything like that 'cause their immune systems were so weak.
>
> (Kantrowitz-Gordon *et al.*, 2016, p. 8)

Factors that protect against psychological distress

Support may protect mothers from psychological distress. High satisfaction with support from any source, whether family or friends or professionals, after admission and prior to discharge is associated with an absence of PTSD at discharge (Eutrope *et al.*, 2014). Greater marital satisfaction may protect against psychological distress in the early years (Evans, Whittingham & Boyd, 2012) as reflected in this quote:

> Every night when we left, [my partner and I] talked about it … I think that was good. It was constant communication. And so we weren't afraid to tell each other how we were feeling or what we were feeling. I think that kind of got us through it.
>
> (Smith, Steelfisher, Salhi & Shen, 2012, p. 347)

Support from staff during hospitalisation and follow-up clinic visits after discharge can be important, and take many forms including providing information and referrals to resources, teaching and coaching to learn infant care, emotional support and reassurance (Ballantyne *et al.*, 2015). The impact of these practices is reflected in qualitative data:

> They [the nurses] talked me through holding my baby for the first time. This meant a lot to me, so I didn't panic. I was so worried that I might hurt my baby, they [the nurses] calmed me down. It made the whole thing a lot easier.
>
> (Lee *et al.*, 2009, p. 331)

A positive supportive relationship with NICU staff can protect mothers from psychological distress and promote involvement with their infant. Better mother–staff communication is associated with more days of maternal visitation and greater provision of skin-to-skin care (Gonya & Nelin, 2013). Parent–staff interactions can either constrain or enable parenting as indicated by a meta-synthesis of qualitative study findings on parenting during the NICU hospitalisation (Gibbs, Boshoff & Stanley, 2015). When staff facilitate parent involvement this enables parents to assume and develop their parental role, confidence and their relationship with the infant. On the other hand, parents who have conflictual interactions with staff experience frustration, anger, and distress, and feel blocked from involvement (Gibbs, Boshoff & Stanley, 2015).

Although the impact of NICU architectural design on infants and parents is currently of interest, few well-designed studies examine parents' well-being and results are not consistent. In one study mothers in single family rooms had lower NICU-stress, felt more involved in infant care, reported greater satisfaction and better family centred care compared to mothers of infants in the open ward (Lester et al., 2014). Moreover, greater maternal involvement during hospitalisation was associated with better infant neurobehavioral outcomes at discharge. In contrast in the second study, mothers of infants assigned to a single family room reported more NICU-stress compared to open ward mothers, and their children had poorer language development as toddlers (Pineda et al., 2012). Mother visitation and holding during hospitalisation were associated with better later child cognitive and language outcomes (Pineda et al., 2012). Thus unit design may influence parent psychological distress and involvement; however, the direction of effects is not yet clear.

What interventions might help mitigate psychological distress and improve infant outcomes?

During hospitalisation many units encourage parents to hold their infant in skin-to-skin care. This involves holding the infant upright against their bare chest for an extended period of time. Skin-to-skin or kangaroo care is associated with important benefits for infants including decreased mortality and risk of sepsis, and lower risk for re-hospitalisation (Boundy et al., 2016). It can also have positive effects on mothers. A systematic review found it reduces symptoms of anxiety and depression and promotes positive mother–infant interaction (Athanasopoulou & Fox, 2014). The benefits are also evident from qualitative studies:

> It felt so good; I was sitting in the chair sleeping while he was lying on my chest … They tried to help me bond with him as early as possible, so that I would not keep my distance from him because he was inside the incubator and this made me feel more confident.
>
> (Fegran, Helseth & Fagermoen, 2008, p. 814)

Family centred care (FCC) is an approach to care that involves partnership between staff and parents in the planning and provision of infant care (Griffin, 2006).

Innovative FCC programmes are being proposed that involve a transformation in typical NICU care, and a shift in the roles of health care professionals and parents. Such programmes aim to minimise parent role restriction, and promote autonomy and the development of the parent–infant relationship. In the *Family Integrated Care* model, parents are primary caregivers for the hospitalised infant (O'Brien *et al.*, 2013). After completing training parents provide most of the infant's care, aside from intravenous procedures and medications, at least eight hours per day. The results of a clinical trial to establish efficacy are forthcoming.

Another interesting approach to address parents' needs is peer-to-peer support. Former NICU parents are trained to provide information and support to parents of infants currently hospitalised (Hall, Ryan, Beatty & Grubbs, 2015). The advantages are that former NICU parents can best understand parents' experience, normalise responses, share coping strategies, and provide hope (Ardal *et al.*, 2011). Peer support may be particularly valuable as family and friends may have difficulty providing the support that parents require. Support can be provided face-to-face, over the telephone, in a group, or Internet forums. There is some evidence in the NICU and other contexts that peer support can decrease stress, anxiety and depressive symptoms (Hall *et al.*, 2015; Preyde & Ardal, 2003); however, more studies are needed testing efficacy in the NICU context.

Programmes have been developed to promote mother's psychological well-being particularly during hospitalisation. A meta-analysis of studies of early intervention programmes found that interventions had positive, clinically significant effects on anxiety, depressive symptoms and self-efficacy (Benzies, Magill-Evans, Hayden & Ballantyne, 2013). Education or training (i.e. information-giving, demonstration and practice of skills) was a component of all effective programmes. However, programmes combining education with support (i.e. counselling) were more effective than those consisting of education alone. Education alone had an effect on anxiety, while the provision of support along with stress reduction (i.e. listening and debriefing) was necessary to reduce depressive symptoms. However, none of these interventions had an effect on NICU or parenting-related stress.

Efficacious programmes typically involve additional services beyond usual NICU care. One example is the Mother–Infant Transaction Program (MITP) which was developed and first tested in the United States two decades ago (Achenbach, Howell, Aoki & Rauh, 1993), and more recently evaluated in two other countries. The MITP and modified MITP combine support and training on how to interact sensitively with preterm infants in eight in-hospital sessions plus four home visits. Compared to mothers receiving usual care, Norwegian mothers who received the modified MITP had lower parenting stress when their children were 6 and 12 months, and 2, 3, 5, 7, and 9 years old (Kaaresen, Ronning, Ulvund & Dahl, 2006). Furthermore, follow-up revealed important outcomes for their children such as fewer behaviour problems and better cognitive development at 5 years, and fewer attention problems and better school adaptation at 7 and 9 years (Landsem, Handegard, Ulvund, Tunby, Kaaresen & Ronning, 2015; Nordhov, Ronning, Dahl, Ulvund, Tunby & Kaaresen, 2010; Nordhov, Ronning, Ulvund,

Dahl & Kaaresen, 2012). Australian mothers who received seven sessions of modified MITP in hospital plus two home visits were more responsive in interactions with their infants, and infants were more attentive and alert (Newnham, Milgrom & Skouteris, 2009). Moreover, magnetic resonance imaging of infant's brains showed better white matter microstructure among MITP infants, suggesting that mothers learned to interact with the infant in a way that minimised infant stress (Milgrom et al., 2010). One disadvantage of MITP is that it is time-consuming for parents and providers, and thus costly. Hence despite evidence of efficacy the programme has not been readily adopted in practice.

Another promising programme is Baby Triple P (Positive Parenting Program) for Preterm Infants (Colditz et al., 2015). Triple P is a well-established programme with demonstrated efficacy for parents of children aged 2 to 12 years and was adapted for parents of preterm infants. Eight sessions during hospitalisation with additional sessions up to two years post-discharge focus on establishing a positive parent–infant relationship and sensitive interactions, enhancing parent support and minimising psychological distress. Although feasibility and acceptability for parents have been demonstrated (Ferrari, Whittingham, Boyd, Sanders & Colditz, 2011), efficacy is only now being evaluated.

Efforts have been made to evaluate programmes to address the PTSD symptoms experienced by mothers. A six-session, trauma-based cognitive behavioural therapy programme was effective in reducing both maternal trauma and depressive symptoms five weeks after birth (Shaw et al., 2013a). Education about PTSD, cognitive restructuring, muscle relaxation, and reframing perceptions of the infant and parenting abilities are the main programme components (Shaw et al., 2013b). Of note, an earlier pilot study of a three-session version failed to show effects (Bernard et al., 2011), suggesting that three may be too few.

Assessment of psychological well-being

The National Perinatal Association in the United States convened experts to develop evidence-based recommendations for psychosocial care for NICU parents (Hynan & Hall, 2015) (www.support4NICUparents.org). They recommend that parents be screened for mental health problems in the first week of hospitalisation and prior to discharge. Recommendations point to the importance of assessing both mothers and fathers for various types of psychological distress (Hynan et al., 2015). NICUs with more than twenty beds should have mental health professionals on staff to oversee screening (Hynan et al., 2015).

A number of screening options are proposed including quick screening with two- to four-item questionnaires for depression and PTSD (Gjerdingen, Crow, McGovern, Miner & Center, 2009; Prins et al., 2003) or longer questionnaires such as the Edinburgh Postnatal Depression Scale (Cox, 1994), or Perinatal PTSD Questionnaire (PPQ) (Callahan, Borja & Hynan, 2006), or clinical interview by trained staff. This first step in screening can be delegated to nurses. Positive screens should be followed by a more complex screening by a mental health professional.

Screening should be implemented if referral mechanisms are in place and resources available for further assessment and treatment. Many NICUs provide specialised follow-up care after discharge to assess infant health and development. Given that some parents might experience psychological distress after discharge, screening should also be conducted at these visits.

Implications for practice

- NICU staff play a pivotal role in fostering parent involvement and the development of the parent–infant relationship, and this can impact positively on parent psychological well-being. Staff need to understand the importance of involvement for infant and parent well-being, and should actively promote involvement in care, decision-making and planning for discharge.
- Skin-to-skin care is a relatively simple intervention that promotes the well-being of infants and parents and should be actively encouraged.
- Most mothers who experience psychological distress will not have a mental health disorder. Nevertheless, they may benefit from additional support and resources. During hospitalisation, the support available to mothers and their satisfaction with such should be assessed. Referrals to resources should be needs-based. Support and counselling may be better utilised if provided as routine care to all and readily accessible so mothers do not have to leave the bedside. This may also decrease the stigma associated with mental health care.
- NICU design must encourage parental presence. There must be adequate space for parents at the bedside. Design also needs to take into account the need for parents to interact with one another.
- Meetings for parents to acquire information, voice their concerns, and support one another should be offered during hospitalisation. Peer support programmes should be introduced, and there are recommendations on how these should be operationalised (Hall *et al.*, 2015).
- Parents could be directed to online resources for support such as:
    - March of Dimes – www.shareyourstory.org
        - Forum for parents to share their stories and worries about prematurity.
    - Canadian Premature Babies Foundation – www.cpbf-fbpc.org
        - Information on skin-to-skin care, what to do in the NICU, preparing for discharge, bereavement, and a support forum.
    - European Foundation of the Care of New-born Infants – www.efcni.org
        - Information on preterm birth, breastfeeding, and the rights of parents and new-borns.

Conclusion

Parent involvement and a positive parent–infant relationship is key to the healthy development of children born preterm. Mothers of infants born preterm are at risk of various types of psychological distress, and they may experience symptoms long after childbirth. It is imperative that NICU staff are cognisant of the critical role they play in promoting the parent-child relationship and parent psychological well-being through their promotion of parent involvement. The organisation of care and the design of units also needs to take into account the need to promote parents' presence and involvement.

We know little about what protects parents from the deleterious effects of NICU hospitalisation. Studies are needed that identify factors that explain positive adjustment. Longitudinal studies are also needed that follow parents beyond the first year. Existing programmes are expensive and time-consuming. Thus, there is a pressing need to develop brief programmes that can be integrated into routine care. Finally, compared to mothers, fathers have been less well studied and often feel neglected. To optimise family well-being, more research on fathers and what interventions might be efficacious for them is warranted.

References

Achenbach, T.M., Howell, C.T., Aoki, M.F, & Rauh, V.A. (1993). Nine-year outcome of the Vermont Intervention Program for low birth weight infants. *Pediatrics, 91*(1), 45–55.

Andersen, L.B., Melvaer, L.B., Videbech, P., Lamont, R.F. & Joergensen, J.S. (2012). Risk factors for developing post-traumatic stress disorder following childbirth: A systematic review. *Acta Obstetricia et Gynecologica Scandinavica, 91*(11), 1261–1272.

Ardal, F., Sulman, J. & Fuller-Thomson, E. (2011). Support like a walking stick: Parent-buddy matching for language and culture in the NICU. *Neonatal Network – Journal of Neonatal Nursing, 30*(2), 89–98.

Athanasopoulou, E. & Fox, J.R.E. (2014). Effects of kangaroo mother care on maternal mood and interaction patterns between parents and their preterm, low birth weight infants: A systematic review. *Infant Mental Health Journal, 35*(3), 245–262.

Ballantyne, M., Benzies, K., Rosenbaum, P. & Lodha, A. (2015). Mothers' and health care providers' perspectives of the barriers and facilitators to attendance at Canadian neonatal follow-up programs. *Child: Care, Health & Development, 41*(5), 722–733. doi:10.1111/cch.12202.

Benzies, K.M., Magill-Evans, J.E., Hayden, K.A. & Ballantyne, M. (2013). Key components of early intervention programs for preterm infants and their parents: A systematic review and meta-analysis. *BMC Pregnancy & Childbirth, 13*(Suppl. 1), S10. doi:10.1186/1471-2393-13-S1-S10.

Bernard, R.S., Williams, S.E., Storfer-Isser, A., Rhine, W., Horwitz, S.M., Koopman, C. & Shaw, R.J. (2011). Brief cognitive-behavioral intervention for maternal depression and trauma in the neonatal intensive care unit: A pilot study. *Journal of Traumatic Stress, 24*(2), 230–234.

Boundy, E.O., Dastjerdi, R., Spiegelman, D., Fawzi, W.W., Missmer, S.A., Lieberman, E., Kajeepeta, S., Wall, S. & Chan, G.J. (2016). Kangaroo mother care and neonatal outcomes: A meta-analysis. *Pediatrics, 137*(1), 1–16. doi:10.1542/peds.2015-2238.

Callahan, J.L., Borja, S.E. & Hynan, M.T. (2006). Modification of the perinatal PTSD questionnaire to enhance clinical utility. *Journal of Perinatology, 26*(9), 533–539.

Centers for Disease Control and Prevention. (2014). *Live births by selected demographic and health characteristics: United States and total of 47 revised states and the District of Columbia, 2014 (Table 5) User guide to the 2014 natality public use file.* Available from: ftp://ftp.cdc.

gov/pub/Health_Statistics/NCHS/Dataset_Documentation/DVS/natality/UserGuide 2014.pdf [Accessed 15 April 2016].

Colditz, P., Sanders, M.R., Boyd, R., Pritchard, M., Gray, P., O'Callaghan, M.J., Slaughter, V., Whittingham, K., O'Rourke, P., Winter, L., Evans, T., Herd, M., Adhern, J. & Jardine, L. (2015). Prem Baby Triple P: A randomised controlled trial of enhanced parenting capacity to improve developmental outcomes in preterm infants. *BMC Pediatrics*, *15*, 15. doi:10.1186/s12887-015-0331-x.

Cox, J. (1994). Origins and development of the 10-item Edinburgh Postnatal Depression Scale. In J. Cox & J. Holden (Eds.), *Perinatal psychiatry: Use and misuse of the Edinburgh Postnatal Depression Scale* (pp. 115–124). London: Gaskell.

Erickson, S.J., Duvall, S.W., Fuller, J., Schrader, R., Maclean, P. & Lowe, J.R. (2013). Differential associations between maternal scaffolding and toddler emotion regulation in toddlers born preterm and full term. *Early Human Development*, *89*(9), 699–704.

Eutrope, J., Thierry, A., Lempp, F., Aupetit, L., Saad, S., Dodane, C., Bednarek, N., De Mare, L., Sibertin-Blanc, D., Nezolof, S. & Rolland, A.C. (2014). Emotional reactions of mothers facing premature births: study of 100 mother-infant dyads 32 gestational weeks. *PLoS ONE*, *9*(8), e104093. doi:10.1371/journal.pone.0104093. eCollection 2014.

Evans, T., Whittingham, K. & Boyd, R. (2012). What helps the mother of a preterm infant become securely attached, responsive and well-adjusted? *Infant Behavior & Development*, *35*(1), 1–11.

Feeley, N., Gottlieb, L. & Zelkowitz, P. (2005). Infant, mother, and contextual predictors of mother-very low birth weight infant interaction at 9 months of age. *Journal of Developmental & Behavioral Pediatrics*, *26*(1), 24–33.

Feeley, N., Zelkowitz, P., Charbonneau, L., Lacroix, A. & Papageorgiou, A. (2010). Post-traumatic stress among mothers of very low birthweight infants at 6 months after discharge from the neonatal intensive care unit. *Applied Nursing Research*, *24*(2), 114–117.

Fegran, L., Helseth, S. & Fagermoen, M.S. (2008). A comparison of mothers' and fathers' experiences of the attachment process in a neonatal intensive care unit. *Journal of Clinical Nursing*, *17*(6), 810–816.

Ferrari, A.J., Whittingham, K., Boyd, R., Sanders, M. & Colditz, P. (2011). Prem Baby Triple P a new parenting intervention for parents of infants born very preterm: Acceptability and barriers. *Infant Behavior & Development*, *34*(4), 602–609.

Garfield, L., Giurgescu, C., Carter, C.S., Holditch-Davis, D., McFarlin, B.L., Schwertz, D., Seng, J.S. & White-Traut, R. (2015). Depressive symptoms in the second trimester relate to low oxytocin levels in African-American women: A pilot study. *Archives of Women's Mental Health*, *18*(1), 123–129. doi:10.1007/s00737-014-0437-0434.

Gibbs, D., Boshoff, K., & Stanley, M. (2015). Becoming the parent of a preterm infant: A meta-ethnographic synthesis. *The British Journal of Occupational Therapy*, *78*(8), 475–487. doi:10.1177/0308022615586799.

Gjerdingen, D., Crow, S., McGovern, P., Miner, M. & Center, B. (2009). Postpartum depression screening at well-child visits: Validity of a 2-question screen and the PHQ-9. *Annals of Family Medicine*, *7*(1), 63–70. doi.org/10.1370/afm.933.

Gonya, J. & Nelin, L.D. (2013). Factors associated with maternal visitation and participation in skin-to-skin care in an all referral level IIIc NICU. *Acta Paediatrica*, *102*(2), e53–56. doi:10.1111/apa.12064.

Gray, P.H., Edwards, D.M., O'Callaghan, M.J., Cuskelly, M. & Gibbons, K. (2013). Parenting stress in mothers of very preterm infants: Influence of development, temperament and maternal depression. *Early Human Development, 89*(9), 625–629.

Grekin, R. & O'Hara, M.W. (2014). Prevalence and risk factors of postpartum post-traumatic stress disorder: A meta-analysis. *Clinical Psychology Review, 34*(5), 389–401.

Griffin, T. (2006). Family-centered care in the NICU. *The Journal of Perinatal & Neonatal Nursing, 20*(1), 98–102.

Hall, S.L., Ryan, D.J., Beatty, J. & Grubbs, L. (2015). Recommendations for peer-to-peer support for NICU parents. *Journal of Perinatology, 35 Suppl 1,* S9–13. doi:10.1038/jp.2015.143.

Holditch-Davis, D., Bartlett, T.R., Blickman, A.L. & Miles, M.S. (2003). Post-traumatic stress symptoms in mothers of premature infants. *JOGNN – Journal of Obstetric, Gynecologic, & Neonatal Nursing, 32*(2), 161–171.

Holditch-Davis, D., Santos, H., Levy, J., White-Traut, R., O'Shea, T.M., Geraldo, V. & David, R. (2015). Patterns of psychological distress in mothers of preterm infants. *Infant Behavior & Development, 41,* 154–163. doi:10.1016/j.infbeh.2015.10.004.

Hsu, H.C. & Jeng, S.F. (2013). Differential effects of still-face interaction on mothers of term and preterm infants. *Infant Mental Health Journal, 34*(4), 267–279.

Huhtala, M., Korja, R., Lehtonen, L., Haataja, L., Lapinleimu, H. & Rautava, P. (2012). Parental psychological well-being and behavioral outcome of very low birth weight infants at 3 years. *Pediatrics, 129*(4), e937-e944.

Hynan, M.T., & Hall, S.L. (2015). Psychosocial program standards for NICU parents. *Journal of Perinatology, 35 Suppl. 1,* S1–4. doi:10.1038/jp.2015.141.

Hynan, M.T., Steinberg, Z., Baker, L., Cicco, R., Geller, P.A., Lassen, S. & Stuebe, A. (2015). Recommendations for mental health professionals in the NICU. *Journal of Perinatology, 35*(Suppl 1), S14–18. doi:10.1038/jp.2015.144.

Kaaresen, P.I., Ronning, J.A., Ulvund, S.E. & Dahl, L.B. (2006). A randomized, controlled trial of the effectiveness of an early-intervention program in reducing parenting stress after preterm birth. *Pediatrics, 118*(1), e9-e19.

Kantrowitz-Gordon, I., Altman, M. & Vandermause, R. (2016). Prolonged distress of parents after early preterm birth. *JOGNN – Journal of Obstetric, Gynecologic, & Neonatal Nursing, 45*(2), 196–209.

Korja, R., Savonlahti, E., Ahlqvist-Bjorkroth, S., Stolt, S., Haataja, L., Lapinleimu, H., Piha, J., Lehtonen, L. & PIPARI study group. (2008). Maternal depression is associated with mother-infant interaction in preterm infants. *Acta Paediatrica, 97*(6), 724–730.

Landsem, I.P., Handegard, B.H., Ulvund, S.E., Tunby, J., Kaaresen, P.I. & Ronning, J.A. (2015). Does an early intervention influence behavioral development until age 9 in children born prematurely? *Child Development, 86*(4), 1063–1079.

Lee, S.N., Long, A. & Boore, J. (2009). Taiwanese women's experiences of becoming a mother to a very-low-birth-weight preterm infant: A grounded theory study. *International Journal of Nursing Studies, 46*(3), 326–336.

Lefkowitz, D.S., Baxt, C. & Evans, J.R. (2010). Prevalence and correlates of post-traumatic stress and postpartum depression in parents of infants in the neonatal intensive care unit (NICU). *Journal of Clinical Psychology in Medical Settings, 17*(3), 230–237.

Lester, B.M., Hawes, K., Abar, B., Sullivan, M., Miller, R., Bigsby, R., Laptook, A., Salisbury, A., Taub, M., Lagasse, L.L. & Padbury, J.F. (2014). Single-family room care and neurobehavioral and medical outcomes in preterm infants. *Pediatrics, 134*(4), 754–760.

Miles, M.S., Funk, S.G. & Carlson, J. (1993). Parental Stressor Scale: Neonatal intensive care unit. *Nursing Research*, *42*(3), 148–152.

Milgrom, J., Newnham, C., Anderson, P.J., Doyle, L.W., Gemmill, A.W., Lee, K, Hunt, R.W., Bear, M. & Inder, T. (2010). Early sensitivity training for parents of preterm infants: Impact on the developing brain. *Pediatric Research*, *67*(3), 330–335.

Montirosso, R., Provenzi, L., Calciolari, G. & Borgatti, R. (2012). Measuring maternal stress and perceived support in 25 Italian NICUs. *Acta Paediatrica*, 101(2), 101(2):136–142.

Mulder, R.T., Carter, J.D., Frampton, C.M. & Darlow, B.A. (2014). Good two-year outcome for parents whose infants were admitted to a neonatal intensive care unit. *Psychosomatics*, *55*(6), 613–620.

Murdoch, M.R. & Franck, L.S. (2012). Gaining confidence and perspective: A phenomenological study of mothers' lived experiences caring for infants at home after neonatal unit discharge. *Journal of Advanced Nursing*, *68*(9), 2008–2020.

Newnham, C.A., Milgrom, J. & Skouteris, H. (2009). Effectiveness of a modified mother-infant transaction program on outcomes for preterm infants from 3 to 24 months of age. *Infant Behavior & Development*, *32*(1), 17–26.

Nordhov, S.M., Ronning, J.A., Dahl, L.B., Ulvund, S.E., Tunby, J. & Kaaresen, P.I. (2010). Early intervention improves cognitive outcomes for preterm infants: Randomized controlled trial. *Pediatrics*, *126*(5), e1088-e1094.

Nordhov, S.M., Ronning, J.A., Ulvund, S.E., Dahl, L.B. & Kaaresen, P.I. (2012). Early intervention improves behavioral outcomes for preterm infants: Randomized controlled trial. *Pediatrics*, *129*(1), e9-e16.

O'Brien, K., Bracht, M., Macdonell, K., McBride, T., Robson, K., O'Leary, L., Christie, K., Galarza, M., Dicky, T., Levin, A. & Lee, S.K. (2013). A pilot cohort analytic study of family integrated care in a Canadian neonatal intensive care unit. *BMC Pregnancy & Childbirth*, *13*(Suppl. 1), S12. doi10.1186/1471–2393–2313-S1-S12.

Office for National Statistics Website. Available from: www.ons.gov.uk/ [Accessed 18 March 2016].

Pierrehumbert, B., Nicole, A., Muller-Nix, C., Forcada-Guex, M. & Ansermet, F. (2003). Parental post-traumatic reactions after premature birth: Implications for sleeping and eating problems in the infant. *Archives of Disease in Childhood Fetal & Neonatal Edition*, *88*(5), F400–F404.

Pineda, R.G., Stransky, K.E., Rogers, C., Duncan, M.H., Smith, G.C., Neil, J. & Inder, T. (2012). The single-patient room in the NICU: Maternal and family effects. *Journal of Perinatology*, *32*(7), 545–551.

Preyde, M. & Ardal, F. (2003). Effectiveness of a parent 'buddy' program for mothers of very preterm infants in a neonatal intensive care unit. *CMAJ Canadian Medical Association Journal*, *168*(8), 969–973.

Prins, A., Ouimette, P., Kimerling, R., Cameron, R.P., Hugelshofer, D.S., Shaw-Hegwer, J., Thrailikill, A., Gusman, F.D. & Sheikh, J.I. (2003). The primary care PTSD screen (PC-PTSD): Development and operating characteristics. *Primary Care Psychiatry*, *9*(1), 9–14.

Public Health Agency of Canada. (2013). *Perinatal health indicators for Canada 2013: A report of the Canadian perinatal surveillance system.* Available from: http://publications.gc.ca/collections/collection_2014/aspc-phac/HP7-1-2013-eng.pdf [Accessed 6 February 2016].

Ross, L.E. & McLean, L.M. (2006). Anxiety disorders during pregnancy and the postpartum period: A systematic review. *Journal of Clinical Psychiatry*, *67*(8), 1285–1298.

Schappin, R., Wijnroks, L., Uniken Venema, M.M. & Jongmans, M.J. (2013). Rethinking stress in parents of preterm infants: A meta-analysis. *PLoS ONE*, *8*(2), e54992.

Segre, L.S., McCabe, J.E., Chuffo-Siewert, R. & O'Hara, M.W. (2014). Depression and anxiety symptoms in mothers of newborns hospitalized on the neonatal intensive care unit. *Nursing Research*, *63*(5), 320–332.

Shaw, R.J., Bernard, R.S., Deblois, T., Ikuta, L.M., Ginzburg, K. & Koopman, C. (2009). The relationship between acute stress disorder and post-traumatic stress disorder in the neonatal intensive care unit. *Psychosomatics*, *50*(2), 131–137.

Shaw, R.J., St John, N., Lilo, E.A., Jo, B., Benitz, W., Stevenson, D.K. & Horwitz, S.M. (2013a). Prevention of traumatic stress in mothers with preterm infants: A randomized controlled trial. *Pediatrics*, *132*(4), e886–e894.

Shaw, R.J., Sweester, C.J., St, John. N., Lilo, E., Corcoran, J.B., Jo, B., Howell, S.H., Benitz, W.E., Feinstein, N., Melnyk, B. & Horwitz, S.M. (2013b). Prevention of postpartum traumatic stress in mothers with preterm infants: Manual development and evaluation. *Issues in Mental Health Nursing*, *34*(8), 578–586.

Smith, V.C., Steelfisher, G.K., Salhi, C. & Shen, L.Y. (2012). Coping with the neonatal intensive care unit experience: Parents' strategies and views of staff support. *Journal of Perinatal & Neonatal Nursing*, *26*(4), 343–352.

Soderquist, J., Wijma, B., Thorbert, G. & Wijma, K. (2009). Risk factors in pregnancy for post-traumatic stress and depression after childbirth. *BJOG: An International Journal of Obstetrics & Gynaecology*, *116*(5), 672–680.

Vigod, S.N., Villegas, L., Dennis, C.L. & Ross, L.E. (2010). Prevalence and risk factors for postpartum depression among women with preterm and low-birth-weight infants: A systematic review. *BJOG: An International Journal of Obstetrics & Gynaecology*, *117*, 540–550.

Watson, G. (2011). Parental liminality: A way of understanding the early experiences of parents who have a very preterm infant. *Journal of Clinical Nursing*, *20*, 1462–1471.

Whittingham, K., Boyd, R.N., Sanders, M.R. & Colditz, P. (2014). Parenting and prematurity: Understanding parent experience and preferences for support. *Journal of Child and Family Studies*, *23*(6), 1050–1061.

Zelkowitz, P. & Papageorgiou, A. (2005). Maternal anxiety: An emerging prognostic factor in neonatology. *Acta Paediatrica*, *94*(12), 1704–1705.

11

THE RIPPLE EFFECTS OF A TRAUMATIC BIRTH

Risk, impact and implications for practice

Gill Thomson, Cheryl Beck and Susan Ayers

Introduction

Childbirth is recognised as a significant life-changing psychological event that can lead to enhanced self-efficacy, mastery and competence. However, over the last two decades a number of studies have identified how childbirth can be a deeply distressing, traumatic event, leading to women experiencing post-traumatic stress disorder symptoms (PTSD) and associated adverse impacts on maternal, infant and family functioning. Recent evidence is also emerging on the negative implications of secondary trauma on partners and clinical providers. In this chapter we provide an overview of key issues to help understand what childbirth-related PTSD is, its prevalence and risk factors and the implications of a traumatic birth on women and others. In recognition of how traumatic events have the potential to create positive outcomes, we also highlight how some women can experience post-traumatic growth following a traumatic birth. Finally we reflect on issues concerning the assessment of risk and PTSD onset, interventions to prevent and ameliorate childbirth-related PTSD as well as implications for practice.

What is PTSD?

The recently updated diagnostic criteria for post-traumatic stress disorder (PTSD) in DSM-5 define this condition as an individual having been exposed to a traumatic event (directly or indirectly) when they feel their own or another's life is threatened, and who experience symptoms that cause significant distress from four different symptom clusters: intrusion, avoidance, negative alterations in cognitions and mood, and alterations in arousal and reactivity (American Psychiatric Association [APA], 2013). While these symptoms can be considered to be a normal and adaptive reaction to trauma (Horowitz, 1979), it is when these symptoms continue long-term that problems ensue. The DSM-5 criteria specify that symptoms should continue for more than a one-month period in order to qualify for a diagnosis of PTSD (APA, 2013).

Theoretical frameworks to help understand PTSD onset have been developed, a number of which are briefly considered here. The work of Janoff-Bulman (1992) (also discussed in Chapter 6) is illuminating as she considers that we generally hold beliefs and assumptions that we will not be subject to misfortune and that the world is 'meaningful', 'benevolent' and that we have positive 'self-worth'. When these beliefs are violated (such as through a traumatic birth), our conception of ourselves and others is destroyed, leading to fundamental and often negative alterations in our self-image and interactions with others (Janoff-Bulman, 1992). A cognitive model developed by Ehlers and Clark (2000) suggests that PTSD onset occurs when the traumatic event is processed in such a way that it creates a 'sense of current threat' for the individual – and that this threat is associated with an individual's level of vulnerability (e.g. beliefs, prior experiences, coping abilities), negative appraisal of the event and disrupted memory processes. Whereas the diathesis stress model considers that negative responses (such as those associated with PTSD) occur due to a combination of an individual's vulnerability and when the level of stress experienced exceeds a certain threshold.

Prevalence of a traumatic birth and PTSD

A recent meta-analysis of 78 studies identified that a PTSD diagnosis was 3.1 per cent in all postnatal women and 15.7 per cent in 'at risk' groups (e.g. experienced previous trauma, history of psychopathology; Grekin & O'Hara, 2014). However, rates of PTSD can depend on the population studied, country of residence (which may also reflect the dominant model of maternity care, i.e. biomedical or midwifery) as well as time of measurement. For example, a study by Olde and colleagues in the Netherlands reported PTSD rates of 2.1 per cent at three months (Olde, van der Hart, Kleber, van Son & Pop, 2005) compared to 17.2 per cent at 6–8 weeks in an Iranian study (Shaban, Dolatian, Shams, Alavi-Majd, Mahmoodi & Sajjadi, 2013). PTSD profiles are also usually higher when measured soon after the birth, for instance, Ayers and Pickering (2001) found that prevalence rates decreased from 2.8 per cent at six weeks to 1.5 per cent at six months postpartum. A further noteworthy point is that while the prevalence of childbirth-related PTSD is low, it has been estimated that between 20 per cent and 48 per cent of postnatal women experience PTS symptoms post-birth (Alcorn, O'Donovan, Patrick, Creedy & Devilly, 2010; Ayers, Harris, Sawyer, Parfitt & Ford, 2009; Polachek, Harari, Baum & Strous, 2012; Soet, Brack & DiIorio, 2003).

Risk factors for childbirth-related trauma and PTSD onset

To date two meta-analytic reviews have been undertaken to identify risk factors (Ayers, Bond, Bertullies & Wijma, 2016; Grekin & O'Hare, 2014) and impact

(Ayers et al, 2016) of childbirth-related PTSD in community and 'at risk' samples. The most recent included 50 studies that examined birth-related PTSD factors at least one-month post-birth (Ayers *et al.*, 2016). Pre-birth risk factors were antenatal depression, fear of birth, poor health/complications, history of PTSD and previous counselling for pregnancy or birth-related factors. Birth-related risk factors were negative experiences of childbirth, an operative birth, lack of support and dissociation (mild to severe physical and emotional detachment from the experience). During the postnatal period, birth-related PTSD was significantly associated with high levels of stress and poor coping skills, and had high co-morbidity with depression (Ayers *et al.*, 2016).

The identification of pre-birth vulnerabilities and risk are obviously important to help direct assessment and treatment (discussed below). However, it is also important to reflect that these risks can be exacerbated by poor care practices and negative experiences during childbirth. For some women, the intra-partum events will be the primary reason for their adverse responses. While an 'operative birth' (caesarean or assisted vaginal birth) is a significant predictor of childbirth-related PTSD, qualitative studies of women who had traumatic birth experiences have revealed similar reports among those who had a 'normal' vaginal birth, as well as those who had emergency and unplanned obstetric interventions (Ayers, 2004; Thomson & Downe, 2008). These findings therefore emphasise that it is not only *what* happens during childbirth, but *how* it happens that is important. A meta-synthesis of women's experiences of a traumatic childbirth (which include women's experiences of various delivery modes) highlighted how a lack of informed consent, poor communication and a lack of a relationship with health professionals, and inhumane and degrading care led women to feel 'faceless', invisible and out of control during the labour (Elmir, Schmied, Wilkes & Jackson, 2010) as reflected in the following excerpts:

> I had to grab the midwives hand, I didn't feel like she was there for me at all. The contractions I was having at that time were horrendous and I was sat there on my own, totally coping on my own.
>
> (Thomson & Downe, 2008, p. 270)

> I was screaming, I'll never forget her [midwife] saying: 'Don't be silly now! Pull yourself together'. All I wanted was some reassurance. I'll never forget her words.
>
> (Moyzakitis, 2004, p. 11)

Impact of trauma on mothers and others

Just as ripples spread out when a stone is dropped into a pond a traumatic birth may have consequences that spread out like ripples not only to mothers but also their infants, partners and healthcare providers (see Figure 11.1). In the following

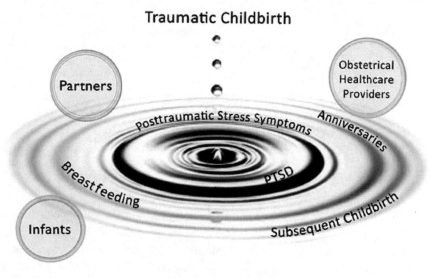

FIGURE 11.1 Ever widening ripple effect of post-traumatic childbirth
Beck, 2015, p. 5.

sections we offer an overview of a series of qualitative studies that illustrate some
of the key impacts of a traumatic birth on these different population groups.

For mothers

In considering the impact on mothers, a number of qualitative studies have
highlighted how women were bombarded with uncontrollable flashbacks and
nightmares of their traumatic births (e.g. Ayers, 2007; Beck, 2004; Beck & Watson,
2008):

> I just kept thinking about it [birth] all the time and I felt like I had some sort
> of car crash or something, I kept getting flashbacks all the time and I found
> it really upsetting.
>
> (Ayers, 2007, p. 17)

Women described the image of their brains having a video recorder in them with
their traumatic births on automatic replay resulting in loop tracks in their brains.
One mother described:

> I lived in two worlds, the videotape of the birth and the 'real' world. The
> videotape felt more real. I lived in my own bubble, not quite connecting
> with anyone. I could hear and communicate, but experienced interaction
> with others as a spectator. The 'videotape' ran constantly for four months.
>
> (Beck, 2004, p. 219)

Women suffering with childbirth-related PTSD explained that due to their numbness they were only a shadow of their former selves. Mothers struggled with a dangerous trio of anger, anxiety, and depression which isolated them from the world of motherhood that they had dreamed of:

> At night I tried to connect/acknowledge in my heart that this was my son and I cried. I knew that there were great layers of trauma around my heart. I wanted to feel motherhood. I wanted to experience and embrace it. Why was I chained up in the vice-like grip of this pain? This was my gethsemane – my agony in the garden.
>
> (Beck, 2004, p. 222)

Beck and Watson's (2008) qualitative study identified how the impact of traumatic childbirth on breastfeeding was found to be one of two possible pathways. One path facilitated breastfeeding as the women turned their traumatic event into a positive experience for themselves and their infants. Women shared how they needed to prove to themselves and to others that they could do something right (i.e. breastfeeding) after 'failing' at giving birth. They were unyielding in their steadfastness to make atonement to their infants:

> Breastfeeding became my focus for overcoming the birth and proving to everyone else and mostly to myself that there was something that I could do right. It was part of my crusade, so to speak, to prove myself as a mother.
>
> (Beck & Watson, 2008, p. 233)

Other women travelled down the second path that hindered their breastfeeding attempts (Beck & Watson, 2008). There were multiple reasons for this. For some mothers their need was to protect their bodies from further violations, and these mothers became vigilant about protecting their breasts. Women did not want clinicians handling their breasts in attempts to initiate breastfeeding. Intrusive thoughts and flashbacks to their birth trauma while breastfeeding caused great distress, and for some women, this led to a difficult decision to discontinue breastfeeding:

> The flashbacks to the birth were terrible. I wanted to forget about it and the pain so stopping breastfeeding would get me a bit closer to my 'normal' self again.
>
> (Beck & Watson, 2008, p. 234)

Difficulties with subsequent pregnancies and births can be another long-term detrimental effect of a previous traumatic birth. Some women delay a further pregnancy following a traumatic birth (Thomson & Downe, 2010) and others make a conscious and difficult decision to not have a further child (Ayers, Eagle & Waring, 2006; Nicholls & Ayers, 2007) thereby disrupting their family ideal.

However, for those women who do become pregnant again, the nine long months of pregnancy can be filled with terror, panic, and denial as women wait for what they fear the most: the possibility of another traumatic birth. One mother who had not planned a second pregnancy recalled the exact moment she knew she was pregnant again:

> I was on my lunch break at work, sitting under a large oak tree, watching cars go by my office, talking with my husband. I suddenly knew ... I am pregnant again! I remember the exact angle of the sun, the shading of the objects around me. I remember looking into the sun, at that tree, at the windows to the office thinking, 'NO! God PLEASE NO!' I felt my chest at once sink inward on me and take on the weight of a 1000 bricks. I was short of breath, my head seared. All I could think of was NOOOOOOOOO!
>
> (Beck & Watson, 2010, p. 245)

For infants

Another ripple effect of a traumatic childbirth is on the mother–infant relationship (also refer to Chapter 10 which discusses the impact of having a premature infant on mother–infant interactions). While some quantitative studies have not found an association between PTSD symptoms and the quality of parent–infant relationships (e.g. Nicholls & Ayers, 2007) qualitative research has suggested otherwise. Some mothers shared how they had disturbing detachment from their infants as reflected in the following quote:

> I didn't feel I was connected with her at all ... I didn't feel anything. That took a very, very long time ... for the actual bonding to occur.
>
> (Moyzakitis, 2004, p. 11)

A long-term impact of traumatic childbirth occurred around anniversary time (i.e. the child's birthday). In Beck's (2006) study mothers revealed that it was not only the actual day but also the weeks leading up to the anniversary which were an agonising time. A recurrence of flashbacks and nightmares could occur, along with an array of distressing emotions such as dread, anxiety, and guilt. Complicating this prologue was the fact that mothers knew it should be a day of celebration. Flare-ups of the mother's detachment towards their infants could also occur, as reflected by a woman recalling her daughter's first birthday:

> I wanted to die. I felt nothing for her and found it hard to celebrate the joy of this child that meant so little to me. I took excellent care of her but it was as if I was babysitting. The emotional bond just wasn't there.
>
> (Beck, 2006, p. 386)

For partners

Other qualitative studies have revealed how birth trauma can have negative implications for women's relationships with their partners, as well as for the fathers themselves. Some women described how they blamed their partners for events that occurred during the birth, as well as how the traumatic event had impacted on their sexual and intimate relationships (Ayers *et al.*, 2006; Nicholls & Ayers, 2007):

> There have been times when I felt I want to leave and just take the baby and not be with him anymore and it's not because I don't love him. It's because I don't feel that I can give him any more.
>
> (Ayers *et al.*, 2006, p. 394)

A synthesis of qualitative findings of father's experiences of a complicated, and potentially traumatic birth undertaken by Elmir & Schmied (2016) revealed accounts of fear, anxiety, and a sense of inadequacy and powerlessness. A father from a study in one of the included papers reported:

> When [my wife] was in there having the operation, it was like, this is not the way it should be … suddenly you've got no real control of what is happening … and you're just completely overwhelmed. You have no control, no input.
>
> (Nicholls & Ayers, 2007, p. 497)

Men recounted a lack of information and miscommunication with health professionals which often exacerbated their negative emotions. Furthermore, following the birth, fathers' experienced flashbacks and nightmares, and disclosed deleterious impacts on their relationships with their partners (Elmir & Schmied, 2016).

For maternity care providers

Secondary traumatic stress in maternity healthcare providers is also starting to be reported. Beck conducted mixed methods studies with labour and delivery nurses (Beck & Gable, 2012) and certified nurse-midwives (Beck, LoGiudice & Gable, 2015) who had attended traumatic births. These studies revealed that 26 per cent of the labour and delivery nurses and 36 per cent of the certified nurse-midwives screened positive for meeting all the diagnostic criteria of the DSM-4 for PTSD (APA, 1994). The first UK-based study to explore this phenomenon also revealed similar rates, with 32 per cent of midwives experiencing PTSD symptoms (Sheen, Spiby & Slade, 2015). Qualitative insights highlight how healthcare providers can be haunted by secondary traumatic stress symptoms as the following quote illustrates:

> Each traumatic birth adds another scar to my soul. Sometimes I tell my husband that I feel like the picture of Dorian Grey. Somewhere my real face

is in a closet and it reveals the awful things I've seen during my labour and delivery career. The face I show the world is of an aging woman who works in this lovely place called a delivery room where happy things happen.

(Beck & Gable, 2012, p. 756)

The vicarious experience of observing and attending a traumatic birth led some maternity professionals: to feel responsible and frustrated with existing maternity services; to have a negative impact on their capacity to provide care to other women; and to a number of professionals either wanting to, or had left maternity care practice (Beck & Gable, 2012; Beck et al., 2015; Rice & Warland, 2013).

Post-traumatic growth in mothers

Post-traumatic growth is the 'positive psychological change experienced as a result of the struggle with highly challenging life circumstances' (Tedeschi & Calhoun, 2004, p. 1). There are five possible dimensions of growth: appreciation of life, relating to others, personal strength, new possibilities, and spiritual change (Tedeschi & Calhoun, 1996). To date three quantitative studies have been conducted on post-traumatic growth in mothers from community samples using the Post-traumatic Growth Inventory (PTGI; Tedeschi & Calhoun, 1996). The findings report that 35 per cent-50 per cent of mothers had experienced small/ moderate levels of growth, with the 'appreciation of life' being the most endorsed dimension (Sawyer & Ayers, 2009; Sawyer, Ayers, Young, Bradley & Smith, 2012; Sawyer, Rados, Ayers, & Burn, 2015).

Beck and Watson (2016) conducted a phenomenological study of 15 mothers who perceived they had experienced some aspects of personal growth after their traumatic childbirth. Four themes explained their experiences. The first theme was 'opening oneself to a new present'. One mother shared that her journey of post-traumatic growth was 'much like the agony a butterfly suffers as it fights through its chrysalis'. Another mother revealed that 'I was broken. Now I am unbreakable'. Women felt that surviving their traumatic childbirth made them stronger due to heightened levels of trust and confidence in themselves. It provided them with a feeling that they can survive anything. The second theme was 'achieving a new level of relationship nakedness' as connections with their partners, children, family, and friends were deepened. 'Fortifying spiritual-mindedness' was the third theme whereby some mothers experienced a stronger faith. One mother disclosed how she had learned to embrace her traumatic birth because it kept her connected to God. The fourth and final theme was 'forging new paths' in their lives. New personal and professional goals developed as a result of women's growth, such as enrolling in universities to seek a new career often in the health care arena, such as nursing. A further area was in devoting themselves to volunteer work as part of mothers' positive life changes. Women felt the need to help other women who have experienced birth trauma through volunteering for organisations such as the Birth Trauma Association (www.birthtraumaassociation.org.uk).

Primary, secondary and tertiary treatment

If we can identify the main risk factors for PTSD following childbirth it should be possible to prevent and treat a large proportion of PTSD. Prevention and intervention can be primary, secondary or tertiary. Primary interventions aim to prevent PTSD by identifying women with key vulnerability and risk factors in pregnancy and adapting their antenatal and intra-partum care to minimise the potential for trauma and PTSD to arise. An example is outlined by Olander, McKenzie-McHarg, Crockett and Ayers (2014) who evaluated a system where vulnerable women had a special sticker attached to the front of their maternity notes and information was put within their notes about their specific needs with regard to emotional well-being and maternity care. Healthcare professionals in the hospital were trained in perinatal mental health and provided trauma-informed care. Thus all healthcare professionals who came in contact with vulnerable women were immediately alerted to their vulnerability and needs. The results showed that the proportion of referrals to psychology services for birth trauma reduced from 34 per cent to 19 per cent over the first seven years of this system being in place.

Secondary interventions aim to reduce the development of PTSD by identifying women at high risk after birth. These might include women who found birth traumatic or who show early symptoms of trauma, such as dissociation during labour or PTSD-like symptoms immediately after birth. An example of this is midwife debriefing where women are offered an opportunity to discuss their birth experiences with a midwife or obstetrician, usually with their medical records available. A randomised control trial of a midwifery-led intervention was undertaken by Gamble, Creedy, Moyle, Webster, McAllister and Dickson (2005). At-risk women received telephone counselling at 72 hours and six6 weeks postnatal, leading to reduced trauma and depression symptoms and feelings of self-blame when compared to those in the control group (Gamble *et al.*, 2005). However, debriefing has attracted some controversy because there is wide variation in what is provided under the title of 'debriefing' and little robust evidence of its effectiveness. A Cochrane review of randomised controlled trials found no evidence that midwife debriefing had a positive or negative effect in preventing psychological trauma following childbirth, but also noted the heterogeneity of research and overall lack of high quality evidence (Bastos, Furuta, Small, McKenzie-McHarg & Bick, 2015). In contrast, a narrative review of the literature on debriefing concluded that, although it might not reduce morbidity, women respond positively to it and value the service (Baxter, McCourt & Jarrett, 2014).

Other possible secondary interventions are the use of self-help techniques. For example, there is emerging evidence that expressive writing might be beneficial after birth. Two studies suggest it might be helpful for mothers of babies needing special care. Barry and Singer (2001) evaluated expressive writing with women whose babies were in intensive care in the USA, and found that severe distress reduced from 37 per cent to 16 per cent in the group who used expressive writing. Similarly, Horsch and colleagues found that expressive writing reduced symptoms of PTSD and depression in mothers of very preterm infants (Horsch, Tolsa, Gilbert, du Chene, Muller-Nix & Graz, 2015). A series of studies in Italy also found that women who wrote expressively about their labour and birth experiences in the first week after birth had fewer PTSD symptoms postpartum (Di Blasio & Ionio, 2002; Di Blasio, Ionio & Confalonieri, 2009; Di Blasio *et al.*, 2015).

Tertiary interventions aim to treat women with PTSD and lead to recovery. Clinical guidelines recommend the use of trauma-focused therapy, such as trauma-focused cognitive behaviour therapy (CBT) or eye-movement desensitisation and reprocessing (EMDR) because of their evidence of effectiveness in other populations (Bisson, Roberts, Andrew, Cooper & Lewis, 2013). However, to date there has been no evaluation of such therapies for postpartum PTSD. Case studies of CBT and EMDR for women with postpartum PTSD have been published that suggest it is acceptable to women, but do not give a measure of efficacy (Ayers, McKenzie-McHarg & Eagle, 2007; Sandstrom, Wiberg, Willman, Wikman & Hogberg, 2008).

Assessment of birth trauma/PTSD

Most primary, secondary and tertiary interventions rely on accurate identification of women at risk or who have PTSD. Assessment is therefore critical but unfortunately this is an area where there is very little research. First, to assess women for risk we need to know what the main risk factors are and how best to assess these. While meta-analytic reviews (Ayers *et al.*, 2016; Grekin & O'Hare, 2014) have identified key risk and vulnerability factors (discussed above), consideration of how these could be used in practice to identify at-risk women have not yet emerged.

One of the barriers to screening for childbirth-related PTSD post-partum is that very few validated questionnaires are available. Research in this area has typically adapted questionnaires designed for other groups, such as war veterans, which may not be as applicable to women after birth. Two questionnaires have been developed specifically for PTSD in pregnancy or post-birth: the Traumatic Events Scale (Wijma, Soderquist & Wijma, 1997) that follows DSM-4 diagnostic criteria (APA, 1994) can be used in pregnancy to measure PTSD symptoms related to the upcoming birth (version A), or after birth to measure postpartum PTSD symptoms (version B). This measure has been widely used in perinatal research and has good face validity but has not been tested psychometrically. Other measures have been developed for specific groups, such as the Perinatal PTSD Questionnaire (Quinnell & Hynan, 1999) for parents of preterm babies and the Childbirth Trauma Index for adolescent mothers (Anderson, 2011) but neither of these follow diagnostic criteria. Recent changes to diagnostic criteria made in DSM-5 (APA, 2014) also mean previous questionnaires used with perinatal women are outdated. Currently only one measure exists that follows DSM-5 and was developed with perinatal women (Ayers *et al.*, in prep). This measure has reasonable psychometric properties but has not yet been validated against clinical interviews, which are seen as the gold standard.

Implications for practice

The best remedy against trauma is to prevent it from happening in the first place. This could be achieved by ensuring that sensitive, woman centred care is provided by known care provider(s) who can provide continuity of care. However, it also requires maternity care providers to be cognisant of how the language they use and the way in which care is provided can have a detrimental impact on women's experiences. Women who are at risk/have experienced a traumatic birth are also often unwilling to disclose their concerns (to professionals or members of their personal networks) due to fears of stigma, judgement and blame; leading women to feel socially isolated, and avoiding contact with healthcare providers. It is therefore imperative that these women receive extra attention and support. Despite the paucity of evidence, we offer a framework of prevention and intervention that could be considered to prevent and protect against PTSD onset following childbirth (Figure 11.2).

A number of implications based on qualitative insights and targeted to women, partners and professionals are detailed below:

- Appropriate assessments should be undertaken with women in the antenatal period to establish any prior history of trauma (birth or otherwise) or psychopathology. As women may struggle in making sensitive disclosures, repeated opportunities to explore these issues should be sought.
- Care pathways (which could incorporate the intervention by Olander *et al.* (2014) described above) should be introduced to alert and ensure that all care providers (antenatal, intra-partum and postnatal) are cognizant of the women's needs.

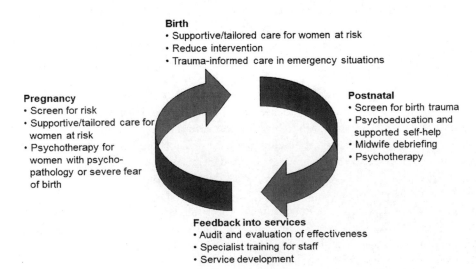

Birth
- Supportive/tailored care for women at risk
- Reduce intervention
- Trauma-informed care in emergency situations

Pregnancy
- Screen for risk
- Supportive/tailored care for women at risk
- Psychotherapy for women with psycho-pathology or severe fear of birth

Postnatal
- Screen for birth trauma
- Psychoeducation and supported self-help
- Midwife debriefing
- Psychotherapy

Feedback into services
- Audit and evaluation of effectiveness
- Specialist training for staff
- Service development

FIGURE 11.2 Prevent and intervention in perinatal care

- To offer non-judgemental opportunities for parents to discuss the birth with maternity providers in the immediate and later postnatal period as well as during a subsequent conception (with validation and recognition of concerns and opportunities to understand what happened during the birth reported to have salutary effects, e.g. Thomson and Downe (2010)).

- Low-level interventions could be introduced by informing parents (verbally and/or in written form) of potential trauma-related responses, and the normalcy of such to help ease their concerns, together with information on where and how to access support should they need it.

- Flexible support pathways should be provided to enable women (including those who are identified as at risk during pregnancy and those who have experienced a traumatic birth) to access different types of support, when they need it, and for as long as they require it. Ideally this could include a range of support options such as:

  - Access to support groups or online forums (such as the Birth Trauma Association in the UK (www.birthtraumaassociation.org.uk/) or Trauma and Birth Stress (TAB) in New Zealand (www.tabs.org.nz/).
  - Encouraging women to engage in self-help options, such as expressive writing or online self-supported counselling treatments.
  - Counselling/psychology services such as CBT.
  - Homeopathic remedies.
  - Care plans to be co-constructed with women and maternity professionals to discuss and consider how relationship-based and maternity care should be provided.
  - Increased antenatal and postnatal contacts with maternity providers.
  - Opportunities to visit/re-visit the birth environment (i.e. delivery suite, operating theatre) – together with appropriate support to discuss their concerns.

- Observations of mother–infant interactions (such as breastfeeding or general interactions) to assess maternal sensitivity and responsivity may prove beneficial to identify concerns.

- Due to implications of secondary trauma for partners, opportunities to engage, involve and inform them at all stages (during their partner's subsequent conception) should be ensured.

- Further training is needed for maternity care providers to raise awareness about how care should be provided (e.g. perinatal mental health, trauma-informed care). Continuing education is also needed regarding their risk for secondary traumatic stress as well as suitable support (such as via peer support, or access to more specialist services) to help decrease stress responses (also refer to Chapter 13 for further insights into how to promote resilience amongst maternity care providers).

Conclusion

Childbirth-related trauma has been described as the 'uninvited birth companion' (Polachek *et al.*, 2012). An apt term when considering how its impact ripples out to all connected to the birth. While there are new insights into the positive psychological growth that can occur following a traumatic birth, this is an area where further research is needed. Overall, the prevalence of childbirth-related PTSD is low, although many more women can experience sub-clinical PTSD symptoms post-birth. On one hand it could be argued that this is due to women's pre-birth vulnerabilities. On the other hand, there is evidence from meta-analytic reviews and qualitative insights that '*how*' the birth occurs plays an important part in women's internalisation of the event and her subsequent responses. These layers of complexity thereby support the need for further work to identify the direct, mediating and unique risk factors that contribute to postpartum PTSD (Grekin & O'Hara, 2014).

Currently, the lack of validated instruments for assessing postpartum PTSD and risk factors is a critical barrier in accurately identifying women at risk or with PTSD. While there are plenty of opportunities for interventions to prevent and treat postpartum PTSD, the evidence to support any particular treatment is sparse. We have offered implications for practice largely based on qualitative accounts of what women/partners/professionals would have or did find beneficial. A number of these, as well as presumably many other possible interventions have yet to be evaluated.

Currently there are multiple areas where further research is needed. A paper written by an international collaboration of clinicians and academics offers numerous recommendations for different directions, such as longitudinal studies to assess the impact of childbirth-related PTSD, interventions to ameliorate stress in maternity care providers and to improve mother-infant bonding (McKenzie-McHarg *et al.*, 2015). Despite this being a relatively new and fast evolving area of study, the fact that childbirth-related trauma/PTSD is recognised as a real phenomenon with widespread negative consequences, the motivation and impetus to prevent and protect against trauma will continue.

References

Alcorn, K.L., O'Donovan, A., Patrick, J.C., Creedy, D. & Devilly, G.J. (2010). A prospective longitudinal study of the prevalence of post-traumatic stress disorder resulting from childbirth events. *Psychological Medicine*, *40*, 1849–1859.

American Psychiatric Association. (1994). *Diagnostic and statistical manual of mental disorders.* 4th edition. Washington DC: American Psychiatric Association.

American Psychiatric Association. (2013). *Diagnostic and statistical manual of mental disorders.* 5th edition. Washington, DC: American Psychiatric Association.

Anderson, C. (2011). Construct validity of the childbirth trauma index for adolescents. *Journal of Perinatal Education*, *20*(2), 78–90.

Ayers, S. (2004). Delivery as a traumatic event: Prevalence, risk factors, screening & treatment. *Clinical Obstetrics & Gynecology, 47*(3), 552–567.

Ayers, S. (2007). Thoughts and emotions during traumatic birth: A qualitative study. *Birth, 34*(3), 253–263.

Ayers, S. & Pickering, A.D. (2001). Do women get post-traumatic stress disorder as a result of childbirth? A prospective study of incidence. *Birth, 28*(2), 111–118.

Ayers, S., Bond, R., Bertullies, S. & Wijma, K. (2016). The aetiology of post-traumatic stress following childbirth: A meta-analysis and theoretical framework. *Psychological Medicine, 46*(6), 1121–1134.

Ayers, S., Eagle, A. & Waring, H. (2006). The effects of postnatal PTSD on women and their relationships: A qualitative study. *Psychology, Health & Medicine, 11*(4), 389–398.

Ayers, S., Harris, R., Sawyer, A., Parfitt, Y. & Ford, E. (2009). Post-traumatic stress disorder after childbirth: Analysis of symptom presentation and sampling. *Journal of Affective Disorders, 119*, 200–204.

Ayers, S., McKenzie-Harg, K. & Eagle, A. (2007). Cognitive behaviour therapy for postnatal post-traumatic stress disorder: Case studies. *Journal of Psychosomatic Obstetrics & Gynaecology, 28*(3), 177–184.

Ayers, S., Wright, D.B. & Thornton, A. (in prep). Validation of a diagnostic measure of postpartum PTSD: The City Birth Trauma Scale (City BiTS).

Barry, L.M. & Singer, G.H. (2001). Reducing maternal psychological distress after the NICU experience through journal writing. *Journal of Early Intervention, 24*(4), 287–297.

Bastos, M., Furuta, M., Small, R., McKenzie-McHarg, K. & Bick, D. (2015) Debriefing interventions for the prevention of psychological trauma in women following childbirth. *Cochrane Library,* doi:10.1002/14651858.CD007194.pub2.

Baxter, J.D., McCourt, C. & Jarrett, P.M. (2014). What is current practice in offering debriefing services to postpartum women and what are the perceptions of women in accessing these services: A critical review of the literature. *Midwifery, 30*(2), 194–219.

Beck, C.T. (2004). Post-traumatic stress disorder due to childbirth: The aftermath. *Nursing Research, 53*, 216–224.

Beck, C.T. (2006). The anniversary of birth trauma: Failure to rescue. *Nursing Research, 55*, 381–390.

Beck, C.T. (2015). Middle range theory of traumatic childbirth: The ever-widening ripple effect. *Global Qualitative Nursing Research, 2*, 1–13.

Beck, C.T. & Gable, R.K. (2012). Secondary traumatic stress in labor and delivery nurses: A mixed methods study. *Journal of Obstetric, Gynecologic, and Neonatal Nursing, 41*, 747–760.

Beck, C.T. & Watson, S. (2008). Impact of birth trauma on breast-feeding: A tale of two pathways. *Nursing Research, 57*, 228–236.

Beck, C.T. & Watson, S. (2010). Subsequent childbirth after a previous traumatic birth. *Nursing Research, 59*, 241–249.

Beck, C.T. & Watson, S. (2016). Post-traumatic growth following birth trauma: 'I was broken. Now I am unbreakable'. *MCN: American Journal of Maternal Child Nursing, 41*(5), 264–271.

Beck, C.T., LoGiudice, J. & Gable, R.K. (2015). A mixed methods study of secondary traumatic stress in certified nurse-midwives: Shaken belief in the birth process. *Journal of Midwifery & Women's Health, 60*, 16–23.

Bisson, J.I., Roberts, N.P., Andrew, M., Cooper, R. & Lewis, C. (2013). Psychological therapies for chronic post-traumatic stress disorder (PTSD) in adults. *Cochrane Library.* doi:10.1002/14651858.CD003388.pub4.

Di Blasio, P.D. & Ionio, C. (2002). Childbirth and narratives: how do mothers deal with their child's birth. *Journal of Prenatal & Perinatal Psychology & Health*, *17*(2), 143–151.

Di Blasio, P.D., Caravita, S.C.S., Ionio, C., Milani, L., Valtolina, G.G. & Camisasca, E. (2015). The effects of expressive writing on postpartum depression and post-traumatic stress symptoms. *Psychological Reports: Mental & Physical Health*, *117*(3), 1–27.

Di Blasio, P.D., Ionio, C. & Confalonieri, E. (2009). Symptoms of postpartum PTSD and expressive writing: A prospective study. *Journal of Prenatal & Perinatal Psychology & Health*, *24*(1), 49–65.

Ehlers, A. & Clark, D.M. (2000). A cognitive model of post-traumatic stress disorder. *Behaviour Research and Therapy*, *38*, 319–345.

Elmir, R. & Schmied, V. (2016). A meta-ethnographic synthesis of fathers' experiences of complicated births that are potentially traumatic. *Midwifery*, *32*, 66–74.

Elmir, R., Schmied, V., Wilkes, L. & Jackson, D. (2010). Women's perceptions and experiences of a traumatic birth: A meta-ethnography. *Journal of Advanced Nursing*, *66*(10), 2142–2153.

Gamble, J., Creedy, D., Moyle, W., Webster, J., McAllister, M. & Dickson, P. (2005). Effectiveness of a counselling intervention following a traumatic childbirth: A randomized controlled trial. *Birth*, *32*(1), 11–19.

Grekin, R. & O'Hara, M.W. (2014). Prevalence and risk factors of postpartum post-traumatic stress disorder: A meta-analysis. *Clinical Psychology Review*, *34*(5), 389–401.

Horowitz, M.J. (1979). Psychological response to serious life events. In V. Hamilton & D.M. Warburton (Eds.), *Human stress and cognition: An information processing approach* (pp. 237–265). Chichester: Wiley.

Horsch, A., Tolsa, J.F., Gilbert, L., du Chene, L.J., Muller-Nix, C. & Graz, M.B. (2015). Improving maternal mental health following preterm birth using an expressive writing intervention: A randomized controlled trial. *Child Psychiatry & Human Development*, *47*(5), 780–791.

Janoff-Bulman, R. (1992). *Shattered Assumptions: Towards a new psychology of trauma*. New York: The Free Press.

McKenzie-McHarg, K., Ayers S, Ford, E., Horsch, A., Jomeen, J., Sawyer, A., Stramrood, C., Thomson, G. & Slade P. (2015) Post-traumatic stress disorder following childbirth: an update of current issues and recommendations for future research. *Journal of Reproductive and Infant Psychology*, *33*, 219-237

Moyzakitis, W. (2004). Exploring women's descriptions of distress and/or trauma in childbirth from a feminist perspective. *Evidence Based Midwifery*, *2* (1), 8–14.

Nicholls, K. & Ayers, S. (2007). Childbirth-related post-traumatic stress disorder in couples: A qualitative study. *British Journal of Health Psychology*, *21*(4), 491–509.

Olander, E.K., McKenzie-McHarg, K., Crockett, M. & Ayers, S. (2014). Think pink! A pink sticker alert system for women with psychological distress or vulnerability during pregnancy. *British Journal of Midwifery*, *22*(8), 590–595.

Olde, E., van der Hart, O., Kleber, R.J., van Son, M.J., Wijnen, H.A. & Pop, V.J. (2005). Peritraumatic dissociation and emotions as predictors of PTSD symptoms following childbirth. *Journal of Trauma Dissociation*, *6*(3), 125–142.

Polachek, I.S., Harari, L.H., Baum, M. & Strous, R.D. (2012) Postpartum post-traumatic stress disorder symptoms: The uninvited birth companion. *The Israeli Medical Association Journal*, *14*(6), 347–353.

Quinnell, F.A. & Hynan, M.T. (1999). Convergent and discriminant validity of the perinatal PTSD questionnaire (PPQ): A preliminary study. *Journal of Traumatic Stress*, *12* (1), 193–199.

Rice, H. & Warland, J. (2013). Bearing witness: Midwives experiences of witnessing traumatic birth. *Midwifery, 29*(9), 1056–1063.

Sandstrom, M., Wiberg, B., Willman, A.K., Wikman, M. & Hogberg, U. (2008). A pilot study of eye movement desensitisation and reprocessing treatment (EMDR) for post-traumatic stress after childbirth. *Midwifery, 24*(1), 62–73.

Sawyer, A. & Ayers, S. (2009). Post-traumatic growth in women after childbirth. *Psychological Health, 24*, 457–471.

Sawyer, A., Ayers, S., Young, D., Bradley, R. & Smith, H. (2012). Post-traumatic growth after childbirth: A prospective study. *Psychology and Health, 27*, 362–377.

Sawyer, A., Rados, S.N., Ayers, S. & Burns, E. (2015). Personal growth in UK and Croatian women following childbirth: A preliminary study. *Journal of Reproductive and Infant Psychology, 33*, 294–307.

Shaban, Z., Dolatian, M., Shams, J., Alavi-Majd, H., Mahmoodi, Z. & Sajjadi H. (2013). Post-traumatic stress disorder (PTSD) following childbirth: Prevalence and contributing factors. *Iranian Red Crescent Medical Journal, 15*(3), 177–182.

Sheen, K., Spiby, H. & Slade, P. (2015). Exposure to traumatic perinatal experiences and post-traumatic stress symptoms in midwives: Prevalence and association with burnout. *International Journal of Nursing Studies, 52* (2), 578– 587.

Soet, J.E., Brack, G.A. & DiIorio, C. (2003). Prevalence and predictors of women's experience of psychological trauma during childbirth. *Birth, 30*(1), 36–46.

Tedeschi, R. & Calhoun, L. (1996). The post-traumatic growth inventory: Measuring the positive legacy of trauma. *Journal of Traumatic Stress, 9*, 455–472.

Tedeschi, R.G. & Calhoun, L.G. (2004). Post-traumatic growth: Conceptual foundations and empirical evidence. *Psychological Inquiry, 15*, 1–18.

Thomson, G. & Downe, S. (2008). Widening the trauma discourse: The link between childbirth and experiences of abuse. *Journal of Psychosomatic Obstetrics and Gynecology, 29*(4), 268–273.

Thomson, G. & Downe, S. (2010). Changing the future to change the past: Women's experiences of a positive birth following a traumatic birth experience. *Journal of Reproductive and Infant Psychology, 28*, 102–112.

Thomson, G. & Slade P. (2015) Post-traumatic stress disorder following childbirth: An update of current issues and recommendations for future research. *Journal of Reproductive and Infant Psychology, 33*, 219–237.

Wijma, K., Soderquist, J. & Wijma, B. (1997). Post-traumatic stress disorder after childbirth: A cross sectional study. *Journal of Anxiety Disorders, 11*(6), 587–597.

12

REPRODUCTIVE LOSS AND GRIEF

Hannah Dahlen

> There is a love that begins before birth. There is a love that is unmarked by
> death. There is a love that never ends. This is the love we have for our children.
> It is untouched by wind, rain and sun. Age has no impact on its ferocity, and life
> with all its beauty and pain cannot distract us from it. We have been privileged
> to know this love four times. But there has been a price to pay for this love. The
> price has been a broken heart.
>
> (Dahlen, 2003)

Introduction

When we think of pregnancy and birth we don't usually think of death, or if we
do, it passes fleetingly through our minds, dismissed in an instant as something that
happens to other people – unlucky people. When we think of reproductive loss we
may not consider things such as infertility, miscarriage and termination of pregnancy
as being a part of this. The loss of hopes and dreams are what underpins all these
losses. When we lose someone we have loved we have memories, photos, a
personality, a voice and a touch we once knew that we can mourn. When we lose
a baby, or even the possibility of a baby, we lose a future – not a past. We mourn
shadows of possibility. We chase fragments of dreams. We are haunted by regret
and we are left with the imagined and not the real – what could have been, not
what has been.

Not all losses are equal to all people, but it is not for us to judge the degree or
meaning a loss will hold for someone. The woman who has a miscarriage can be
utterly devastated at losing a much-wanted baby or secretly relieved that an
unplanned pregnancy has not become a reality she was not prepared for. Our
responsibility and our privilege as health providers is to walk the journey with
families, to hold the space and not be the cause of further pain, so that when the

time comes for them to be built back up and to hope again they are not battling scars we have inflicted on them.

When a women and her partner experience loss it creates ripples that impact significantly on family, friends and the community they inhabit. De Frain and colleagues (1991) said, 'the death of a baby is like a stone cast into the stillness of a quiet pool; the concentric ripples of despair sweep out in all directions, affecting many, many people' (De Frain, Jakub & Mendoza, 1991, p. 165). As health workers, and particularly as midwives, we get to witness the despair; we are honoured to wipe the tears; we are privileged to hold those shaking shoulders and we learn to walk through a fog that grief and loss creates in lives. However, knowing what to do and say, and more importantly what not to do and say, is not always so intuitive to us. In this chapter I will explore the experience of loss from my perspective as a mother and a midwife. I examine the definitions and prevalence of loss as well as the research on optimal care. Tips and strategies to help families cope with perinatal loss will also be given.

When the thing you fear most happens to you

For so much of my life when I contemplated the one thing I feared most, that I was sure would crush me beyond redemption, I would know in an instant it was the loss of a child, but I knew it would not happen to me. This was not just based on my imagination or some premonition. At the age of seven and a half I watched my mother's and father's heart break as my only little sister died in their arms at the tender age of three and a half. Death struck such fear into my soul from that time onwards. It broke me down in unimaginable ways. I feared losing everything on the one hand, and yet I felt like nothing more could happen on the other, as I rationalised that I had had my bad luck and the cold finger of fate would now leave me alone and touch another. When I was 22 years of age my brother Sam was electrocuted at work. He was only 21. My world fell apart again. The unthinkable had happened once again. Surely, now I was done with tragedy – and death would look elsewhere for the next unwitting victim.

When I became a mother for the first time at the age of 34 I knew the fear that snakes anew around the heart of a parent. I experienced the subtle stripping away of my protective chest wall and the exposure of my vulnerable heart forever to the potential terrible loss of child. I had never loved so completely and terrifyingly and I could not envisage my life without her. Lydia my firstborn was perfect, she was strong and she was given to us first so we could bear what was to come.

Four years later in 2002 our son Luke was born after a very long labour and an emergency caesarean. He arrived and did not breathe. Two days later we held him in our arms as the ventilator was switched off and I knew there was no celestial tally; there was no justice when it comes to loss, and all the impossibilities so logically dismissed were now possible. Following an autopsy that gave us no answers as to the cause we embarked on another pregnancy three short months later. The desire to fill one's arms defies all logic. You would pluck out your eyes and sever a limb if it meant holding a healthy baby in your arms again – if it meant your only child would have a sibling. One year to the day after we had buried Luke, at almost the same time precisely we gave birth to our second son. Ethan was to be the redemption and reward for our pain but by now I knew what I could no longer communicate in the face of reassuring ultrasounds, that something was very wrong. Ethan was born and also did not breathe. For 11 days as my perfect-looking full-term baby was ventilated he along with my husband and I got tested for every possible condition. Eventually a rare disorder was discovered, one that had an appropriately trained perinatologist undertaken the autopsy on Luke, would have been picked up. While my body told me again and again that things were not right with both boys, numerous ultrasounds told me I was wrong. But I was not wrong – I have learned to trust that voice now. The pain of holding two babies in your arms as they die cannot be communicated adequately. It is a place you never want to be and yet, at that moment, there is no other place you can be. I wrote the following in my diary when reflecting on this:

> My story is not unique. Millions of women through history have walked this road of pain before me, and many will walk the road after me. Their untold stories are not less valuable than mine because they have been lost in the immensity of time. Each story would hold a unique message of pain, guilt, longing, sorrow and at times utter despair. Yet each would also tell us of possibilities, of hope and a love that never ends. Each story would teach us an important lesson – children are not our right in life but a privilege and a blessing. Mostly that blessing is one of joy, but sometimes that blessing is in the form of sorrow. And it is a sorrow like no other. It is a sorrow that unravels your very soul. It leaves you bleeding out the essence of your being until you no longer know where you begin and end, or who you really are.
>
> (Dahlen, 2003)

This story has a happy ending, though all are not as lucky as we were. Following several miscarriages, failed IVF and a termination of pregnancy for yet another abnormality I gave birth to Bronte in 2005. Just before Bronte was born Lydia painted a beautiful picture for her sister (Figure 12.1). It was a sign of hope, as the rainbow is only possible when the sun shines through the rain. It will forever symbolise the journey one takes through grief and loss when supported through one of the hardest times of human suffering.

The facts about perinatal loss

The World Health Organisation (WHO) defines perinatal mortality as the number of stillbirths and neonatal deaths in the first week of life per 1,000 births (from 22 weeks to seven days after the birth) (WHO, 2016). When gestational age is missing then a fetal weight of 500gms and more is taken. These definitions vary around the world. In Australia for example we use 20 weeks and 400gms or more and within

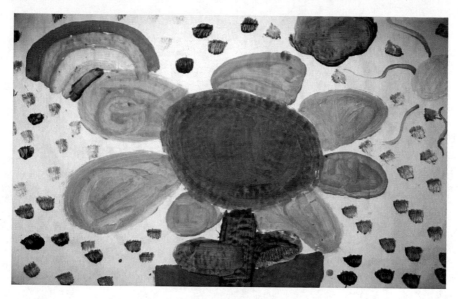

FIGURE 12.1 Lydia's (age 7) picture of hope painted for Bronte

the first 28 days. Germany, Austria, Poland and Slovenia only record fetal deaths with a birthweight >500gms or more. In Hungary and Ireland fetal deaths are registered from 24 weeks of gestation or birthweight >500gms. In Portugal and the UK, while fetal deaths before 24 weeks of gestation are not legally registered, there is voluntary notification of late fetal deaths at 22 and 23 weeks. Greece registers fetal deaths from 24+ weeks. Spain and Catalonia register fetal deaths from 180+ days and 26+ weeks, respectively (Australian Bureau of Statistics, 2013, Euro-Peristat, 2013).

Definitions and prevalence

- *Infertility* – infertility rates are difficult to determine but WHO estimates the rate to be 1:4 couples (WHO, 2016).
- *Miscarriage (15–25 per cent of pregnancies)* – baby born dead before 20 weeks of pregnancy, or weighing <400 g in Australia. In the UK and Europe <22 weeks, or weighing <500gms.
- *Therapeutic termination of pregnancy (TOP)* – pregnancy medically terminated e.g. fetal abnormality incompatible with viability/reasonable quality of life; maternal mental health significantly threatened. Laws around termination of pregnancy vary hugely around the world.
- *Stillbirth (around 7–8 per 1,000 births)* – baby born after 20 completed weeks gestation, or birthweight >400gms, who shows no sign of life at birth in Australia. In the UK and Europe, the cut off is >22 weeks, or weighing >500gms with no signs of life at birth.

- *Sudden unexpected death in infancy (SUDI) – previously sudden infant death syndrome (SIDS) (around 0.5 per 1,000 births)* – death of a neonate or an infant where the post-mortem fails to diagnose cause of death.
- *Infant mortality rate (4 per 1,000 births)* – deaths of babies from birth to one year of age.
- *Perinatal mortality rate (around 10 per 1,000 births)* (Australian Bureau of Statistics 2013; Euro-Peristat 2013):
  - in Australia, measured as rate of babies who die from age 20 weeks' gestation to 28 days after birth, out of 1,000 live and stillborn babies, per year;
  - in New Zealand, rate of babies who die from age 20 weeks' gestation (or 400gms birthweight) to 168 completed hours (7 days) after birth (early neonatal deaths), out of 1,000 live and stillborn;
  - in the UK and much of Europe this is from 22 weeks but another adjusted rate of 28 weeks or birthweight of >1,000gms is used in international reports.

Caring for parents who have suffered a loss

When you cannot take your baby home you may not want to take them into your heart and this is the great dilemma parents face. When I held my dying boys in my arms it was the last place I wanted to be and the only place I could be. It is impossible to explain the pain you experience in doing this. It is almost unbearable but the human spirit is amazing in its capacity to survive. When parents seek to avoid holding their baby and appear to want to move on quickly we need to remember avoidance is simply survival and we should not judge them for it nor do I believe should we force them to do something that at that time does not feel safe for them. Even when they can't be there parents want to know their baby is being cared for and you can reassure them about this with conversations and photos. You need to give parents time to emerge from the shock into the reality. Try to walk their pace rather than at what you think is the right or expected pace as this can help them avoid regret in the long run.

The changing face of perinatal loss care

> Research into perinatal loss shows the aftermath of death includes shock, blame, guilt and hardship; the desperate need to remember; the utility of autopsies and funerals; the burden of irrational and terrifying thoughts; the necessity for adequate support; issues surrounding surviving siblings and subsequent pregnancies; the long journey to healing and the need to reach out and help others in distress.
>
> (De Frain, Martens, Stork & Store, 1990 – cited in
> Donnelly & Dahlen, 2015, p. 1211)

While stories are powerful when it comes to perinatal loss for helping us walk in the shoes of those who have experienced it, it is important we underpin our care with the best scientific evidence. There is no doubt there still remains controversy over how best to care for parents who have experienced a perinatal loss. Before the 1970s health professionals thought it best to shield parents from the pain and trauma by restricting contact between parents and their dead or dying baby (Turton, Evans & Hughes, 2009). Following the 1970s there was a move to letting or even encouraging parents to hold their baby in order to facilitate the grief process (Condon, 1987; Lewis, 1979). Emmanuel Lewis very vividly described how stillbirth was once managed as, 'the rugby pass management of stillbirth ... the catching of a stillbirth after delivery, the quick accurate back-pass through the labor room door to someone who catches the baby' (Lewis, 1979, p. 303). Research followed in the 1980s that demonstrated lower psychological complications six months after the birth if the parents were able to see and hold their stillborn baby (Forrest, Standish & Baum, 1982) encouraging further practice change. The WHO (2003) have also supported this change saying, 'parents of a stillborn baby still need to get to know their baby' and 'separating the woman and baby too soon can interfere with and delay the grieving process'. A survey undertaken through 37 organisations and published in 2008 identified that 90 per cent of parents were now holding their stillborn baby (Cacciatore, Rådestad & Frøen, 2008).

A Lancet *paper raises concerns*

In 2002 a paper was published in the *Lancet* showing women who held and had contact with their stillborn babies had more severe anxiety and depression 12 months following the birth. They also had more disorganised attachment with the next baby following the stillbirth (Hughes, Turton, Hopper & Evans, 2002) (further insights into maternal mental health are discussed in Chapter 2). This paper was published the year I lost Luke and from a personal perspective I agree and disagree with the findings. I agree that holding your baby and walking into the pain of loss unshielded and undenying does lead to worse pain and suffering in the short term. Twelve months is, however, far too early in the grief journey to look at outcomes from this. While initially the pain is so much worse I think in the long run there are fewer regrets and an ability to move on incorporating the pain not fighting it. The publication of the *Lancet* study led organisations such as the National Institute for Health and Clinical Excellence (NICE) in the UK to advise health professionals that women should not be encouraged to hold their baby if they did not want to (NICE, 2007). NICE went further advising parents that 'it is now considered unhelpful for women to see and hold their babies, unless they particularly wish to do so' (NICE 2007). Many health professionals intuitively felt this was wrong as did many of us parents who had experienced the loss of a baby. I did not observe a significant change in practice and this was good because when the seven-year follow up study was undertaken in 2009 we gained more insight into the vulnerabilities that might exacerbate problems. The researchers found that women who held their stillborn baby and had poor perceived support from their partner at the time of the loss were more likely to have a subsequent breakdown in the relationship but no differences in anxiety levels were observed between those who did/did not hold their baby (Turton et al., 2009). The authors themselves recognised the NICE advice had created conflict between established practice and emerging research and that parental characteristics and aspects of care associated with different outcomes required further research so these tensions can be better addressed (Turton et al., 2009). There is no doubt that the loss of a baby increases the risk that the couple's relationship will break down and that men and women may follow different trajectories when it comes to grief. The expansion of support groups for men, such as *Pillars of Strength* (www.pillarsofstrength.com.au/) in Australia following the loss of a baby will hopefully give men the support they need on their own unique journey.

Recent research getting the balance right

In 2008 a study examined effects of women seeing and holding their stillborn baby on the risk of anxiety and depression in a subsequent pregnancy and in the long term (Cacciatore et al., 2008). Over 2,000 women from the USA, UK, Australia and Canada were asked about the contact they had with their baby. Almost 90 per cent of women had held their baby and of these women 99.5 per cent were happy that they did so. The women who did not hold their baby were also asked how they felt about their decision and nearly 80 per cent said they wish they had held the baby. In the Cacciatore et al. (2008) study the researchers found that women who were not pregnant when they answered the survey had lower anxiety symptoms and fewer symptoms of depression when they had held their baby compared to those who were pregnant. Those who were pregnant when they undertook the survey had fewer symptoms of depression but higher anxiety. The authors concluded that seeing and holding a stillborn baby was associated with fewer anxiety and depression symptoms than not doing so, though a subsequent pregnancy may temporarily reverse this (Cacciatore et al., 2008).

Currently there is no level 1 evidence such as from a Cochrane Systematic Review as no eligible trials were found for inclusion (Koopmans, Wilson, Cacciatore & Flenady, 2013). Despite the lack of randomised controlled trials, which one could argue would be unethical in the first place, the authors identified three themes that should be considered when providing care to families following the death of a baby: a deep respect for the individuality and diversity of grief, respect for the deceased child, and recognition of the healing power and resilience of the human spirit.

How should midwives care for a grieving family?

Midwives have a privileged role as they walk beside parents during this very sad time. Judith Murry at a conference in 2008 said 'We [health professionals] sit at the moment when the potential sets in'. This is an incredible responsibility that we need to take seriously. Lundqvist, Nilstun and Dykes (2002) found that a sense of empowerment emerged when health professionals 'saw through the mother's eyes' and 'felt with the mother's feelings' (Lundqvist *et al.*, 2002, p. 192). Women reported feeling empowered when they experienced a sense of nearness, a sense of encouragement and a sense of empathy. They felt powerless when there was a sense of distance, a sense of violation and a sense of disconnection (with similar insights reflected by mothers of premature infants in Chapter 10). While we can never become expert when it comes to death we can learn to become comfortable with being in its presence.

> When birth and death meet we mix two of life's most powerful emotions. Our job is to protect the natural process, to 'midwife' the grief and not to attempt to cure it. We have the choice to be an outsider or insider in grief. Women will know which choice you have made.
>
> (Dahlen, 2003)

Relationships provide safety as they facilitate trusting and respectful relationships between mother/family and midwife (also refer to Chapter 13). In my case I cannot imagine how much more terrible the experience and trauma of the loss of our boys would have been without the wonderful continuity of midwifery care I had. In the pregnancies that followed these losses, not having those same midwives on the journey with us could have meant I would not be here today with the strength to write about this and help others through it. We need more research to show how powerful this relationship potentially is when women lose a baby. The personal stories certainly provide a glimpse into the therapeutic effect.

In a study by Fenwick and colleagues (2007) midwives reported that the most satisfying aspect of midwifery when caring for parents who had experienced perinatal loss was 'connecting with families' and providing what was seen as the 'very best' care. Care was defined as optimal when it included sensitive supportive care, flexible care, response to individual needs, facilitating understanding, creating special memories, listening to and sharing grief, making a positive difference and creating a supportive environment. Midwives found least satisfying the personally challenging experiences, being emotionally overwhelmed, feeling unsure and feeling unsupported (Fenwick, Jennings, Downie, Butt & Okanaga, 2007). A number of top tips (Box 12.1) and do and don't (Box 12.2) to help when engaging with bereaved parents are offered below.

There have been several studies examining critical components of perinatal loss care. Säflund, Sjögren and Wredling (2004) reported on six qualities of care that were important and these were: support in chaos; support in meeting with and separation from the baby; support in bereavement; explanation of the stillbirth; organisation of care of parents and understanding the nature of grief (Säflund *et al.*, 2004). The support from and the emotional attitudes of caregivers was seen as very important in helping parents move through their grief.

BOX 12.1 TOP TIPS IN ENGAGING WITH PARENTS FOLLOWING A PERINATAL LOSS

- Every experience is unique and you can never hope to really understand what someone is going through.
- There is comfort for women in being with those who have gone through what they have, so support groups can help, but this may not be something done straight away.
- Grief paralyses you and families need you to suggest options to them like bathing the baby, taking photos, hand prints and foot prints. Help them create memories (see below for more information).
- When you lose a baby you blame yourself and think others blame you too. You feel like a leper. Don't avoid people who have lost a baby because you don't know what to say. Walk into their grief, wrap them in your arms and tell them you have no words because there really are none.
- Tell women and their partners their baby is beautiful. It does not make it hurt more, it honours their baby.
- Continuity of care is vital and consistency of information is essential.
- You don't ever get over the loss of a baby. There is no expiry date on grief. It will wash over you like a Tsunami at the oddest times.
- Couples don't go on the same journey and the journey may get more diverse as time goes on, not less. This is possibly why marriages are so vulnerable afterwards.
- Fear is a real part of loss and you fear losing everything – it is normal.

BOX 12.2 DO'S AND DON'TS FOR MIDWIVES (DONNELLEY & DAHLEN, 2015, P. 213)

- Make sure you have the time.
- Sit down at the couple's level and use their names.
- Don't be defensive.
- Watch your body language.
- Find out the baby's name first and use it.
- It's okay to cry and touch women as your tears honour the baby, your touch connects you to another and soothes, and your comments reinforce and establish the baby's existence.
- Watch out for technical language.
- Use diagrams.
- Don't hide behind social workers; you are important.

- Don't avoid women as they will think they have done something or that you are trying to hide something, or that nobody cares and this breeds distrust.
- Try and get one person to give the information and make it consistent.
- Don't be positive if you're not and don't be devastating.
- Take your time and don't rush the process.
- It is okay to say 'we don't know'. In the long run this will be respected more than answers forced into the yawning gaps in order to make it better.
- Allow them the opportunity to think about what you have said and offer a contact number or time for a further visit.
- Always ask and don't make decisions on their behalf.

Other research by Kavanaugh and Hershberger (2005) found parents cherished the time they spent with their babies. One woman described the scene as 'a room full of love' (Kavanaugh & Hershberger, 2005, p. 60). It appeared that the creation of memories of their babies, being physically close to them, noticing family resemblances and obtaining keepsakes of the baby were valued highly. Some tips on how to help bereaved parents are detailed in Box 12.3.

BOX 12.3 HELPING TO MAKE MEMORIES (DONNELLEY & DAHLEN, 2015, P. 1214)

To avoid prescribing the parents' grief, use the concept of 'guided participation' (Kobler, Limbo & Kavanaugh, 2007) to quietly do or suggest activities the couple might want to consider which other grieving parents have found helpful:

- Hold their baby's hand. We suggest the midwife consciously behave *as though the baby were alive* (Culling, 2005), gently and courteously taking the baby's hand or holding the baby herself. Seeing this can give the parents confidence and offers a chance to say 'hello' before saying 'goodbye'.
- Hold the baby, lie down with the baby.
- Bathe and dress the baby.
- Take photographs.
- Arrange to take the baby to a place which is special to the family.

Remember, whatever you suggest may be declined, and it can be useful to say to parents that they can slow down, and that in time they may wish to do something they previously felt uncomfortable about doing (Kobler *et al.*, 2007).

Photographs:

- Seek consent before taking any photographs.
- Take lots of photographs with different combinations of family members, e.g. parents and baby; parents, siblings and baby; mother and baby; mother, siblings and baby, etc.
- Digital images have now largely replaced the instant Polaroid photos that fade over time.
- Consider what the baby wears, e.g. make sure the clothes fit or, in the case of a second trimester miscarriage, use a piece of soft material as a wrap.
- Be aware that the skin of babies less than around 24 weeks is translucent (the veins are visible because there is little subcutaneous tissue), red and sticky, so handle the baby carefully.
- Think about where the baby is photographed, e.g. inside a room, outside in the garden, in a Moses basket of a suitable size, lying or propped on a pillow, holding a toy/stuffed animal.
- Avoid having too much white in photographs – it can emphasise the pallor or redness of their skin, e.g. white sheets and a flash-lit exposure can create a stark photograph.
- Think about having a professional photographer, which parents might do to celebrate the arrival of a live baby.

Post-mortems

Raising the issue of post-mortems can be difficult. Sometimes they are a legal requirement if requested by a coroner (e.g. following a sudden unexpected death in infancy). Some families will have cultural and religious considerations we must be aware of. It is important to include interpreters if needed in the discussion when English is not the first language. It is important to address concerns families have about post-mortem as it is a very distressing concept for them and informed consent must be given before it is undertaken. There are often delays in getting reports back to parents and they may need to be prepared that it will not always happen quickly. While ideally the results should be available within six weeks it can be much longer than this. Families often want to know two main things: Why do a post–mortem and what happens in a post–mortem? The answer to these questions is, we do post-mortems in order to try and find out the cause and this may impact other family members and future children, especially if there is a genetic reason as there was in our case. I heard someone once saying to a parent, if you had a family member who needed an operation to help them get better you would not hesitate.

You need to think of a post-mortem as an operation that may help others you love in the future. Post-mortems are undertaken by a skilled doctor and involve incisions to the chest (partial post-mortem) and/or back of the head (full post-mortem). Tissues are examined macro and microscopically with some samples sent for analysis if families give consent. The baby's organs are examined and weighed. These organs are then replaced unless consent has been given for them to be examined further. The incisions are then sutured and covered with a dressing.

Caring for parents in a following pregnancy and birth

One to one care from a known midwife and obstetrician are ideal when caring for couples following a loss. Expect high anxiety, extra visits, concerns over fetal movement, fear and guilt. These are all normal feelings parents experience when they have lost a baby. Often no cause is found and this can make things even worse because it implies it could happen again which of course it could. Don't try and take away the concerns or negate them. Listen, comfort and be there. Don't expect once the baby is born and everything is okay that the worry will stop. It often does not as there is a feeling that something else might go wrong. Fear of sudden unexpected death in infancy may well become the next anxiety. Our job as health professionals is to walk the journey, not to understand it or to grasp it but to accept it is what the parents tell us it is and to provide consistent responsive multidisciplinary care. When I look back at my experience of losing two babies so close together and I know I would not be here strong and well as I am without the continuity of care I received through the pregnancies and births of all four children. Below is an extract from my diary about the care I received:

> Our midwives of life and death came on four incredible journeys with us. The first full of innocence and joy, our Lydia, the second full of worry and sorrow, our Luke, the third full of terror and horror, our Ethan, and the last full of strength and love, our Bronte. I would not take back one laugh or one tear, for mingled together they honour the memories of those who brought them and they define an incredible journey. That journey would have been so much harder without the strength and love that flowed from these two amazing women. They did not claim the joy over the sorrow but fully embraced both. This is a rare gift in a world dedicated to running from pain. My mother called them "the faithful ones". There is no higher honour than this. These incredible women were unafraid to see life in its most raw moments and embrace it all with us, when twice for us 'life and death tripped.' I saw how these experiences undid them both. I felt their pain and numbness as they felt ours. These women taught me much about being a woman, a mother and a midwife – for that I am forever grateful. My memories with them are of tissues and touches, laughter and love, sorrow and serenity, trust and torture, pain and purity, fairies and friendship and beginnings and endings. As we parent our two daughters and cherish the

memories of our sons, we hope the young women we raise will contribute to the universe with the same beauty that these amazing women do.

(Dahlen, 2003)

You don't forget but you do live again

You never forget the losses but you do live again and the moment where this begins is the moment we discover the true meaning of hope. Below is an extract from my diary about how and why we survive a broken heart:

> How do you survive a broken heart? This is a question I have asked myself many times since the deaths of our two sons Luke and Ethan, only a year apart. How do you survive a heart broken, not yet healed and broken again so soon? We survive because there are others we need to survive for – our beautiful daughters, Lydia and Bronte. We survive because of what may be. We survive because as humans we are eternally hopeful in a future we cannot see. We survive because birth and death are forces that move us from the dermis of our superficial half-lives into the deep life-giving marrow of our existence. We survive because that existence has meaning. We survive because not to is a worse option.
>
> (Dahlen, 2003)

Conclusion

Perinatal loss is a reality that has always and will always be with us as humans. When our hearts are breaking we need the soft arms, gentle words and patience of the health providers that go on the journey with us. There is no wrong or right way to grieve and no book that will ever be able to give you the script about how to act. Your role is to walk next to women and their families and guide them and protect them to ensure they have a safe and respectful care while they create precious memories of their baby. We do this best with continuity of care, consistent information and supporting choices along the way. Don't rush grief or the decisions that need to be made. There is no expiry date on grief but we do know with good care, time and understanding most people can have full and meaningful lives following the death of a baby.

> The reality is that you will grieve forever. You will not 'get over' the loss of a loved one; you will learn to live with it. You will heal and you will rebuild yourself around the loss you have suffered. You will be whole again but you will never be the same. Nor should you be the same nor would you want to.
>
> (Kubler-Ross & Kessler, 2005, p. 230).

Future research will hopefully focus on what aspects of care are most effective and what characteristics in parents make them more or less resilience. We also need to understand more about how to care for couples in a future pregnancy and what models work best.

References

Australian Bureau of Statistics. (2013). *Causes of death 2011.* Canberra: ABS.

Cacciatore, J., Rådestad, I. & Frøen, F. (2008). Effects of contact with stillborn babies on maternal anxiety and depression. *Birth, 35*(4), 313–320.

Condon, J.T. (1987). Prevention of emotional disability following stillbirth: The role of the obstetric team. *Australian and New Zealand Journal of Obstetrics & Gynaecology, 27,* 323–329.

Culling, V. (2005) What can midwives learn from bereaved parents? A presentation from SANDS fifth National Conference. Wellington: SANDS.

Dahlen, H. (2003). Personal diaries.

De Frain, J.D, Jakub, D.K. & Mendoza, B.L. (1991). The psychological effects of Sudden Infant Death on grandmothers and grandfathers. *Journal of Death and Dying, 24*(3), 165–182.

Donnelley, N. & Dahlen, H. (2015). Grief and loss during childbearing: The crying times. In S. Pairman, J. Pincombe, J.C. Thorogood & S. Tracy (Eds.), *Midwifery preparation for practice* (pp. 1203–1223). Chatswood, NSW: Elsevier.

Euro-Peristat. (2013). *European perinatal health report: Health and care of pregnant women and babies in Europe in 2010.* Available from: www.europeristat.com/ [Accessed 12 May 2016].

Fenwick, J., Jennings, B., Downie, J., Butt, J. & Okanaga, M. (2007). Providing perinatal loss care: Satisfying and dissatisfying aspects for midwives. *Women and Birth, 20,* 153–160.

Forrest, G.C., Standish, E. & Baum, J.D. (1982). Support after perinatal death: A study of support and counselling after perinatal bereavement. *British Medical Journal, 285,* 1475–1479.

Hughes, P., Turton, E., Hopper, C.D. & Evans, C.D.H. (2002). Assessment of guidelines for good practice in psychosocial care of mothers after stillbirth: A cohort study. *The Lancet,* 360(9345), 114–118.

Kavanaugh, K. & Hershberger, P. (2005). Perinatal loss in low-income African American parents. *Journal of Obstetric, Gynecologic, & Neonatal Nursing,* 34(5), 595–605.

Kobler, K., Limbo, R. & Kavanaugh, K. (2007). Meaningful moments: The use of ritual in perinatal and pediatric death. *American Journal of Maternal Child Nursing,* 32, 288–295.

Koopmans, L., Wilson, T., Cacciatore, J. & Flenady, V. (2013). Support for mothers, fathers and families after perinatal death. *Cochrane Database of Systematic Reviews,* Issue 6. Art. No.: CD000452. doi:10.1002/14651858.CD000452.pub3.

Kubler-Ross, E. & Kessler, D. (2005) *On grief and grieving: Finding the meaning of grief through the five stages of loss.* New York: Scribner Publishers.

Lewis, E. (1979). Mourning by the family after a stillbirth or neonatal death. *Archives of Disease in Childhood, 54*(4), 303–306.

Lundqvist, A, Nilstun, T. & Dykes, A.K. (2002). Both empowered and powerless: Mothers' experiences of professional care when their newborn dies. *Birth, 29*(3), 192–199.

National Institute for Health and Clinical Excellence. (2007). *Antenatal and postnatal mental health: The NICE guideline on clinical management and service guidance.* London: The British Psychological Society and the Royal College of Psychiatrists.

Säflund, K., Sjögren, B. & Wredling R. (2004). The role of caregivers after a stillbirth: Views and experiences of parents. *Birth*, *31*(2), 132–137.

Turton, P., Evans, C. & Hughes, P. (2009). Long-term psychosocial sequelae of stillbirth: Phase II of a nested case-control cohort study. *Archives of Women's Mental Health*, *12*, 35–41.

World Health Organisation. (2016). *Global prevalence of infertility, infecundity and childlessness*. Available from: www.who.int/reproductivehealth/topics/infertility/burden/en/ [Accessed 9 June 2016].

World Health Organisation. (2003). *Managing complications in pregnancy and childbirth: A guide for midwives and doctors*. Available from: http://apps.who.int/iris/bitstream/10665/43972/1/9241545879_eng.pdf [Accessed 9 June 2016].

13

RESILIENCE AND SUSTAINABILITY AMONGST MATERNITY CARE PROVIDERS

Susan Crowther

Introduction

The preceding chapters have explored a variety of complexities experienced by women. This chapter turns to the maternity care providers who provide care in this social, political and emotional milieu on a daily basis. The emotional work of maternity care provision cannot be underestimated (Hunter & Deery, 2009). Contemporary maternity environments have an accumulative psychosocial and biomedical complexity and acuity which create increasing stress for perinatal health providers when supporting women. This is coupled with the growing desire for technological interventions from mothers and families who use the services (McAra-Couper, Jones & Smythe, 2010). With raising birth rates juxtaposed to financially stretched local services and frequent unrealistic staffing ratios in many services, the potential for unhealthy practices and low levels of resilience in order 'to cope' arise in practice reality. There is evidence of increasing burnout, emotional fatigue, depression and subsequent reduction in work satisfaction in the perinatal health workforce (Beaumont, Durkin, Hollins Martin & Carson, 2015; Curtis, Ball & Kirkham, 2003; Govardhan, Pinelli, & Schnatz, 2012; Yoon, Rasinski & Curlin, 2010). This is becoming more evident; for example, the increasing number of midwives choosing part-time work and leaving the profession (Hunter & Warren, 2014). Turning our attention to the psychosocial well-being of the perinatal health workforce is relevant.

The focus needs to be on developing healthy resilient behaviours that nurture and protect the individual and how maternity systems/organisations can both support staff to be resilient to facilitate long-term sustainability. Although the focus in this chapter is largely on midwives the content, suggestions and implications have parallel concerns with other professionals engaged in the perinatal period. This chapter therefore argues for more trans-disciplinary long-term strategies.

Drawing on several studies involving midwives and medical staff the notions of resilience and sustainability are explored. Case studies, based on lived experiences, highlight the tensions in practice which draw out what is within and beyond the everyday practice realities and gesture to best practice that nurtures and sustains optimal psychosocial resilience in maternity care providers.

Background

In contemporary maternity practice there is a relentless expectation for health professionals to provide more and more with seemingly less and less. This is taking its toll on perinatal health providers to the point where newly qualified midwives report that they are 'surviving and not thriving' in their chosen vocation (Fenwick et al., 2012). To address this, there is now a focus on understanding and researching resilient or protective factors across disciplines. The concept of resilience is difficult to define (also discussed in Chapter 2) and there are challenges in understanding the ineffability of how this aspect of human nature reveals itself in individuals and organisations. It is often a quality only appreciated after it has revealed itself and can rarely (if ever) be predicted. Applied to organisations, businesses and individuals, resilience implies that an individual or system needs to be prepared to respond to whatever surprise and disturbance occurs (Folke, 2006).

Sustainability and resilience are emergent notions in maternity care discourse (Crowther et al., 2016). Two midwifery workforce studies have recently defined resilience and sustainability; a United Kingdom (UK) study defines resilience as 'the ability of an individual to respond positively and consistently to adversity, using effective coping strategies' (Hunter & Warren, 2014, p. 927) and a New Zealand (NZ) study defines sustainability as enabling 'something to continue to exist, whilst maintaining the mental and physical wellbeing of the agent' (Gilkison et al., 2015; McAra-Couper, Gilkison, Crowther, Hunter, Hotchin & Gunn, 2014). Hunter and Warren's (2014) study found that being resilient is concerned with dynamism and stability and the capacity to bounce back from times of adversity; qualities regarded as a strength in midwifery. However, this raises concerns.

Workforce interventions to promote resilience are becoming popular. Some criticise these programmes, such as 'resilience training', as a quick-fix solution that does not address fundamental concerns with maternity systems. Leitch & Bohensky (2014) caution that resilience could be an 'aspirational rhetorical device'. I would contend that the constant need to accommodate, adapt and recover from vulnerable situations in terms of personal well-being needs further exploration. Care is required to ensure constructive help is available when required and is not replaced with a set of formulaic principles in the hope that recovery from times of practice adversity is possible. The subsequent expectation could be construed as exploitative as the message could be 'toughen up and get on with your job then you are a real midwife'. This obviously is not the intention of the current growth in resilience training workshops yet this interpretation may have negative implications that cannot be ignored. The 'I can do' stoic mood of many maternity care practitioners may be commendable to a degree but comes at a cost. To cope with whatever one is 'thrown' into without choice and little opportunity for a reprieve is unsustainable and has the potential for propagating adverse psychosocial consequences amongst maternity care providers.

Resilience amongst maternity care providers

Currently there is no agreement on the notion of resilience as applied to the professional workforce. For the purposes of this chapter several case studies using Coutu's (2002) three principal qualities of resilience provide a starting point for discussion:

- Ability and capacity to accept the harshness of reality.
- An ability to improvise and make the best of what resources are available in a given situation.
- The tendency to find meaning in times of adversity.

These qualities are illustrated through the use of experiential examples taken from various studies (Crowther, 2014, 2015; Hunter & Warren, 2014; McAra-Couper et al., 2014). Following this section suggestions for individual and maternity care system psychosocial resilience are offered.

Ability and capacity to accept the harshness of reality

To face the reality of whatever confronts one demands self-awareness and being prepared to meet the worst and deal with it. Childbirth and consequently midwifery is immersed in a world that is inherently unpredictable. Most of the time this is an experience of joy and delight, but on occasions there are traumatic perinatal events which can be harrowing, disruptive and sorrowful (Crowther, 2014). Midwives, for example, have reported post-traumatic stress symptoms (Sheen, Spiby & Slade, 2015) (also refer to Chapter 11) and the effects of exposure to perinatal trauma are exacerbated when there is an unsupportive infrastructure (Calvert & Benn, 2015; Crowther, 2015).

Here Deepa (rural GP) describes how she is thrown into the unpredictable suddenness of a childbirth situation with little expert help nearby:

> By the time I got there this wee one didn't have a line in, they'd actually failed on two attempts. The umbilical vein catheter I tried didn't actually work because the umbilical cord had been cut quite short. I did get a line into the back of the hand and we resuscitated the baby and the chopper did come about an hour later after doing major resus. We were 3 hours away from secondary care. Once I'd got the line in I was really quite thankful. She was only 2.3 kilo baby. I have to say that was probably my closest call for a neonatal resus in this area.
>
> (Crowther, 2015, p. 31)

The 'can do' mood of rural living often serves communities of practice well. It is about using all the skills and help to hand, as another participant in the same study states it is 'all hands on deck'. Yet this is dependent on a willingness to work together in teams locally, be focused and recognise and appreciate what expertise is nearby. This is equally true of other environments and with different outcomes including those that are not as positive as the above example. Simone (midwife working with a mother in hospital) narrates her story with a very different outcome:

> The mother went to the bathroom and didn't come back [long pause] then it was just like white lightening and bright lights and people … [cries]. I just didn't think it would come back like this [crying, interview stopped for 10 minutes]. But when you contextualize it in relation to the beauty of birth and new life and then death enters. The joy was there because the baby was coming; there was no hint that kind of thing was going to happen … the baby could've died, but it didn't. It's almost like it wasn't the baby's time to die, [whispers] but it was the mother's time.
>
> (Crowther, 2014, p. 174)

To face the reality of a situation is contrary to ignoring or/and unquestioningly persevering in adversity despite personal costs. Unhealthy resilience is a bouncing back and coping strategy that does not promote personal well-being. Such 'just keep going' behaviour despite personal consequences is unsustainable long-term. Simone later described how she continued to provide care to the mother's partner and their new-born and spoke about the initial support she received from peers and other members of the hospital team. This interview was six months after the event yet it is evident that the distress of the events remained unresolved and continued to affect her.

Deepa and Simone learn to face the situations confronting them and step up to what is required. This is not possible when that demand is unrelenting and support from others is insufficient or not available. The harshness of the practice reality in maternity care, that can often take an emotional toll on the individual, must be acknowledged and appreciated by the team of professionals and the organisation. The constant need to accept and be competent to meet the unpredictability within maternity services is dependent on trusted local processes, good communication pathways and local support structures.

Ability to improvise and make the best of what resources are available

The ability to continually improvise is another quality of resilience. Chris, a New Zealand midwife, finds herself thrown into a situation requiring immediate improvisation during a lengthy transfer to hospital:

> The car in front just stopped. I was following them in my own car. She got out leaned on the car and pushed and pushed. So there we were on the side

of the road with baby coming. Cars driving past and her bum out to the world! So I throw what I had in my car on the back seat of her car and got her to climb back in onto her knees where she birthed … in some privacy. I just grabbed whatever I had to hand. No way can you plan for that type of thing I just had to deal with it.

(Crowther, 2015, p. 30)

Resilience requires the capacity to accept and face the realities of practice, be realistic and optimise outcomes by whatever is available. This requires flexibility and resourcefulness. Chris is able to improvise on the spot, making the most of what is at hand and delivers the safest skilled care possible in the unexpected situation that she is thrown into. Likewise, the practitioner rushing from one task to the other on a busy yet understaffed labour or postnatal ward needs to improvise and keep care as safe as possible.

As with Deepa above Chris rises to the challenge and adapts. Chris and Deepa have maintained perspective in the face of potential adverse outcomes and demonstrate a level of skill and expertise. To improvise requires a supportive infrastructure and a leadership that cares and acknowledges these times of heightened stress imposed on the team. It is not clear, however, how effective the support is that midwives receive from managers. Particularly when they are working in continuity of care models. Here Sally, another New Zealand rural midwife, shares her story:

So if I am really exhausted I'll pull off the road and have a sleep in the car. Once you've had your birth you're all kind of hyped up and busy and you've got so much to do and then you get in the car and drive; then tiredness hits. I've got a sleeping bag in the car for when this happens. I am set up for this. I've woken up with all sorts of people staring into the car at me. There was a dustbin man at one small town. I had obviously parked my car in front of someone's drive. I was in a pub carpark at one point, I had no idea, but I was so tired I didn't care.

(Crowther, 2016, p. 29)

Sally's story draws attention to the question of personal safety and self-care. Her ability to improvise is not questioned. Sally wants to provide continuity of carer for members of her community. Yet is it sustainable for Sally to be sleeping in the back of her car on the way home from providing intrapartum care? The time, inconvenience, disruption to her personal life and the effects on her psychosocial well-being need addressing. It is important to ask what the manager's role is in this context. Does the manager even know this is occurring?

It is plausible to assume that perinatal health workers practising in different practice settings strive to provide the best care within their local contexts. Sally's story highlights the significance of models of maternity care and service philosophies and how they directly influence the experience of those that work within them.

The drive to make a particular model of care function and remain philosophically aligned to the current discourse in a region is unrealistic when practitioners are sanctioning unsustainable practices. This is not to undermine continuity of carer provision and its proven benefits. It is about ensuring sustainable psychosocial and physical well-being for all perinatal health workers wherever they practice.

Maternity care providers in all settings, models of care and regions constantly need to adapt and meet the unexpected. It is vital that the individual sacrifice and expertise is not invisible to the organisations that regulates, manages and pays them. If these organisations/institutions lack compassion, insight and appreciation of what practitioners do it becomes a recipe for fatigue and system breakdown leaving communities and practitioners vulnerable threatening long-term sustainability of perinatal care provision.

The skills and aptitude of perinatal professionals to cope, even when exposed to adversity and challenge is impressive. They appear to always be on the way to new ways of doing things, developing systems that work better for their communities; even when support from organisations and institutions appears not to be forthcoming, such as lack of individual control over workloads and staff finding ways to ensure breaks on a busy labour ward. To be resourceful, adaptive and have the skill to improvise are certainly qualities worthy of nurturing but balance is required. Self-care, self-awareness and determining what works and does not work locally is crucial. There needs to be recognition by practitioners and those that manage them to be aware of when healthy resilience turns into unhealthy resilience. Alexandra (2013) stated that 'One person's resilience may be another's vulnerability, and one would not want the concept to be used as a means of reinforcing unethical practices or hegemonies' (p. 2714). Persistent unhealthy coping strategies need addressing. Constantly trying to keep up with demands without a pause for reflection may lead to a rigidity of practice that is then unable to adapt and improvise when needed. The consequence of this may be an inability to find meaning in the work they do when times are challenging.

Tendency to find meaning in times of adversity

As previously stated maternity care is unpredictable, there is always going to be unavoidable times of adversity. Coutu (2002) describes how we need to build bridges over present hardships and times of adversity in order to make better futures. The result is making the present moment of adversity feel more manageable and less overwhelming. As human beings we continually interpret and make meaning out of all our experiences (Gadamer, 2008/1967). The following example is taken from my personal reflective diary written in the late 1990s following an adverse outcome:

> I've been involved in an unexpected neonatal death at 3 days old whilst providing postnatal care in the community. It was obviously devastating for all involved. That evening I was called to another birth. It was like swimming

through treacle to attend that birth yet I found solace in the mystery of life as another baby arrived. I relished the depth of relationship I had with these new parents. Joy and sorrow danced around me that night yet somehow I was able to remain grounded in the reality of my work. I desperately wanted to know 'why' and seek some meaning. Later colleagues came to my home and supported me, the next day I sat with the grieving parents and we hugged, cried and spoke of the precious time we shared with their baby before he died. I had never known such a depth of connection with other families. The significance of being alive profoundly touched my soul in new ways. I plan to attend the funeral.

The neonatal death provided me with a depth of understanding about childbirth not previously encountered. That baby boy's death has taken on a rich and lasting meaning for me professionally and personally. I keep a picture of that baby as a remainder of the significance of being with others in this life and the significance of being a midwife. The event strengthened me and made me less vulnerable to the uncertainties that can meet me as a midwife and revealed deeper layers of sensitivity that made me feel stronger. I realised that whatever I do, however honed my skills are, 'things' happen beyond my control and that is bearable. Gaining perspective, seeking out social support and using reflection for self-awareness contributed to my ability to continue and nurture my joy of midwifery practice; attributes that have since been identified in the midwifery sustainability and resilience literature (Crowther et al., 2016; Hunter & Warren, 2014; McAra-Couper et al., 2014).

Creating and nurturing meaning helps practitioners survive professionally and personally. Here Brenda (obstetrician) speaks about the joy of being at an emergency high-risk caesarean section for twins and the meaning of that experience has for her:

> Seeing that baby surviving in a sack and in an instant changing to being an independent little human being was amazing. It is more than the medical stuff to me it's spiritual. There's no laboratory you could cook that up in! It's the gesture or the action that shows us that there is continuity, there's more purpose to life. The fact that it keeps happening with such continuity is a good symbol to us to keep hoping for better things. Birth is a symbol of the continuity of life and gives us value for our lives, giving birth value.
>
> (Crowther, 2014, p. 203)

Despite the emergency nature of the events unfolding Brenda finds meaning. To be working at the start of life gifts Brenda insight and purpose in the work she does. Birth for Brenda is informed by spiritual values that may seem surprising to the outsider. Yet it is deeply felt meaningfulness that inspire and sustain maternity care professionals.

For Lisa, a community-based midwife working in an area of high social deprivation the rewarding part of midwifery practice is supporting and making a difference to women:

> I as one individual can't make a huge difference … and I think you have to
> have an acceptance that you're not going to change the world, but that you
> may be able to make a little bit of a shift and a dent in it.
>
> (Griffiths, McAra-Couper, Nayar, 2013, pp. 226–227)

Lisa accepts her limitations and finds purpose in the small contributions she can
provide to the women in her care despite the enormity of the psychosocial concerns
in her caseload. Finding and having purpose is arguably a psychosocial spiritual
need nurturing positive resilience individually and organisationally. An aligned
philosophical approach amongst midwifery colleagues may provide meaning when
times are challenging (McAra-Couper et al., 2014). However, what remains largely
hidden is the philosophy and 'what matters most' that provides meaning and
inspiration to all individual members of the perinatal health team beyond the
medical and midwifery rhetoric (Crowther, 2014).

Building and sustaining psychosocial resilience

This section focuses on building and sustaining psychosocial resilience in the
perinatal workforce through relationships and shared resonance.

Relationships

Drawing on the studies cited in this chapter, it is apparent that resilience in
maternity care is fundamentally built upon a rich tapestry of relationships attuning
in a way distinctly different to other aspects of healthcare. The joy experienced in
reciprocal relationships with women and families contributes to the meaning of
maternity practice and thus promotes healthy psychosocial resilience. When
reciprocity in relationships is not possible and challenged, either by models of care
or/and workloads the significance of that part of maternity care is brought into the
light. Carol, an obstetrician, who had moved from one model of care to another
(from private obstetric-led caseload practice in the USA to a hospital consultant in
a state hospital without a personal caseload in New Zealand) shares her experience:

> I don't know the women I don't have that relationship with them. So it is a
> much more clinical; someone calls me, I need to assess the situation, I need
> to make a recommendation and get the baby delivered. It's much more
> clinical and the emotional part of it for me about being excited or happy or
> satisfied about a birth, that's much less now, it's changed. It was that
> relationship part of it that was important for me to feel much more
> emotionally involved in births. Whereas now I would say it's much more
> clinical; it's my job to get this baby delivered and as safely as possible.
> Sometimes I feel sad about that sometimes not. I mean it's sort of easier
> emotionally to just walk in, get my job done and go. But, I sort of miss that

emotional part of it too when you have much more invested in these women's lives.

(Crowther, 2014, p. 192)

The loss of reciprocal relationships with the families she works with is missed. She remembers how those relationships were important to her in private practice. Relationships allowed Carol to be more touched by the meaning of birth. Likewise, professional relationships (both inter- and intra-professional) are equally crucial as exemplified by a midwife in Hunter and Warren's study:

> I love being a midwife and learned very early in my career to seek out like minded individuals and also other individuals who I knew would be supportive in certain situations. I also know that others use me for support and that mutuality helps build resilience.
>
> (Midwife 9, Hunter & Warren 2014, p. 931)

Building and sustaining resilience is multifaceted and requires healthy trusting functional relationships. When these relationships break down and professional disputes unfold, it is challenging. Living with conflict between maternity professional groups leads to resentment and potential care being unsafe. Stress and potential for burnout amongst perinatal health providers has been shown to be exacerbated by lack of support and isolation (Patterson, Skinner & Foureur, 2015).

It is apparent that whatever the regional situation, maternity care provision is about creating trust and good working team relationships. One person or professional group cannot retain all information or have all skills required in every situation. The need to work together is essential. Undoubtedly isolated practitioners are developing unhealthy resilient strategies that worsen the situation. Any false dichotomies, battles, conflicts, territorial disputes and boundary protection strategies would appear to impede any chance of resilience building.

Challenging communications and professional disputes create potential for misunderstandings and undermines accessibility to supportive local networks. Good communication and collegial rapport are key to ensuring integrated maternity services that maintain the safety of mothers and babies (Bar-Zeev, Barclay, Farrington & Kildea, 2011). Not addressing discord locally, regionally and nationally, gestures towards unsustainability and unhealthy resilience. The consequences of ongoing discord in communities of practice result in professional burnout (Crowther, 2015). Collaboration and cooperation is needed (also refer to Chapter 14) whilst acknowledging professional agendas, local risks and complexities.

Shared resonance

There is a special resonance or shared mood in maternity that is rarely experienced elsewhere in human life that sustains those involved (Crowther, Smythe & Spence, 2014, 2015). Empathic resonance, in other words, how we 'catch the moods of others' filters through organisations because moods are contagious. Relationality and mood are closely linked. For example reciprocal relationships between women and midwives appear to affect and influence the atmosphere at a birth (Berg, Ólafsdóttir & Lundgren, 2012). Indeed, moods in maternity can spread rapidly creating barriers and facilitators, rousing intense fear and overwhelming moments of joy (Crowther *et al.*, 2014). To be resilient in these tides of emotional changes requires individuals to be self-aware and have the ability to manage how they feel and what they do.

Organisations that resonate with a positive yet down to earth realistic agenda can galvanise those that work within them providing the potential for optimising worker performance even when confronted by adversity. Hierarchical structures that do not resonate with local and individual needs are not useful and impede progress. The mood of organisations and the individuals who manage them thus determine how integrated a service is and how engaged its members feel. According to Goleman (2014) this requires resonant leadership with a long-term sustainable vision for an organisation. Unfortunately, this is not always the case in maternity organisations. A midwife in the UK resilience study acknowledges that it is the organisational system that is failing, not her:

> No matter how busy or stressful it can be it is important to acknowledge that we are dealing with a 24/7 situation and others will pick up where I have left off. Part of the price for aiming high and 'giving your all' while on duty is that occasionally you can't do the impossible, we must tell ourselves that it is the system that is failing, not us!
>
> (Hunter & Warren, 2014, p. 931)

Feeling continually overburdened in a poorly staffed organisation does not provide the opportunity for practice to be meaningful and joyful. 'Giving your all' and remaining optimistic despite the odds is not sustainable. The harsh reality is that sometimes it is not possible to provide the service you wish to.

I would contend that discordant resonance weakens the long-term sustainability of a service. When dissonance from organisational values arises, tension and emotional exhaustion can occur (Hunter, 2004; Murphy-Lawless, 1998; Yoon *et al.*, 2010). Equally, misaligned practice philosophies amongst midwifery colleagues have been shown to be unsustainable (McAra-Couper *et al.*, 2014). Even highly motivated practitioners may choose to leave in order to ensure their own well-being if their work becomes overly busy, purely rule-based, meaningless and lacking congruence in what they value. This could leave a service bereft of healthy resilient role models and the potential for unhealthy resilience to become the norm and contaminate an entire organisation.

Self-assessment and identification of risk

Crowther *et al.* (2016) describe how sustainability in midwifery requires the environment and the individual to be in a reciprocal relationship. Resilience is thus about balance between the organisation and personal; one cannot flourish without the other. Examine the maternity service in your region and ask yourself:

- Is there any inter-professional conflict?
- Is there any fear of discord and censure?
- Are there maternity care provider retention/recruitment issues in your service or region?
- Are service-users excluded from local and national maternity policy/guideline decisions?
- Are some maternity care providers excluded from local and national maternity policy/guideline decisions?
- Is any single professional group dominating others in policy, guideline and protocol development?
- Are maternity care providers treated with disrespect and unappreciated for their contributions?
- Is there a paucity of locally accessible emotional and psychosocial support to help practitioners?
- Is the service constantly busy and/or set up in a way that restricts opportunities for conversations among colleagues?

If the answer to any (or all) of the above is 'yes' then urgent work is required to ensure a sustainable healthy psychosocial resilient service. The following questions are focused on (you) the individual maternity care provider:

- Are you self-directed, self-determined in the way you work and how you work?
- Do you share the core values of maternity care provision in your hospital or region?
- Do you have healthy self-care strategies?
- Do you have passion and enjoy the work you do?
- Do you nurture/build relationships (social and professional, including across professional groups)?

If the answer to any of these is 'no' then self-exploration of your personal current working practices and situation is necessary. The above exercises would be beneficial to do with others, preferable a multi-professional discussion group.

Recommendations for practice and research

Various individual practice and service system characteristics and qualities need addressing to ensure psychosocial healthy resilience. Table 13.1 summarises the psychosocial resilience qualities and two principal attributes for building resilience.

Some techniques/approaches have been reported to promote healthy psychosocial resilience: self-determination, self-care, self-awareness and nurturing the love, joy and passion for practice. The foundations for these are relationality and shared resonance requiring a transdisciplinary approach.

Relationality builds psychosocial resilience

Reciprocal relationships are crucial; this includes multi-professional collegial networking. Developing strategies that promote collaborative working, for example local multi-disciplinary meetings that include GPs, obstetricians, midwives and other members of the perinatal team are essential. Nurturing cross-professional sharing could include development of optimal communication pathways using technology (e.g. tele-emergency systems) for more remote members of the team. Other strategies can include peer group support, and clinical supervision which provides opportunities for debriefing in a safe context away from the situation or employment structures (Deery, 2005).

Professional isolation and a tendency to build individual professional territories serve neither women and families or members of any professional group. Collaborative multi-disciplinary approaches are required locally and at secondary level, along with collaborative learning opportunities. Such initiatives allow cohesive common understandings and contextual meanings (McDonald, Jackson, Wilkes & Vickers, 2012). The process of sharing and collaborative learning engenders transformative learning and reflexivity. Another strategy to promote well-being and reduce burnout is the use of mindfulness techniques. Mindfulness is being explored in relation to healthcare providers and shows promise (Goodman & Schorling 2012), yet may not be acceptable to everyone. What is clear is that one strategy will not be suitable in all contexts and for all individuals.

TABLE 13.1 Qualities and attributes for building and sustaining psychosocial resilience

Qualities of psychosocial resilience	Attributes for building and sustaining psychosocial resilience
Ability and capacity to accept the harshness of reality An unusual ability to improvise and make the best of what resources are available in a given situation and The tendency to find meaning in times of adversity	Reciprocal healthy relationships Shared resonance

The starting point is simply getting to know one another and oneself and honouring differences. This holds the possibility to be powerful and transformative bringing meaningful interpretations to perinatal health professionals across working and personal lives. Each member of the perinatal team has their own concerns, values and needs who may feel unappreciated and misunderstood. These are equally significant. What is called for is a focus that is not polarising. For example, the indeterminate psychosocial and spiritual dimensions to childbirth are often left silenced in contemporary maternity, yet they are ever present (Crowther & Hall, 2015). Examining meaningful holistic experiences in and around childbirth reveals how obstetricians and midwives are not so different (Crowther et al., 2014).

Relationships matter

The centrality of relationships in maternity are indeterminate and not easily measurable. The midwifery holistic model of care that is built upon relationships is often at odds with the structured determinate knowing that provides kudos to medical disciplines. This can leave midwives feeling marginalised and vulnerable and out of synchronisation with the dominant 'mood' of contemporary maternity organisations. This can produce discordance in an already stressful clinical environment. Nurturing relationships and a shared resonance requires a new approach to perinatal health care, an approach that engenders collaborative decision-making and working beyond the containment of individual professional groups – an approach that requires all stakeholders, both at local and national levels, to sit together and work through the issues. This is not a new idea. Robertson (2008) argued for a more collaborative model in maternity. She contended that functional teams of practitioners of more than one discipline would provide higher-quality services. Stock and Burton (2011) contend 'sustainability is also inherently transdisciplinary' (p. 1091). Transdisciplinarity through emergent co-participative conversations breaks down barriers and may lead to strength-based improvements in retention and recruitment. Although this approach is more challenging in the short term, the long-term gains in terms of safety, sustainability, optimal childbirth experiences, well-being and psychosocial resilient communities of practice is a possibility worth pursuing and requires further examination.

Conclusion

The intention of this chapter is not to further problematise the situation but contribute to a more transdisciplinary thinking and development of services. Maternity care providers face a host of challenges – it is imperative that their individual needs are recognised, identified and appropriate strategies employed. Maternity care providers need to be treated fairly, be heard, be valued, enjoy open non-hierarchical communications, feel safe and experience well-being. This chapter does not present all there is to know about psychosocial resilience amongst maternity care providers. The insights and suggestions presented are from personal and professional experiences as well as involvement in several of the studies cited. The examples and subsequent recommendations provide no guarantee of healthy psychosocial resilience; they do, however, offer possibility for it to flourish. Finally, the focus has been on the concerns related to maternity care providers working and living in high- and medium-income regions of the world. The realisation of psychosocial resilience amongst maternity care providers within low-income regions remains little understood. Those maternity care provider's perspectives and daily practice realities remain largely hidden behind significantly harsher complex challenges than those highlighted in this chapter.

References

Alexandra, D.E. (2013). Resilience and disaster risk reduction: An etymological journey. *Natural Science and Earth System Sciences*, *13*, 2707–2713.

Bar-Zeev, S.J., Barclay, L., Farrington, C. & Kildea, S. (2011). From hospital to home: The quality and safety of a postnatal discharge system used for remote dwelling Aboriginal mothers and infants in the top end of Australia. *Midwifery*, *28*, 366–373.

Beaumont, E., Durkin, M., Hollins Martin, C.J. & Carson, J. (2015). Compassion for others, self-compassion, quality of life and mental well-being measures and their association with compassion fatigue and burnout in student midwives: A quantitative survey. *Midwifery*, *34*, 239–244.

Berg, M., Ólafsdóttir, O.A. & Lundgren, I. (2012). A midwifery model of woman-centred childbirth care: In Swedish and Icelandic settings. *Sexual and Reproductive Healthcare*, *3*(2), 79–87.

Calvert, I. & Benn, C. (2015). Trauma and the effects on the midwife. *International Journal of Childbirth*, *5*(2), 100–112.

Coutu, D.L. (2002). How resilience works. *Harvard Business Review*, *80*(5), 46–55.

Crowther, S. (2014). Sacred joy at birth: A hermeneutic phenomenology study. PhD, Auckland University of Technology. Available from: http://hdl.handle.net/10292/7071. [Accessed 10 January 2016].

Crowther, S. (2015). *All is not as it first may seem: Experiences of maternity in rural and remote rural regions in New Zealand from the perspectives of families and health care providers*. Funded study report. Auckland: AUT University.

Crowther, S. (2016). Providing rural and remote rural midwifery care: An 'expensive hobby'. *New Zealand College of Midwives Journal*, *52*, 26–34.

Crowther, S. & Hall, J. (2015). Spirituality and spiritual care in and around childbirth. *Women and Birth: Journal of the Australian College of Midwives*, *28*(2), 173–178.

Crowther, S., Smythe, L. & Spence, D. (2014). Mood and birth experience. *Women and Birth: Journal of the Australian College of Midwives*, *27*(1), 21–25.

Crowther, S., Hunter, B., McAra-Couper, J., Warren, L., Gilkison, A., Hunter, M., Fielder, A. & Kirkham, M. (2016) Sustainability and resilience in midwifery: A discussion paper. *Midwifery*, *40*, 40–48.

Crowther, S., Smythe, L. & Spence, D. (2015). Kairos time at the moment of birth. *Midwifery*, *31*, 451–457.

Curtis, P., Ball, L., & Kirkham, M. (2003). *Why do midwives leave? Talking to managers*. London: Royal College of Midwives.

Deery, R. (2005). An action-research study exploring midwives & support needs and the affect of group clinical supervision. *Midwifery*, *21*(2), 161–176.

Fenwick, J., Hammond, A., Raymond, J., Smith, R., Gray, J., Foureur, M., Homer, C. & Symon, A. (2012). Surviving, not thriving: A qualitative study of newly qualified midwives. *Journal of Clinical Nursing, 21,* 2054–2063.

Folke, C. (2006). Resilience: The emergence of a perspective for social–ecological systems analyses. *Global Environmental Change, 16*(3), 253–267.

Gadamer, H.G. (2008/1967). *Philosophical hermeneutics* (D.E. Linge, trans.). London: University of California Press.

Gilkison, A., McAra-Couper, J., Gunn, J., Crowther, S., Hunter, M., Macgregor, D. & Hotchin, C. (2015). Midwifery practice arrangements which sustain caseloading lead maternity carer midwives in New Zealand. *New Zealand College of Midwives Journal, 51,* 11–16.

Goleman, D. (2014). Leading for the long future. *Leader to Leader, 72,* 34–39.

Goodman, M.J. & Schorling, J.B. (2012). A mindfulness course decreases burnout and improves well-being among healthcare providers. *The International Journal of Psychiatry in Medicine, 43*(2), 119–128.

Govardhan, L., Pinelli, V. & Schnatz, P.F. (2012). Burnout, depression and job satisfaction in obstetrics and gynecology residents. *Connecticut Medicine, 76*(7), 389–395.

Griffiths, C., McAra-Couper, J. & Nayar, S. (2013). Staying involved 'because the need seems so huge': Midwives working with women living in areas of high deprivation. *International Journal of Childbirth, 3*(4), 218–232.

Hunter, B. (2004). Conflicting ideologies as a source of emotion work in midwifery. *Midwifery, 20,* 261–272.

Hunter, B., & Deery, R. (Eds.). (2009). *Emotions in midwifery and reproduction.* New York: Palgrave Macmillan.

Hunter, B., & Warren, L. (2014). Midwives' experiences of workplace resilience. *Midwifery, 30*(8), 926–934.

Leitch, A.M. & Bohensky, E.L. (2014). Return to 'a new normal': Discourses of resilience to natural disasters in Australian newspapers 2006–2010. *Global Environmental Change, 26,* 14–26.

McAra-Couper, J., Gilkison, A., Crowther, S., Hunter, M., Hotchin, C. & Gunn, J. (2014). Partnership and reciprocity with women sustain lead maternity carer midwives in practice. *New Zealand College of Midwives Journal, 49,* 27–31.

McAra-Couper, J., Jones, M. & Smythe, E. (2010). Rising rates of intervention in childbirth. *British Journal of Midwifery, 18*(3), 160–169.

McDonald, G., Jackson, D., Wilkes, L. & Vickers, M.H. (2012). A work-based educational intervention to support the development of personal resilience in nurses and midwives. *Nurse Education Today, 32*(4), 378–384.

Murphy-Lawless, J. (1998). *Reading birth and death.* Indianapolis, IN: Indiana University Press.

Patterson, J., Skinner, J. & Foureur, M. (2015). Midwives decision making about transfers for 'slow' labour in rural New Zealand. *Midwifery, 31*(6), 606–612.

Robertson, A.M. (2008). Rural women and maternity services. In J. Ross (Ed.), *Rural nursing: Aspects of practice* (pp. 179–197). Dunedin: Rural Health Opportunities, Available from: ruralhealthopportunities@xtra.co.nz. [Accessed 10 January 2016].

Sheen, K., Spiby, H. & Slade, P. (2015). Exposure to traumatic perinatal experiences and post-traumatic stress symptoms in midwives: Prevalence and association with burnout. *International Journal of Nursing Studies, 52*(2), 578–587.

Stock, P. & Burton, R.J.F. (2011). Defining terms for integrated (multi-inter-trans-disciplinary) sustainability research. *Sustainability, 3*(8), 1090–1113.

Yoon, J.D., Rasinski, K.A. & Curlin, F.A. (2010). Conflict and emotional exhaustion in obstetrician-gynaecologists: A national survey. *Journal of Medical Ethics*, *36*(12), 731–735.

14

INTERPROFESSIONAL COLLABORATION

A crucial component of support for women and families in the perinatal period

Kim Psaila and Virginia Schmied

Introduction

Chapters in this edited volume have highlighted the impact of both fetal life and early childhood experiences on later life achievements, social adjustments, mental health, physical health and longevity of individuals. Intervening early in life either during pregnancy and or in the early childhood period is therefore considered critical. However, many women and families who are marginalised or experiencing complex life situations have difficulty accessing the services they need because the services are not well connected or integrated (Schmied *et al.*, 2015; Sutherland, Yelland, & Brown, 2012). To address the increasingly complex problems faced by families, commentators, including authors in this book, emphasise that effective service collaboration and interprofessional relationships are required so that women and families can benefit most from the expertise of a variety of professionals. Development of successful interprofessional relationships requires a clear understanding of the concept of collaboration (D'Amour & Oandasan, 2005).

In this chapter our aim is to examine collaborative practice as a way to address the challenges women and families face when trying to access appropriate services within a fragmented system of health and social care. First, the literature related to the concept of collaboration within healthcare is discussed. This is followed by an examination of the prerequisites and facilitators of collaborative practice. To demonstrate collaborative practice, we draw on exemplars from the Child Health: Researching Universal Services (CHoRUS) study, an Australian study investigating the feasibility of implementing a national approach to child and family health (CFH) services in Australia (Schmied, Fowler, Rossiter, Homer, Kruske & CHoRUS team, 2014; Schmied *et al.*, 2015). A model for collaboration by D'Amour and colleagues (D'Amour, Goulet, Labadie, San Martin-Rodriguez & Pineault, 2008) is used to discuss the levels at which collaborative practice is required.

What is collaboration?

While the concept of collaboration is complex and difficult to define, it refers to a variety of strategies that facilitate individuals working together (Petri, 2010). Collaboration is not a new concept to health care. The World Health Organisation (WHO) initially acknowledged interprofessional collaboration as being essential to primary health care in 1978 (WHO, 1978). A key message recently put forward by WHO states that health systems and outcomes are strengthened by collaborative practice (WHO, 2010). Ineffective collaboration between professionals increases difficulties for women and families in accessing the information they require to navigate perinatal health services (Psaila, Schmied, Fowler & Kruske, 2014a).

Collaboration has been described as developing along a continuum of increasing interdependency with simple networking on one end and collaboration on the other (refer to Figure 14.1) (Schmied, Homer, Kemp, Thomas, Fowler & Kruske, 2008; Thistlethwaite, 2008).

At one end of the continuum individual practice is essentially autonomous, and although a degree of cooperation may exist there is no coherence or shared philosophy of care. As the relationship advances a cooperative network develops with some communication between services, but sharing of information is ad hoc rather than planned. In the next point along the continuum some alignment of policy making, management and practice exists, there is a shared commitment and

Autonomous	Cooperative	Coordinated	Collaborative
Organisations operate independently	Remain independent but network and share information	Some joint planning	Shared culture, visions, values and resources
	Low commitment	Often project-based coordination	Joint planning and delivery of some services
	Informal arrangements	Medium commitment	High commitment
		Semi-formal partnerships	Formal partnerships

NO INTEGRATION   **INTEGRATION**

FIGURE 14.1 Depicts movement from autonomous practice to full collaborative practice
Adapted from Department of Education, Training and Employment, 2013.

shared decision-making. Finally integration develops in services in which a cohesive relationship exists with formal arrangements based on common philosophy and a clear focus on the needs of service-users (Schmied, Mills, Kruske, Kemp, Fowler & Homer, 2010).

Researchers have identified a number of key characteristics of effective collaboration. A summary of these are presented in Box 14.1 below (Darlington, Feeney, & Rixon, 2004; Huxham & Vangen, 2004; Katz & Hetherington, 2006; Roberts, 2007; Scott, 2005; Valentine, Katz, & Griffiths, 2007).

BOX 14.1 KEY CHARACTERISTICS OF SUCCESSFUL COLLABORATION

- Shared vision and values.
- Agreement on common goals and clearly stated aims.
- Inspirational and energetic leadership.
- Build on the enthusiasm and commitment of others.
- Sound governance, clarity of leadership and assessment of risks.
- Recognition of and valuing diverse professional contributions.
- Capacity to address issues of power and achieve an equitable distribution of resources.
- A willingness to share risks and problems as well as any positive outcomes.
- Mechanisms in place to deal with conflict.
- Recognising all contributions.
- Public recognition of worth.
- Evaluations to assess effectiveness and cost-effectiveness.
- The need for frequent and effective communication.
- Time and resources particularly to have time to spend in building relationships with other professionals.
- Mechanisms to facilitate sharing of information and administrative data as appropriate.
- Understand participants' practice, philosophy, culture, ideas and beliefs.

These characteristics are also reflected in the experiences of health and social care professionals working with families with complex needs. For example, in the CHoRUS study, a Child Family Health (CFH) nurse (also known as maternal and child health nurses in some States and Territories of Australia, a health visitor in the UK, family health nurse in Europe or public health nurse in USA) highlighted the importance of developing respect, trust and building relationships to be able to share information and using multiple modes of communication:

> She [perinatal mental health worker] and I get together at least weekly. We talk on the phone. And I think there's been a lot of just sharing between us

just what our challenges are within our organisation and what we do, so I think over the twelve months that I've worked with her we've developed respect for each other and once you've got that relationship you can start to branch it out a bit further into, 'okay, well now, with confidence, I can bring you into my organisation to get you to talk … but we're at a place now where we could actually really go, 'yep now we really can focus on this,' because we've built the trust.

(Schmied *et al.*, 2015, p. 166)

A model of collaboration

The capacity for collaboration is influenced by human interaction, organisational and systemic (factors external to the organisation) constraints (D'Amour & Oandasan, 2005). D'Amour, Ferrada-Videla, San Martin-Rodriguez & Beaulieu (2005) initially developed a typology of collaboration which was later progressed to a model of collaboration (D'Amour, Goulet, Labadie, San Martin-Rodriguez & Pineault, 2008). This four-dimensional model is based on the idea that collective action results from a series of interactions and behaviours of professionals. D'Amour *et al.* (2008) have used their model to analyse collaboration at three ecological levels: macro, meso and micro.

The macro (system) level

Systemic factors (factors external to the organisation) from the macro level influencing collaborative practice include the professional system which refers to the separate 'silos' of professional practice (Lahey & Currie, 2005). The social and cultural values of health care providers, consumer groups and the general public also impact on collaborative practice. Professional education is a major determinant of interprofessional collaboration, as the fostering of collaborative practice values is influenced by the educational framework within which future health care professionals are trained (Oandasan *et al.*, 2004). Government policies (medico-legal liability, professional regulatory frameworks, etc.) have significant flow on effects on the capacity of organisations and professionals to develop collaborative relationships.

The meso (interorganisational) level

Indicators of collaboration at the meso level refer to the organisational factors which are needed to achieve collaborative practice. The quality of organisational collaboration is influenced by the collaborative history and environment of each service (D'Amour, *et al.*, 2005). Here 'environment' refers to the service culture, quality of leadership and available resources that support collaboration. These factors include attributes of the work environment such as structure, philosophy, resources and support, information transfer and coordination processes (McDonald, Powell Davies & Fort Harris, 2009).

The micro (interprofessional) level

Indicators of collaboration at the micro level refer to the components of interpersonal relationships such as mutual trust, respect and communication and their willingness to collaborate. The components of interpersonal relationships are influenced by a variety of factors such as professional education, previous collaborative experience, emotional maturity, available time and resources, communication skills, and each professional's knowledge and recognition of the contributions of other professionals.

What is known about the effectiveness of collaborative models of care?

Reported advantages of interprofessional collaboration include improved planning and policy development, more clinically effective services, enhanced problem solving, reduced duplication and service fragmentation, as well as increased job satisfaction for health care professionals (Schepman, Hansen, de Putter, Batenburg & de Bakker, 2015). Schepman *et al.* (2015) undertook a systematic review of studies that tested outcomes of multidisciplinary collaboration in primary care in high-income countries. These authors contend that successful collaboration is dependent upon context – the quality of the relationship between the groups, the sectors involved (e.g. child welfare, mental health, child health) and the strategies utilised by the agencies.

Internationally, there are several well-known whole-of-government models of integrated service delivery for children and families including Sure Start in the UK and Toronto First Duty in Canada. These models bring together a range of services in one centre (collocation), including midwifery services, health visiting, public health nursing, parenting support, early childhood education, and employment support. In Australia, national policy initiatives (e.g. Communities for Children) have supported integrated service delivery and professional collaboration in disadvantaged communities (Moore & Skinner, 2010). At state government level, initiatives have included Families New South Wales, a service coordination programme that attempted to integrate planning for services at government and local levels.

While there is a general consensus that integrated service models with strong collaboration amongst professionals are the best way to deliver services to women and children, currently there is limited evidence of direct benefits for women and children. Evaluations of these models have found a range of indirect benefits for children, families and professionals. Sure Start in the UK (Belsky, Barnes & Melhuish, 2007; Melhuish, Belsky & Barnes, 2010) showed modest benefits in social and emotional development for children living in Sure Start Local Programme areas with a health service hub, compared to children living in similar areas that did not have a health service hub. Evaluations of the Toronto First Duty program found children benefited socially and developed pre-academic skills (Corter, Patel,

Pelletier & Bertrand, 2008). Moore and Skinner (2010) also reported positive outcomes from other projects including, better resourcing of services, parent satisfaction, improved well-being and quality of life, and reduced impact of social exclusion.

Further evidence is presented in a systematic review of collaboration in perinatal mental health services (Myors, Schmied, Johnson & Cleary, 2013) and in a review (Niccols, Milligan, Smith, Sword, Thabane & Henderson, 2012) and metasynthesis (Sword, Jack, Niccols, Milligan, Henderson & Thabane, 2009) of parents with substance use problems. Myors *et al.* (2013) reported benefits for women with mental health problems including individualised client care; flexible multidisciplinary services offering a range of interventions and more thorough assessment and case planning. The benefits for the professional and organisations included enhanced confidence and increased communication with other professionals and minimised service overlaps and wasted resources (Myors *et al.*, 2013).

Niccols *et al.* (2012) compared integrated programmes to addiction treatment-as-usual for parents with substance use disorders. The integrated treatment programmes included on-site pregnancy, parenting, or child-related services with addiction services. Small benefits were identified in the parent-infant relationship and maternal mental health (Niccols *et al.*, 2012). Women reported increased sense of self; development of personal agency; giving and receiving of social support; engagement with programme staff and recognising patterns of destructive behaviour (Sword *et al.*, 2009) (also refer to Chapter 8 for further insights into women who misuse substances).

The central point however is that service integration can only benefit children and families if it results in higher quality intervention (Valentine *et al.*, 2007). Some commentators have questioned whether it is the collaboration and integrated models that influence outcomes or whether the most direct benefit comes from the nature of the relationship between the professional/service provider and the woman/family that leads to direct benefits.

Prerequisites for collaborative practice

Researchers have studied prerequisites needed to ensure collaboration in practice. The prerequisite most often described *is interprofessional education (IPE)*. IPE can build effective communication, mutual trust and respect among different professional groups (Petri, 2010). It offers exposure to the worldview of other professionals promoting understanding and acknowledgment of the value of others' contributions (D'Amour & Oandasan, 2005; McCallin & McCallin, 2009; Petri, 2010). The implementation of ongoing professional IPE programmes was one strategy put forward by participants in the CHoRUS study to improve collaboration (Psaila, Schmied, Fowler & Kruske, 2014b).

Role awareness is also a prerequisite for collaborative practice. This refers to the thorough understanding of one's own role in addition to an understanding of the roles of others. One of the most important prerequisites for collaboration is a strong professional identity (Bronstein, 2003; Hall, 2005). Professional identity reflects an individual's self-definition as a member of a profession and is associated with the enactment of a professional role (Chreim, Williams & Hinings, 2007). However, with professional identity come group norms that professionals use to guide their own behaviour and assess the behaviour of other professionals. Professional associations and governments through indoctrination and regulation greatly influence professional identity (Chreim *et al.*, 2007). The shared values of the professional group are often valued over personal characteristics of the individuals with whom they work (Kreindler, Dowd, Star & Gottschalk, 2012).

Despite this, several authors recommend that innovations are best facilitated when there is diversity of experience and expertise of personnel within the team (Mitchell, Parker & Giles, 2011; West & Sacramento, 2012; Xyrichis & Lowton, 2008). However, the tendency for each profession to defend their professional boundary combined with the differences in professional cultures and values, may contribute to interprofessional tensions resulting in role conflict, overlap and ambiguity (Gray, Hogg & Kennedy, 2011). For example, we found in the CHoRUS study that professional tensions and limited understanding of others roles led to negative perceptions of other professionals. Each professional group expressed concern that their contribution to the well-being of children and families was not known or appropriately valued by the other groups. The phrase 'they don't know what we do' reflected the perspective of CFH nurses, GPs (general practitioner/family doctor), practice nurses and midwives alike:

> Contribution to health not appreciated, our strengths not seen by other health professionals ... [General practice] is often viewed from a deficit model – that is acute services only see what has gone wrong – the failures.
> (GP e-conversation – Schmied *et al.*, 2014, p. 165)

> The GPs do not refer back to Child Health Services regularly enough. They sort of think of us as something that isn't really available. They just forget that we're there sometimes, depending on where you are.
> (CFH nurse – Schmied *et al.*, 2014, p. 165)

The *interpersonal relationship skills* of mutual respect, trust and effective or open communication discussed previously are both prerequisites and characteristics of collaborative practice. (D'Amour & Oandasan, 2005; Petri, 2010).

Deliberate action: This prerequisite for collaboration is described as teambuilding or relationship building (also refer to Chapter 13). Various strategies such as professional communication, shared goal and commitment, and relational agency to promote teambuilding and relationship building are central to teambuilding (Lindeke & Sieckert, 2005; Schmied *et al.*, 2010). Relational agency refers to the capacity of professionals to work with others to explore the focus of interest that one is working on and trying to transform by recognising and accessing resources that others bring to bear as they interpret and respond to the focus of interest. It is argued that relational agency leads to an enhanced form of professional agency which is of benefit to the objects of practice (Edwards, 2005).

Finally, '*support*' is a prerequisite for collaboration and encompasses individual and organisational support. Support from one's organisation is realised in the form of education, resources and commitment to the process (D'Amour & Oandasan, 2005b; McCallin & McCallin, 2009). Lack of organisational support is commonly reported to obstruct attempts at developing collaborative relationships (Psaila, Schmied, Fowler & Kruske, 2013).

Service innovation to facilitate collaboration

In the following section, we draw on case examples and the experience of professionals to illustrate how services and professionals worked collaboratively to design and implement new models of service delivery. The data exemplars come from CHoRUS study (Olley, Psaila, Fowler, Kruske, Homer & Schmied, 2016; Psaila et al., 2013; Psaila et al., 2014a, 2014b; Psaila, Schmied, Kruske, Fowler & Homer, 2014c). In phase three of this mixed methods study, we examined innovations in the delivery of CFH services, a total of 21 sites/services across five Australian States and Territories and 121 professionals participated. Data were collected via one-to-one interviews, small group interviews and focus groups (Psaila et al., 2014c; Schmied et al., 2015). These 21 sites were selected because they had made a change at the level of policy, service design or professional practice [macro, meso, micro level] (D'Amour et al., 2008) to improve continuity of care for children and families by ensuring effective collaboration between services and or professionals. Thematic analysis of the data identified a range of motivations for change.

Primarily, professionals had two key concerns that motivated change. First, some services were not able to engage all families in the universal CFH services either because the service system was so fragmented that they did not receive information about new-borns from the maternity service or they did not have the resources to reach out to all families. Second, some sites had identified poor developmental and health outcomes for children in their community with many children not ready for school.

Five different approaches to innovation were identified; 'Streamlining information exchange processes' (see below), 'Roles supporting co-ordination of care' (see Box 14.2), 'Using funding and resources in innovative ways' (see Box 14.3), 'Joint working', and 'Co-locating services' (see Box 14.4). Participants at several sites reported using a combination of these strategies to engage families.

Streamlining information exchange

One state level (macro) site focused on improving the electronic transfer of information from all publicly funded maternity services to the community-based CFH nursing services. The main concern was related to the provision of comprehensive referrals for women and new-borns following birth, who had been identified to have additional physical, social and emotional health needs. The maternity database was redesigned to provide an automatic email notification linked via the woman's postcode to the relevant CFH nursing service centralised email account. A predetermined list of maternal and or infant physical, mental or social health risk factors was included in the woman's notes as part of the routine discharge data collection. In another site, the service managers and data custodians worked collaboratively to ensure access by CFH nursing service to the maternity database. This facilitated informational continuity for the CFH nursing service.

BOX 14.2 ROLES SUPPORTING CO-ORDINATION OF CARE

Liaison roles (meso and micro levels)

Liaison roles are increasingly being used to improve communication between health services and professionals, and to facilitate access to support for children and families.

Collaborative service model: HealthOne General Practice Liaison Nurse (GPLN), New South Wales, Australia.

HealthOne is a government initiative. It aims to provide integrated care for children and families with complex needs, by linking GPs, CFH nurses and other professionals in community, maternity and acute care services (Hanley, Doyle, Fagan & Mulligan, 2014).

The role of the GPLN is central to the enactment of the HealthOne approach. The GPLNs have been described as the 'lynchpin' (McNab, Mallit & Gillespie, 2013), acting as *'the bridge'* linking local services to support pregnant women, children and families and *'holding'* or *'supporting'* families as they move between services and professionals. While the GPLN identifies and establishes the best service pathway for the family, often the liaison nurse will have to *'untangle'* the array of diverse and sometimes overlapping services connected to each family. The GPLNs also provide support and education of other clinicians (Schmied *et al.*, 2015).

Case example: (Hanley *et al.*, 2014)

Within days of delivery, a mother and baby were referred by the hospital social worker to an early intervention programme. Following the universal health home visit, the allocated CFH nurse raised concern about parental capacity, including learning disabilities, and initiated contact with the HealthOne CFH GPLN. On a subsequent home visit, the CFH nurse identified that the baby required medical attention which, after prompt examination by the family GP, resulted in referral and a week-long admission to hospital during which time concerns were raised with the child protection unit within the hospital. Post-discharge, the family were admitted to a Family Residential Care Unit for another week. During liaison with this unit, the GPLN became aware that the child protection unit had arranged a teleconference with the hospital's paediatrician and social worker. The GPLN intervened to include the family's GP in the feedback loop from the teleconference, since the GP knew the extended family and their clinical history. In the GP's opinion, it was unnecessary to remove the baby from the family, citing the extended family support, the practical nature of the support, and the close proximity of this support to the family and the family's readiness to accept the support. The GPLN then organised a further multidisciplinary case conference, where a care plan was developed with the GP, to ensure ongoing monitoring and support. This alleviated the concerns of the child protection unit, placed the GP as the primary care provider, and facilitated integrated care.

BOX 14.3 USING FUNDING AND RESOURCES IN INNOVATIVE WAYS

Developing partnerships (macro and meso levels – linking organisations and sectors)

In this model of community-based care, partnerships were developed between the health and local council sectors to create a new role for community midwives.

Collaborative service model: West Heildelburgh, Community Midwifery (health service) and Maternal and Child Health (CFH) Nursing Service (local council)

The CFH nurses in this local council site were not able to reach new mothers particularly refugee women in their community and these children were vulnerable for poor developmental outcomes.

A new CFH nurse manager recognised an opportunity for service improvement by utilising the skills of community midwives working in the state government funded health service. This nurse manager worked collaboratively with the manager of the community health service to share their human resources by merging the existing community-based midwifery role and a CFH nursing role into a single role. The purpose of the new role was to provide continuity of care for vulnerable families who engaged in pregnancy with the community midwives employed by community health but who often did not engage post-birth with the CFH nursing service.

The two services developed a memorandum of understanding (MOU) regarding salary allocation to enable community midwives to work across two services – state government community health and local government CFH nursing service. In this joined-up role, the midwives with CFH nursing qualifications were able to provide both antenatal and postnatal midwifery care and to continue to see the woman, her new baby and family in her capacity as a CFH nurse. Without continuity of carer, vulnerable families would most likely have disengaged from the service. The MOU enabled the CFH nursing service to access rooms within the community health centre. This provided the CFH nurses with an opportunity to develop working relationships with a range of professionals and services working from the premises including GPs, speech therapists, dieticians, housing support, financial support, adult education etc. The benefits of continuity for women were highlighted:

> It's been great, because we build the relationship antenatally, and it's just seamless, it just flows straight through. Rather than other CFH nurses, we go and do the first home visit, so it just kind of continues on.
>
> (CFH 1– Psaila & Schmied, 2013)

BOX 14.4 JOINT WORKING AND CO-LOCATING SERVICES

Place-based services: Joint working and collocation of services and professionals – new ways of working at the micro level.

Collaborative service model: Benevolent Society Child and Family Centre, Browns Plains, Queensland, Australia

CFH nurse participants described 'working differently' in early childhood education and care settings. This involved nurses moving away from a traditional, structured, clinic-based model of 'health surveillance' in one-on-one appointments to what participants termed a 'place-based' service and 'play-based' approach, focused on building parenting capacity and facilitating child development and school readiness in a community setting such as a preschool or school. The term 'place-based, play-based work' reflects the importance of the setting for nurses' work as well as the skills they use to work with in partnership with parents.

In this 'place-based' service CFH nurses partner with other professionals such as, early childhood education teachers, speech therapists and family support workers, to provide a safe and open environment for parents to play and interact with their children. This 'play-based' work involves CFH nurses observing and assessing children in their natural environment and being 'down on the floor' with children and parents. This facilitates and enhances the CFH nurse's role in early intervention particularly promoting attachment, referral and tailoring services to meet the needs of parents and the community.

One nurse stated:

> It's a partnership in so much as there's an education component, there's a health component and often a family support component as well. And so the planning is done together, the presentation, the cleaning up, the reflecting.
>
> (CFH nurse – Psaila & Schmied, 2013)

CFH nurses indicated that this was a new way of working:

> I work quite differently. Before I worked on my own. So now to move to this kind of hub where there are two nurses working closely with a lot of the support services around this area it's been working really well.
>
> (CFH nurse – Psaila & Schmied, 2013)

Implications for practice: lessons from the CHoRUS study

Participants in phase three in the CHoRUS study identified the factors that facilitated collaborative models and new ways of working, including some of the prerequisites required for collaborative practice. In this final section of the chapter we address the implications for practice by applying D'Amour's model of collaboration (D'Amour *et al.*, 2008).

Macro level (e.g. policy directives)

Government policies have a significant effect on the capacity of organisations and professionals to collaborate effectively. In the CHoRUS study policy directives were used by services to support changes in practice. For example, in NSW the 'HealthOne' policy brought a range of CFH professionals together to ensure that children and families were linked to appropriate services. In other sites partnerships were developed between federal and state governments, between health and education sectors, between local government and health and between public and non-government organisations. In clinical practice, these collaborations most commonly occurred through the establishment of multidisciplinary case meetings. These partnerships required *funding commitments, leadership and a shared vision and a clear understanding of roles* and resulted in positive interprofessional relationships and better knowledge by all professionals of the services available:

CFH nursing service is smack bang in the middle of the [local council] Early Years Plan, we're on every section, there is an action for CFH or we are mentioned, CFH is central to all the other services.

(CFH nurse manager – Psaila & Schmied, 2013)

Meso level

Effective collaboration at the meso level requires organisational factors such as service structure and governance mechanisms and explicit direction to guide collaborative efforts, as well as leadership support for innovation and connectivity through interprofessional education and networking. Since these functions are influenced by the values, beliefs, norms and regulations of multiple stakeholders, integration requires an understanding of the existing interdependent relationships between the organisation and professionals (Mohler, 2013). In the CHoRUS study strategies to enhance organisational collaboration were identified. For example, deliberate action and leadership was needed to bring health services together with early education and community services to coordinate care for families. One midwife stated, 'we had a leader with a "can do" attitude and we took the initiative'. Leadership is also illustrated in the case studies above and in the following quote from the coordinator of a 'place-based' service for children and families:

It's about joining up and forming partnerships, the majority are just locating with us, signing an MOU and having this as a place based approach. Families see they can come here and all their needs will be met.

(Psaila & Schmied, 2013)

Micro level

Collaboration at the micro level refers to the interactional/relational factors or conditions required to achieve interprofessional collaboration (D'Amour & Oandasan, 2005). This includes *sharing common goals (deliberate action)* and *taking a client centred approach* as well as developing *mutuality* that is, knowing one another well and building trust. In the CHoRUS study different disciplines came together because each was believed to contribute specific skills, enabling them to support families. Professionals emphasised the need for awareness of each other's roles and communication within the multidisciplinary team:

I think there has to be very clear understanding between the partners. They have to know what the goals are, the partners always being on the same page.

(CFH nurse – Psaila & Schmied, 2013)

Professionals found that as they became more familiar with one another, they were able to recognise the skills of other professionals and work well as a team:

There's just no division. We've got very good GPs to work with, they're very happy to work with all us nurses or all Allied Health, and I just think we work really well as a team, we do support each other.

(CFH nurse – Psaila & Schmied, 2013)

For CHoRUS participants, collaborative practice had made a positive change for women, children and families:

Improved our service dramatically, now it's a continuum, we have built a good link with the maternity unit and midwives and our council provides a lot of services, but there's this continuum right through from birth to the school nursing system and to the primary school.

(CFH nurse – Psaila & Schmied, 2013)

Conclusion

Internationally concerted efforts are being made to strengthen interprofessional collaboration and build integrated models of care. To date there is limited empirical evidence of benefits for children and families; however, practice examples and evaluations demonstrate some benefits for families and for services and professionals. Further research is needed to demonstrate the benefits of collaborative practice. Capacity for collaborative practice needs to be developed through a combination of policy, lobbying by professional and client groups, and modifications to existing education and training programmes at undergraduate and postgraduate levels to include interprofessional education strategies.

Collaboration between the various disciplines and services is required to deliver continuity of care and solve complex healthcare problems to prevent adverse outcomes. Professional relationships, however, are less important than a partnership approach to care which involves developing a supportive relationship with parents and families and working with them to develop parental confidence and their capacity to manage their own problems in the longer term is required.

References

Belsky, J., Barnes, J. & Melhuish, E. (2007). *The national evaluation of sure start: Does area-based early intervention work?* Bristol: Policy Press.

Bronstein, L.R. (2003). A model for interdisciplinary collaboration. *Social Work, 48*(3), 297–306.

Chreim, S., Williams, B. & Hinings, C. (2007). Interlevel influences on the reconstruction of professional role identity. *Academy of Management Journal 50*(6), 1515–1539.

Corter, C., Patel, S., Pelletier, J. & Bertrand, J. (2008). The early development instrument as an evaluation and improvement tool for school-based, integrated services for young children and parents: The Toronto First Duty Project. *Early Education and Development, 19*(5), 773–794.

D'Amour, D. & Oandasan, I. (2005). Interprofessionality as the field of interprofessional practice and interprofessional education: An emerging concept. *Journal of Interprofessional Care, 1*, 8–20.

D'Amour, D., Ferrada-Videla, M., San Martin-Rodriguez, L. & Beaulieu, M. (2005). The conceptual basis for interprofessional collaboration: Core concepts and theoretical frameworks. *Journal of Interprofessional Care, 1*, 116–131.

D'Amour, D., Goulet, L., Labadie, J., San Martin-Rodriguez, L. & Pineault, R. (2008). A model and typology of collaboration between professionals in healthcare organisations. *BMC Health Services Research, 8*(188). doi:1186/1472-6963-8-188 T.

Darlington, Y., Feeney, J.A. & Rixon, K. (2004). Complexity, conflict and uncertainty: Issues in collaboration between child protection and mental health services. *Children and Youth Services Review, 26*, 1175–1192.

Department of Education, Training and Employment. (2013). *A framework for integrated early childhood development*. Australia: Government of Queensland. Available from: http://apo. org.au/node/35372. [Accessed 15 March 2016].

Edwards, A. (2005). Relational agency: Learning to be a resourceful practitioner. *International Journal of Educational Research, 43*, 168–182.

Gray, C., Hogg, G., & Kennedy, C. (2011). Professional boundary work in the face of change to generalist working in community nursing in Scotland. *Journal of Advanced Nursing, 67*(8), 1695–1704.

Hall, P. (2005). Interprofessional teamwork: Professional cultures as barriers. *Journal of Interprofessional Care, 19* (Suppl. 1), S188–S196.

Hanley, E., Doyle, T., Fagan, N. & Mulligan, J. (2014). Facilitating integrated care: An approach to child and family health in primary health care. *Australian Journal of Child and Family Health Nursing, 11*(1), 25–29.

Huxham, C. & Vangen, S. (2004). Doing things collaboratively: Realising the advantage or succumbing to inertia. *Organisational Dynamics, 33*(2), 190–201.

Katz, I. & Hetherington, R. (2006). Co-operating and communicating: A European perspective on integrating services for children. *Child Abuse Review, 15*, 429–439.

Kreindler, S., Dowd, D., Star, N. & Gottschalk, T. (2012). Silos and social identity: The social identity approach as a framework for understanding and overcoming divisions in health care. *Milbank Quarterly, 90*(2), 347–374.

Lahey, W. & Currie, R. (2005). Regulatory and medico-legal barriers to interprofessional practice. *Journal of Interprofessional Care*, (Suppl. 1), 197–233.

Lindeke, L.L. & Sieckert, A.M. (2005). Nurse–physician workplace collaboration. *The Online Journal of Issues in Nursing, 10*(1). Available from: http://nursingworld.org/ MainMenuCategories/ANAMarketplace/ANAPeriodicals/OJIN/TableofContents/ Volume102005/No1Jan05/tpc26_416011.html [Accessed 16 June 2016].

McCallin, A. & McCallin, M. (2009). Factors influencing team working and strategies to facilitate successful collaborative teamwork. *New Zealand Journal of Physiotherapy, 37*(2), 61–67.

McDonald, J., Powell Davies, G., & Fort Harris, M. (2009). Interorganisational and interprofessional partnership approaches to achieve more coordinated and integrated primary and community health services: The Australian experience. *Australian Journal of Primary Health, 15*, 262–269. doi:10.3912/OJIN.Vol10No01Man04.

McNab, J., Mallit, K. & Gillespie, J. (2013). *Report of the evaluation of HealthOne Mount Druitt, Menzies Centre for Health Policy*. Sydney. Available from: http://hdl.handle. net/2123/8988 [Accessed 10 March 2016].

Melhuish, E., Belsky, J. & Barnes, J. (2010). Evaluation and value of Sure Start. *Archives of Disease in Childhood, 95*, 159–161.

Mitchell, R., Parker, V. & Giles, M. (2011). When do interprofessional teams succeed? Investigating the moderating roles of team and professional identity in interprofessional effectiveness. *Human Relations, 64*(1321). doi:10.1177/0018726711416872.

Mohler, M. (2013). Collaboration across clinical silos. *Frontiers of Health Service Management, 29*(4), 36–44.

Moore, T. & Skinner, A. (2010). *An integrated approach to early childhood development.* New South Wales: The Benevolent Society.

Myors, K., Schmied, V., Johnson, M. & Cleary, M. (2013). Collaboration and integrated services for perinatal mental health: An integrative review. *Child and Adolescent Mental Health, 18*(1), 1–10.

Niccols, A., Milligan, K., Smith, A., Sword, W., Thabane, L. & Henderson, J. (2012). Integrated programs for mothers with substance abuse issues: A systematic review of studies reporting on parenting outcomes. *Child Abuse & Neglect, 36*(4), 308–322.

Oandasan, I., D'Amour, D., Zwarenstein, M., Barker, K., Purden, M., Beaulieu, M., Reeves, S., Nasmith, L., Bosco, C., Ginsburg, L. & Tregunno, D. (2004). *Interdisciplinary education for collaborative, patient-centred practice.* Ottawa: Health Canada.

Olley, H., Psaila, K., Fowler, C., Kruske, S., Homer, C. & Schmied, V. (2016). 'Being the bridge and the beacon': A qualitative study of the characteristics and functions of the liaison role in child and family health services in Australia. *Journal of Clinical Nursing.* doi:10.1111/jocn.13373. [Epub ahead of print].

Petri, L. (2010). Concept analysis of interdisciplinary collaboration. *Nursing Forum, 45*(2), 73–82.

Psaila, K. & Schmied, V. (2013). *A plea for connectivity: Perspectives of child and family health nurses on continuity of service.* Paper presented at the AAMCFHN: 5th Biennial National Conference, Canberra.

Psaila, K., Schmied, V., Fowler, C. & Kruske, S. (2013). Discontinuities between maternity and child and family health services: Health professional's perceptions. *BMC Health Services Research, 14*(4), 1–12. doi:10.1186/1472-6963-14-4.

Psaila, K., Schmied, V., Fowler, C. & Kruske, S. (2014a). A qualitative study of innovations implemented to improve transition of care from maternity to CFH services in Australia. *Women and Birth, 27*(4), e51–60.

Psaila, K., Schmied, V., Fowler, C. & Kruske, S. (2014b). Interprofessional collaboration at transition of care: Perspectives of child and family health nurses and midwives. *Journal of Clinical Nursing, 24*(1–2), 160–172.

Psaila, K., Schmied, V., Kruske, S., Fowler, C. & Homer, C. (2014c). Smoothing out the transition of care between maternity and child and family health services: Perspectives of child and family health nurses and midwives. *BCM Pregnancy & Childbirth, 14*(151). doi:10.1186/1471-2393-14-151.

Roberts, H. (2007). *What works in collaboration.* Telstra Foundation Community Development Fund. West Perth: Australian Research Alliance for Children and Youth.

Schepman, S., Hansen, J., de Putter, I.D., Batenburg, R.S. & de Bakker, D.H. (2015). The common characteristics and outcomes of multidisciplinary collaboration in primary health care: A systematic literature review. *International Journal of Integrated Care, 15*(2).

Schmied, V., Fowler, C., Rossiter, C., Homer, C., Kruske, S. & CHoRUS team. (2014). The nature and frequency of services provided by child and family health nurses in Australia: Results of a national survey. *Australian Health Review, 38*(2), 177–185.

Schmied, V., Homer, C., Fowler, C., Psaila, K., Barclay, L., Wilson, I., Kemp, L., Fasher, M. & Kruske, S. (2015). Implementing a national approach to universal child and family health services in Australia: Professionals' views of the challenges and opportunities. *Health and Social Care in the Community, 23*(2), 159–170.

Schmied, V., Homer, C., Kemp, L., Thomas, C., Fowler, C. & Kruske, S. (2008). The role and nature of universal health services for pregnant women, children and families in Australia. *Australian Health Review, 38*(2), 177–185.

Schmied, V., Mills, A., Kruske, S., Kemp, L., Fowler, C. & Homer, C. (2010). The nature and impact of collaboration and integrated service delivery for pregnant women, children and families. *Journal of Clinical Nursing, 19*, 3516–3526.

Scott, D. (2005). Inter-organisational collaboration in family-centred practice: A framework for analysis and action. *Australian Social Work, 58*(2), 132–141.

Sutherland, G., Yelland, J. & Brown, S. (2012). Social inequalities in the organisation of pregnancy care in a universally funded public health care system. *Maternal and Child Health Journal, 16*, 288–296.

Sword, W., Jack, S., Niccols, A., Milligan, K., Henderson, J. & Thabane, L. (2009). Integrated programs for women with substance use issues and their children: A qualitative meta-synthesis of processes and outcomes. *Harm Reduction Journal, 6*. doi:10.1186/ 1477-7517-6-32.

Thistlethwaite, P. (2008). *Bringing the NHS and local government together: A practical guide to integrated working.* Available from: http://networks.csip.org.uk/_library/ICNdocument. pdf [Accessed 15 January 2016].

Valentine, K., Katz, I. & Griffiths, M. (2007). *Early childhood services: Models of integration and collaboration.* Sydney: University of New South Wales. Australian Research Alliance for Children and Youth. Available from: www.sprc.unsw.edu.au/media/SPRCFile/5_ Report_ARACY_EarlyChildhood.pdf [Accessed 10 January 2016].

West, M. & Sacramento, C. (2012). Creativity and innovation: The role of team and organisational climate. In M. Mumford (Ed.), *Handbook of organisational creativity* (pp. 359–386). Amsterdam: Elsevier.

WHO. (1978). *Declaration of Alma-Ata.* Available from: www.euro.who.int/AboutWHO/ [Accessed 10 March 2016].

WHO. (2010). *Framework for action on interprofessional education & collaborative practice.* Available from: www.who.int/hrh/nursing_midwifery/en/ [Accessed 10 March 2016].

Xyrichis, A. & Lowton, K. (2008). What fosters or prevents interprofessional teamworking in primary and community care? A literature review. *International Journal of Nursing Studies, 45*, 140–153.

15

DRAWING THE THREADS TOGETHER

Gill Thomson and Virginia Schmied

In this chapter we reflect on a number of issues addressed in the chapters; to highlight the difficulties and challenges that women can face in the perinatal period, as well as how best to provide optimum care delivery.

Difficulties and challenges

Childbirth, and becoming a mother, is a liminal and transformative life experience, a psychological and social experience with impacts for women, infants and family members. While becoming a parent can bring overwhelming joy and life fulfilment for some, for others it can lead to the onset, continuation or exacerbation of stressors, adversity and complications. In this book, it is these more challenging situations that we have focused on. As we highlight at the start of the book (Chapter 1), it has not been our intention to problematise or stereotype 'certain' women and their families – rather to raise awareness of risk factors and consequent psychosocial issues that can be faced due to the women's life histories and/or the healthcare available to them. As identified throughout the majority of chapters, women from chaotic and marginalised backgrounds as well as those who face unexpected maternity experiences (such as through a traumatic birth (Chapter 11), having a premature baby (Chapter 10) or stillbirth (Chapter 12)) experience high levels of morbidity (such as anxiety, stress, depression, post-traumatic stress disorder (PTSD); with negative implications for infant health (e.g. prematurity, infections) and development outcomes (e.g. refer to Chapters 7 and 9). Others, such as women who are asylum seekers or refugees (Chapter 3), from Indigenous communities (Chapter 4), lesbian parents (Chapter 5) and women with a disability (Chapter 6) can also face prejudice and discrimination from care providers as well as from their wider social networks.

In reality it is too simplistic and risks 'Othering' women if we try to assign certain features, traits or areas of adversity to individual groups. For example, as discussed in the context of the Social Ecological Model (Chapter 1) there are multifaceted and interactive effects of personal, family and environmental factors that determine behaviours and outcomes. Angela Taft and Leesa Hooker (Chapter 7) highlight there are many factors that influence the perpetration and victimisation of domestic and family violence (such as socioeconomic status, culture-related issues, substance abuse, self-esteem, level and quality of social networks) as well as how these factors intersect to make woman more susceptible or resilient to domestic and family violence. The consideration of multiple and intersecting factors apply to many of the different life situations considered. So, for instance, women with a disability (Chapter 6) are able to embrace motherhood more readily when they originate from a supportive family environment – whereas those who have experienced marginalisation and disapproval fare worse in their parenting transition. Other women face more unique challenges. For example, as Marie-Clare Balaam and colleagues discuss in Chapter 3, asylum seekers and refugees may have experienced high levels of trauma and distress prior to and/or during their transition to a new country. These stressors can be exacerbated by uncertainty, fear and a lack of cultural sensitivity, or ameliorated by continuity, social support and sensitive needs-led care. Therefore, an important starting position for any healthcare professional, as stipulated by Julie Jomeen and colleagues in Chapter 2, is how a woman's needs should be defined in the context of her life.

Offering a salutogenic perspective

It was also important for this book to offer a more salutogenic (Antonovsky, 1987) perspective: to focus on the positive aspects of health, and to question what gives women the capacity or strength to maintain well-being despite the stressors they face. Resilience, as considered by Julie Jomeen and colleagues in Chapter 2, is as yet a poorly defined construct, and cautions against a deficit based approach that perceives resilience to be an absence of risk. However, the 'positive psychology' focus on positive health and well-being – human flourishing – has been growing in interest over the last few decades. In the chapter by Gill Thomson and colleagues (Chapter 11) they consider the current, albeit limited evidence, into post-traumatic growth following a traumatic birth – women were able to forge new relationships and spiritual beliefs, and held altered world-view perspectives. Denise Lawler (Chapter 6) describes how women with a disability were able to develop strength and sense of purpose through motherhood. Susan Crowther (Chapter 13) also provides illuminating examples of how professionals display resilience in a high-pressured healthcare context. While it may be difficult as this stage to differentiate between a resilience-informed framework of care or 'modifiable risk factors' (Chapter 2), certain qualities of care and support that have/may have salutary outcomes have been highlighted. We summarise these here.

Social support

The positive impact of social support, or potential for such, for women, families and professionals is highlighted throughout all the included chapters. This is reflected within the group-based parenting interventions provided to incarcerated women (Chapter 9), through the close and supportive family support to women with a disability (Chapter 6), a community-based midwifery model of care for Indigenous women (Chapter 4) and peer support for parents of premature infants (Chapter 10), with suggestions for mother-to-mother based support also recommended by others (e.g. Chapters 2, 7, 11). Social support is widely recognised as an important mechanism to buffer against stress and to enhance psychological well-being (Cohen & Wills, 1985; Pearlin, 1989; Umberson & Montez, 2010).

Woman-centred care

Unsurprisingly, a targeted, individualised needs-led approach was a recurrent theme to emerge. The identification and assessment of psychosocial issues is complicated due to the availability (e.g. Chapter 11) or efficacy (e.g. Chapters 2, 4) of suitable screening measures and/or women's reticence to disclose their concerns (e.g. Chapters 2, 4, 6, 7, 8, 11). A study by Shakespeare, Blake and Garcia (2003) into the acceptability of the Edinburgh Postnatal Depression Scale (EPDS) also reported that women preferred to talk about their concerns rather than completing forms. However, what is called for across the chapters is a trust-based relationship with care providers; a woman-centred approach that provides continuity in care provision, positive interpersonal behaviours, sensitivity and empathy. In Hannah Dahlen's Chapter (12) into reproductive loss and grief she tells us her own personal journey, and how supportive, flexible and responsive care should be provided. The chapter by Angela Taft and Leesa Hooker (Chapter 7) also discusses how professionals need to understand, and have the appropriate skills and attitudes to effectively work with women's Stages of Change to leave an abusive partner.

A woman-centred approach should also encompass culturally sensitive and non-judgemental care. The need for culture-specific care (which incorporates language and interpreter services) is discussed by Marie-Clare Balaam and colleagues (Chapter 3) in relation to asylum seekers and refugees and Donna Hartz and Leona McGrath (Chapter 4) in regards to Indigenous women. The community-based midwifery model (Chapter 4) that incorporated Indigenous and non-Indigenous approaches to childbirth reported to have provided a 'platform for cultural regeneration, greater family cohesion and the intergenerational exchange of traditional knowledge'. Other authors, such as Brenda Hayman (Chapter 5) and Denise Lawler (Chapter 6) also urge professionals to use non-discriminatory language, assumptions and/or documentation in their interactions with lesbian parents and women with a disability respectively.

One feasible approach to achieve needs-led support is person-centred care or communication (PCC). McCormack and McCance (2010) describe PCC as a model of care which includes developing therapeutic relationships built on mutual trust and understanding, treating the person as an individual, shared decision-making and providing holistic care. An approach that considers:

> People's desires, values, family situations, social circumstances and lifestyles; seeing the person as an individual, and working together to develop appropriate solutions.
>
> (Health Innovation Network, n.d., p. 2)

Research into PCC has identified how it can improve individual's experience of care, encourage individuals to engage in healthier lifestyles, enable individuals to be more involved in their care decisions and to access appropriate support, and reduce healthcare utilisation and improve job satisfaction for providers (Mead & Bower, 2002; McMillan *et al.*, 2013).

A further consideration is the Family Partnership Model (FPM) (Davis & Day, 2010; Davis, Day & Bidmead, 2002). The FPM focuses on building professionals skills to work in partnership with parents and families, to help them to overcome adversities and to build strengths and resilience. This approach has been reported to improve parenting skills and parent and child outcomes (e.g. Barlow, Davis, McIntosh, Jarrett, Mockford & Stewart-Brown, 2007; Puura *et al.*, 2005).

Workforce development

The requirement for professionals to comprehend the life situations of different population groups of women is repeatedly highlighted by the chapter authors. Gill Thomson and colleagues (Chapter 11) report how professionals should be cognisant of how maternity care can impact on women's birth experiences, as well as how to identify women who are suffering adverse emotional responses post-birth. Overall, training is considered to be important to raise professionals' awareness of the care that women require (e.g. cultural) and/or issues that they face (i.e. psychosocial complexities), in the premise that this will facilitate a more connected and empathic woman-provider relationship. An approach which resonates with these requirements is a trauma-informed approach; an approach that engages with histories of trauma (such as emotional, physical or sexual abuse, witnessing/ experiencing violence, neglect or maltreatment) to enable recognition of trauma symptoms, and awareness into how trauma affects the individual. Moses, Reed and Mazelis (2003, p. 19) define a trauma-informed approach as involving:

> Understanding, anticipating, and responding to the issues, expectations, and special needs that a person who has been victimized may have in a particular setting or service. At a minimum, trauma-informed services endeavour to do no harm – to avoid retraumatizing or blaming [clients] for their efforts to manage their traumatic reactions.

Trauma-informed interventions have been found to be effective when engaging with more vulnerable/marginalised population groups, such as women with co-occurring mental health problems (Gatz, Brown, Hennigan & Rechberger, 2007; Morrissey, Jackson, Ellis, Amaro, Brown & Najavits, 2005) and domestic violence (Chetwin, 2013). As many women discussed in this book have a history of trauma and ongoing complexities, a trauma-informed training approach that considers and raises awareness of women's vulnerabilities and triggers, and to facilitate more sensitive care, may well be beneficial.

A further area of development concerns how professionals should adopt a strength-based approach when engaging with women (e.g. Chapters 2, 4, 7–9 and 14). This is an assets-based, empowerment approach that concentrates on the inherent strengths of individuals and families and operates to strengthen a woman's sense of self-worth and capabilities (Fontein-Kuipers, van Limbeek, Ausems, de Vries & Nieuwenhuijze, 2015). Lucinda Burns and colleagues (Chapter 8) when discussing the needs of women who abuse substances, describe the utility of motivational interviewing in engaging with service-users. This is a non-judgemental person-centred technique that recognises and accepts the individual's readiness to change, and works with the individual to help change their perceptions of their behaviour and to identify strategies and approaches for positive change (Rollnick & Miller, 1995). A number of interventions discussed in the chapters also offer promising models of practice. For example, Cathrine Fowler and Chris Rossiter (Chapter 9) describe intensive relational-based parenting programmes that aim to reverse the intergenerational transmission of poor parenting practices. Nancy Feeley in her chapter on mothers with premature infants (Chapter 10) also identifies the positive impact of targeted, needs-led interventions on mother-infant relationships and infant outcomes.

Opportunities to develop and sustain the resilience of professionals, as posited by Susan Crowther (Chapter 13) also need careful consideration, to empower professionals in order that they can do the same for others. Crowther discusses how current healthcare systems have the potential for unhealthy practices due to 'financially stretched local services and frequent unrealistic staffing ratios', leading to burnout, fatigue and depression (Beaumont, Durkin, Hollins Martin, & Carson, 2015). She identifies a number of resilience-informed strategies to help ameliorate these tensions, such as through developing reciprocal, collegial networks, peer support and clinical supervision. Mindfulness – a meditative, self-reflective psychological process that involves focusing on intrinsic and extrinsic experiences occurring in the present moment – is another strategy reported to be effective in decreasing burnout and increasing well-being for some healthcare providers (Goodman & Schorling, 2012).

Multi-agency collaboration

Multi-agency support is reported as essential for women with challenging life situations (e.g. Chapters 2, 3, 4, 7, 8). As Julie Jomeen and colleagues argue

(Chapter 2), the focus of interventions on uni-dimensional outcomes, such as depression or anxiety, is insufficient to resolve the complexities of issues that women face. The call by Jomeen and colleagues for sufficient support (professional and social) via multi-disciplinary staff being reflected in the work presented by Marie-Clare Balaam and colleagues (Chapter 4) and Kim Psaila and Virginia Schmied (Chapter 14). Psaila and Schmied provide insights into the essential qualities of collaborative practice including interpersonal education, role awareness and interpersonal skills. They also use case examples to illustrate how targeted, integrated service provision achieved collaboration at the meso, micro and macro levels. A number of these insights are also echoed in the work of Susan Crowther (Chapter 13) into how transdisciplinary practice, built on nurturing relationships and a shared resonance amongst service providers is required. As reflected by Jomeen and colleagues (Chapter 2), effective service provision requires seamless, joint working between various healthcare providers (e.g. midwifery, obstetrics, family nurses/health visitors, mental health, paediatrics), other statutory services (such as social workers, housing) and the voluntary sector.

In summary

The work presented in this book has highlighted how risk, psychosocial consequences and the implications of such have costs (emotional and otherwise) for women, infants, families, healthcare providers and society in general. We also recognise that the voices of others from complex psychosocial backgrounds such as women who are trafficked, women who are care leavers and/or those with child protection requirements/orders have not been included. While fathers' needs and issues have only been touched on in some of the chapters (e.g. Chapters 2, 11), we appreciate that research and suitable interventions to ensure fathers are included and supported during the perinatal period are essential. Some of the chapter authors highlight the need for further research into the impact of adversity on women and infant outcomes (e.g. Chapters 3, 9, 10). Fowler and Rossiter (Chapter 9) also propose how a more 'appreciative inquiry' approach should frame future research to enable identification of an individual's strengths, rather than deficits. Such an approach may also help to define the underlying components and features of resilience – a discourse that is currently lacking (refer to Chapter 2). Further work to identify effective evidence-based interventions is also required, such as interventions that move beyond parenting programmes for incarcerated women (Chapter 9) and prevent and/or mitigate against the impact of having a premature infant (Chapter 10) and/or PTSD following childbirth (Chapter 11).

Our starting position, and as reflected in many of the included chapters, is that maternity and early years' services tend to cater for mainstream provision, which does not always accept or adequately respond to diversity. While recommendations and guidelines to optimise care for vulnerable/disadvantaged women are highlighted across the chapters, in the UK and elsewhere, there is evidence of little or no suitable service provision. This in turn creates further inequalities for those who may arguably need the care the most. Indeed, Marmot (2010) calls for a system of proportionate universalism, in which actions (such as care provision) are population-based 'but with a scale and intensity that is proportionate to the level of disadvantage' (p. 10). While areas of good practice have been identified, what appears from across the work presented is the need for person-centred, strength-based care from skilled multi-agency providers who have an understanding of the issues faced by the target population, provided by seamless, sufficiently resourced organisations/services that value and nurture the resilience of their workforce, and who demonstrate true collaborative practice. Pregnancy and early motherhood can present physical and psychological challenges – it is a vital window of opportunity, and one which has far-reaching implications. A perinatal model of empowerment that resonates on an individual, provider and organisational basis should therefore be the goal to aim for.

References

Antonovsky, A. (1987). *Unraveling the mystery of health: How people manage stress and stay well.* London: Jossey-Bass.

Barlow, J., Davis, H., McIntosh, E., Jarrett, P., Mockford, C. & Stewart-Brown, S. (2007). Role of home visiting in improving parenting and health in families at risk of abuse and neglect: Results of a multicentre randomised controlled trial and economic evaluation. *Archives of Disease in Childhood, 92,* 229–233.

Beaumont, E., Durkin, M., Hollins Martin, C.J. & Carson, J. (2015). Compassion for others, self-compassion, quality of life and mental well-being measures and their association with compassion fatigue and burnout in student midwives: A quantitative survey. *Midwifery, 34,* 239–244.

Chetwin, A. (2013). *A review of the effectiveness of interventions for adult victims and children exposed to family violence.* New Zealand: Ministry of Social Development.

Cohen, S. & Wills, T.A. (1985). Stress, social support, and the buffering hypothesis. *Psychological Bulletin, 98,* 310–357.

Davis, H. & Day, C. (2010). *Working in Partnership with Parents.* 2nd edition. London: Pearson.

Davis, H., Day, C. & Bidmead, C. (2002). *Working in partnership with parents: The parent adviser model.* London: Harcourt Assessment.

Fontein-Kuipers, Y., van Limbeek, E., Ausems, M., de Vries, R., & Nieuwenhuijze, M. (2015). Using intervention mapping for systematic development of a midwife-delivered intervention for prevention and reduction of maternal distress during pregnancy. *International Journal of Women's Health and Wellness,* 1:008. Available from: http://clinmedjournals.org/articles/ijwhw/international-journal-of-womens-health-and-wellness-ijwhw-1-008.pdf.

Gatz, M., Brown, V., Hennigan, V. & Rechberger, E. (2007). Effectiveness of an integrated, trauma-informed approach to treating women with co-occurring disorders and histories of trauma: The Los Angeles Site experience. *Journal of Community Psychology, 35*(7), 863–878.

Goodman, M.J. & Schorling, J.B. (2012). A mindfulness course decreases burnout and improves well-being among healthcare providers. *The International Journal of Psychiatry in Medicine, 43*(2), 119–128.

Health Innovation Network. (n.d.) *What is person centred care and why is it important*. Available from: www.hin-southlondon.org/system/ckeditor_assets/attachments/41/what_is_per son-centred_care_and_why_is_it_important.pdf [Accessed 9 February 2017].

McCormack, B. & McCance, T. (2010). *Person-centred nursing: Theory, models and methods.* Oxford: Blackwell Publishing.

McMillan, S.S., Kendall, E., Sav, A., King, M.A., Whitty, J.A., Kelly, F. & Wheeler, A.J. (2013). Patient-centered approaches to health care: A systematic review of randomized controlled trials. *Medical Care Research and Review, 70*(6), 567–596.

Marmot, M. (2010). *Fair society, healthy lives: The Marmot Review.* A strategic review of health inequalities in England. Available from: www.instituteofhealthequity.org/ projects/fair-society-healthy-lives-the-marmot-review [Accessed 9 February 2017].

Mead, N. & Bower, P. (2002). Patient-centred consultations and outcomes in primary care: A review of the literature. *Patient Education and Counseling 48*(1), 51–61.

Morrissey, J.P., Jackson, E.W., Ellis, A.R., Amaro, H., Brown, V. & Najavits, L. (2005). Twelve-month outcomes of trauma-informed interventions for women with co-occurring disorders. *Psychiatric Services, 56*(10), 1213–1222.

Moses, D.J., Reed, B.G. & Mazelis, R. (2003). *Creating trauma services for women with co-occurring disorders: Experiences from the SAMHSA women with alcohol, drug abuse, and mental health disorders who have histories of violence study.* Delmar, NY: Policy Research Associates.

Pearlin, L.I. (1989). The sociological study of stress. *Journal of Health and Social Behavior, 30,* 241–256.

Puura, K., Davis, H., Cox, A., Tsiantis, J., Tamminen, T., Ispanovic-Radojkovic, V., Paradisiotou, A., Mantymaa, M., Roberts, R., Dragonas, T., Layiou-Lignos, E., Dusoir, T., Rudic, N., Tenjovic, L. & Vizacou, S. (2005). The European early promotion project: Description of the service and evaluation study. *International Journal of Mental Health Promotion, 7,* 17–31.

Rollnick, S. & Miller, W.R. (1995). What is motivational interviewing? *Behavioural and Cognitive Psychotherapy, 23,* 325–334.

Shakespeare, J., Blake, F. & Garcia, J. (2003). A qualitative study of the acceptability of routine screening of postnatal women using the Edinburgh Postnatal Depression Scale. *British Journal of General Practice, 53*(493), 614–619.

Umberson, D. & Montez, J.K. (2010). Social relationship and health: A flashpoint for health policy. *Journal of Health and Social Behavior, 51,* S54–S66.

INDEX

Page numbers in **bold** refer to figures, page numbers in *italic* refer to tables.

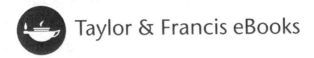